Hans Suter

Paul Klee
and His Illness

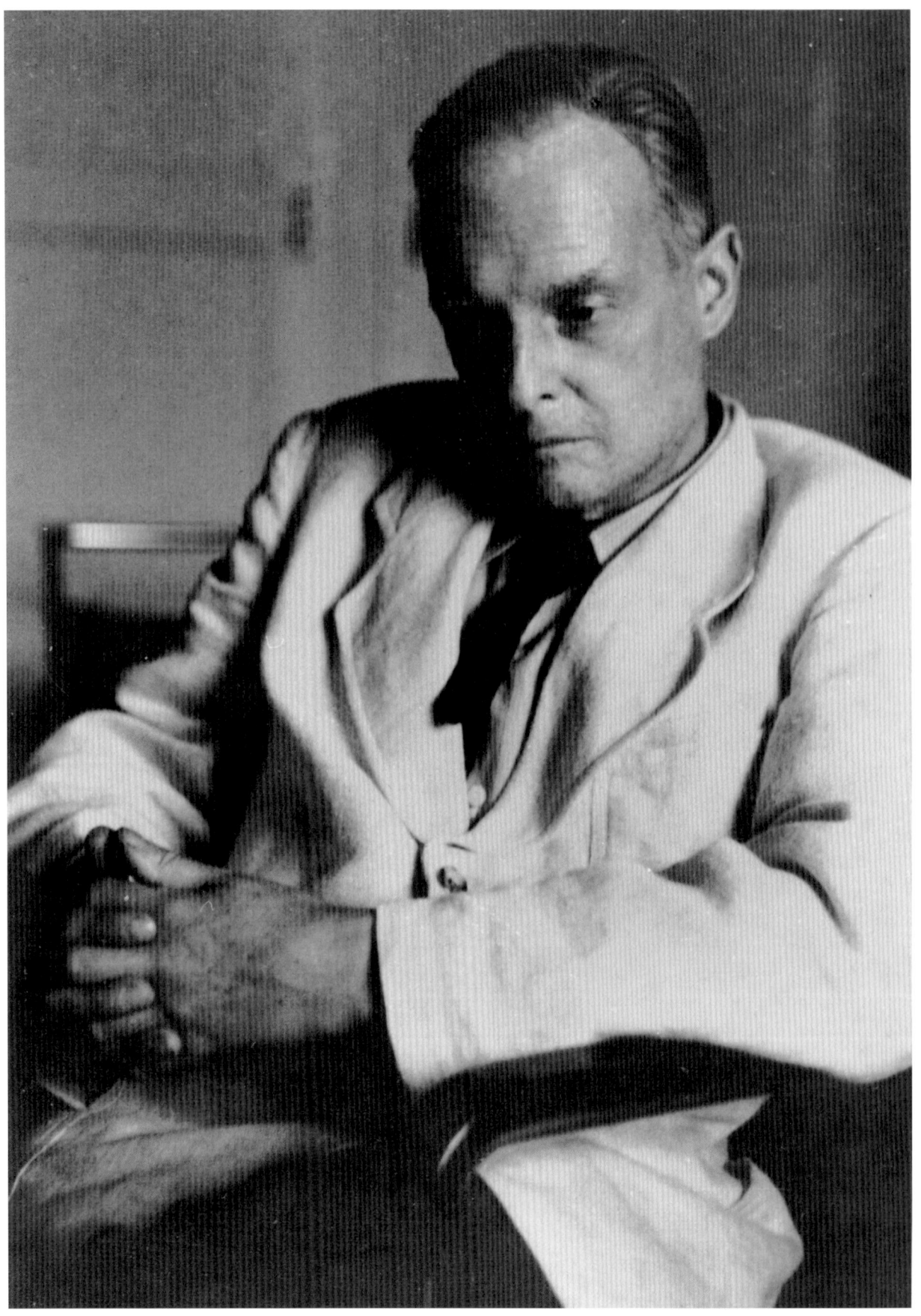

Hans Suter

Paul Klee and His Illness

Bowed but Not Broken by Suffering and Adversity

Translated from the German
by Gill McKay and Neil McKay

186 figures, 77 in color, and 2 tables, 2010

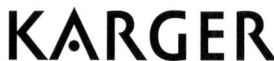

Basel · Freiburg · Paris · London · New York · Bangalore ·
Bangkok · Shanghai · Singapore · Tokyo · Sydney

Contents

7	**Preface**	Aljoscha Klee
8	**Foreword**	Hans Christoph von Tavel
11	**Introduction**	
16	Notes on Interpreting the Works of Art	

19	**1**	**Paul Klee's Life – Major Milestones**
19		Early Years in Bern
19		Artistic Training in Munich and Italy, Sojourns in Bern and Munich
20		Trip to Tunisia, Military Service during World War I, Teaching, Journey to Egypt
21		Dismissal, Return to Bern, Isolation
29		Klee Exhibitions in Switzerland: Attracting Little Interest
31		'And My Sole Remaining Wish Is to Be a Citizen of This City'

39	**2**	**Paul Klee's Illness**
39		First Symptoms – Persistent Bronchitis, Pneumonia, Pleurisy and Permanent Fatigue
40		Measles?
45		Long Convalescence, Debility, Heart and Lung Complications
48		A Possible Diagnosis: Scleroderma
51		Overview of the Forms of Scleroderma
52		Skin Disorders
59		Mucous Membrane Disorders
60		Raynaud's Syndrome
62		Internal Organ Disorders
		Digestive Tract Disorders • Lung Disorders • Cardiac Disorders • Renal Disorders
73		Death in Ticino
78		Discussion of the Symptoms and Course of Paul Klee's Illness
80		How Was Paul Klee's Illness Treated?
86		Other Medical Opinions on Paul Klee's Illness
		F.-J. Beer • Lisbet Milling Pedersen and Henrik Permin • Philip Sandblom • Brigitta Danuser • Michael Reiner • Christoph Morscher • E. Carwile LeRoy and Richard M. Silver • Gabriele Castenholz
104		A Final Assessment of Paul Klee's Illness
108		Paul Klee's Doctors

3 Paul Klee's Personality   115

4 The Effects of Adversity and Illness on Paul Klee's Mind and Work   127
    Robust Psyche   127
    What Could Have Caused Such a Serious Illness?   153
    Great Fortitude   154
    Powers of Intuition, Conserving Energy, Concentrating on the Essentials   156
    Belated Accolades   176
    The Final Works   177

5 Klee's Late Work as a Reflection of His Personality, Social Environment, Illness and Proximity to Death   185
    Isolation and Solitary Internalization   185
    'Death Is Nothing Bad'   186
    Work Full of Spirituality   193
    'Art Is a Parable of Creation'   201
    His Illness as a Constant Companion   203
    A New Style of Extraordinary Intensity and Spontaneity   210
    Meeting with Pablo Picasso   214
    'His Creation Breathes Lightness and Grace'   216
    'Productivity Is Increasing and the Tempo Is Accelerating'   220
    Illness as Opportunity   223

6 Summary and Conclusion   237

    'Paul Klee and His Illness', Exhibition, Bern, 2005   240
    Special Medical Terms   242
    Index of Terms   244
    Index of Names   244
    Biographical Details of People Referred to in the Text   246
    Bibliography   253
    List of Illustrations   259
    Alphabetical Index of Illustrations of Works of Paul Klee   260
    Abbreviations for Document Locations   262
    Photographic Credits   263
    Appendices   264
    Acknowledgements   270
    World Scleroderma Association   271

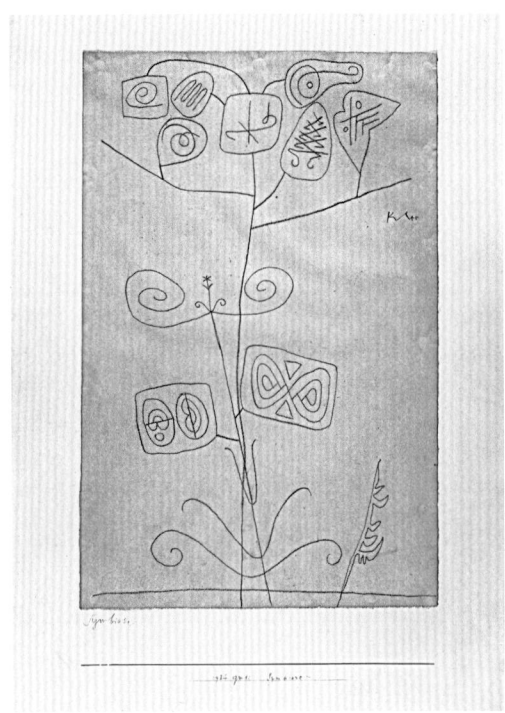

Fig. 1. Symbiosis, 1934, 131

For my wife Marlis Suter-Trächsel
and our daughters Maja Wassmer-Suter
and Christa Zaugg-Suter

In loving memory of our son and brother
Gerhard Suter (1963–1986)

And for my teacher and friend
Professor Dr. med. Alfred Krebs

Preface

As the grandson of Paul Klee, faced with writing a preface to such a meticulously researched and written book and commenting on the tragedy contained in its pages, I find myself delving into a story that is really only relevant to me from a historical perspective. Sadly, I never had the chance to know my grandfather personally, but I have been able to draw on a whole latticework of personal memories. These memories are not directly linked to Paul Klee's illness, but they are a product of my parents' recollections and reflections on what they experienced. They were forced to stand by helplessly, watching and sharing in the artist's inevitable decline towards death. As a child growing up, I was not really able to fully understand my parents' stories and conversations about 'Buzzi'. But I gained a realization of the mystery of death and the artist's awareness of his own mortality, and this made an impression on me and preoccupied me during my formative years. For example, I was impressed by his determination to continue to achieve as much as his remaining time on earth would allow. Paul Klee still had so much more to say, and he knew it.

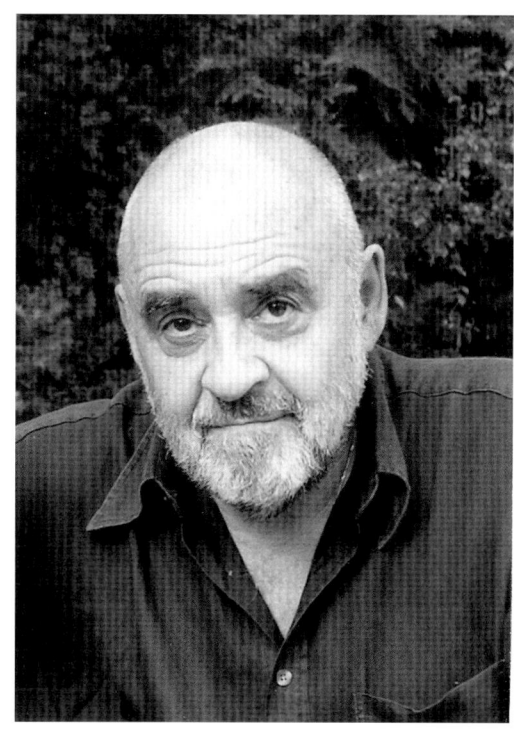

Fig. 2. Aljoscha Klee

His later work, which was not only influenced by his illness, but which was done in defiance of that illness, is surely one of the most brilliant demonstrations of how suffering and sadness can be overcome through art and imagery, and in which, despite everything, irony can still shine through. I welcome this book as an important and sensitive contribution towards the appreciation of Klee's later work.

Aljoscha Klee

Foreword

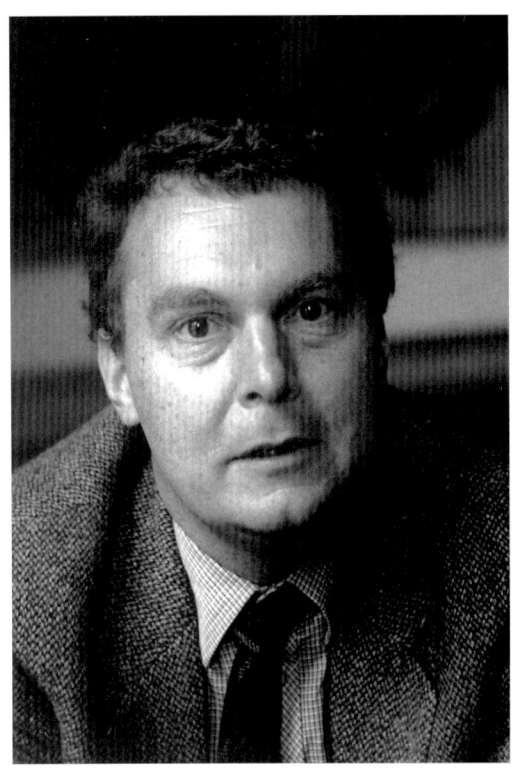

Fig. 3. Dr. Hans Christoph von Tavel, PhD

This publication occupies a special place amongst the many scholarly works on Paul Klee, as it fills a big gap in the studies done so far on an artist who is considered so important in the artistic and intellectual history of the 20th century. The subject of his illness has been brought up regularly in discussions of his later work, but for the most part without any specialist medical knowledge. Conversely, medical studies on the final years of the artist, who died in 1940 aged 60, often suffer from a lack of accurate research into the fateful progress of his illness and from a lack of knowledge about Klee's artistic work. The latter has only recently been catalogued in its entirety.

Hans Suter, who worked in Thun and its surrounding area as a specialist in dermatology and venereology, has been a collector and patron of the visual arts for decades. He began his research into the nature and development of Klee's illness more than 30 years ago. The lack of a medical history and the fact that the artist's death happened several decades earlier meant it was necessary to undertake extensive research. This was made particularly onerous by the fact that most of Klee's doctors, friends and collectors, as well as those who witnessed his illness, had by then also died. The artistic and human isolation that Klee suffered in Bern even before the outbreak of his illness – he was forced to leave Germany in 1933 – complicated matters even more. The author meets these challenges with profound medical knowledge, a comprehensive study of relevant literature and original source material, careful historical research and interviews with Klee's son Felix, other surviving contemporaries, and descendants of Klee's circle.

Doctors and local historians will be fascinated by this book's new insights into everyday medical practices in the university city of Bern in the 1930s, while art historians and art lovers will be absorbed by the newly discovered links and may make further links between the artist's work and his illness.

Hans Christoph von Tavel

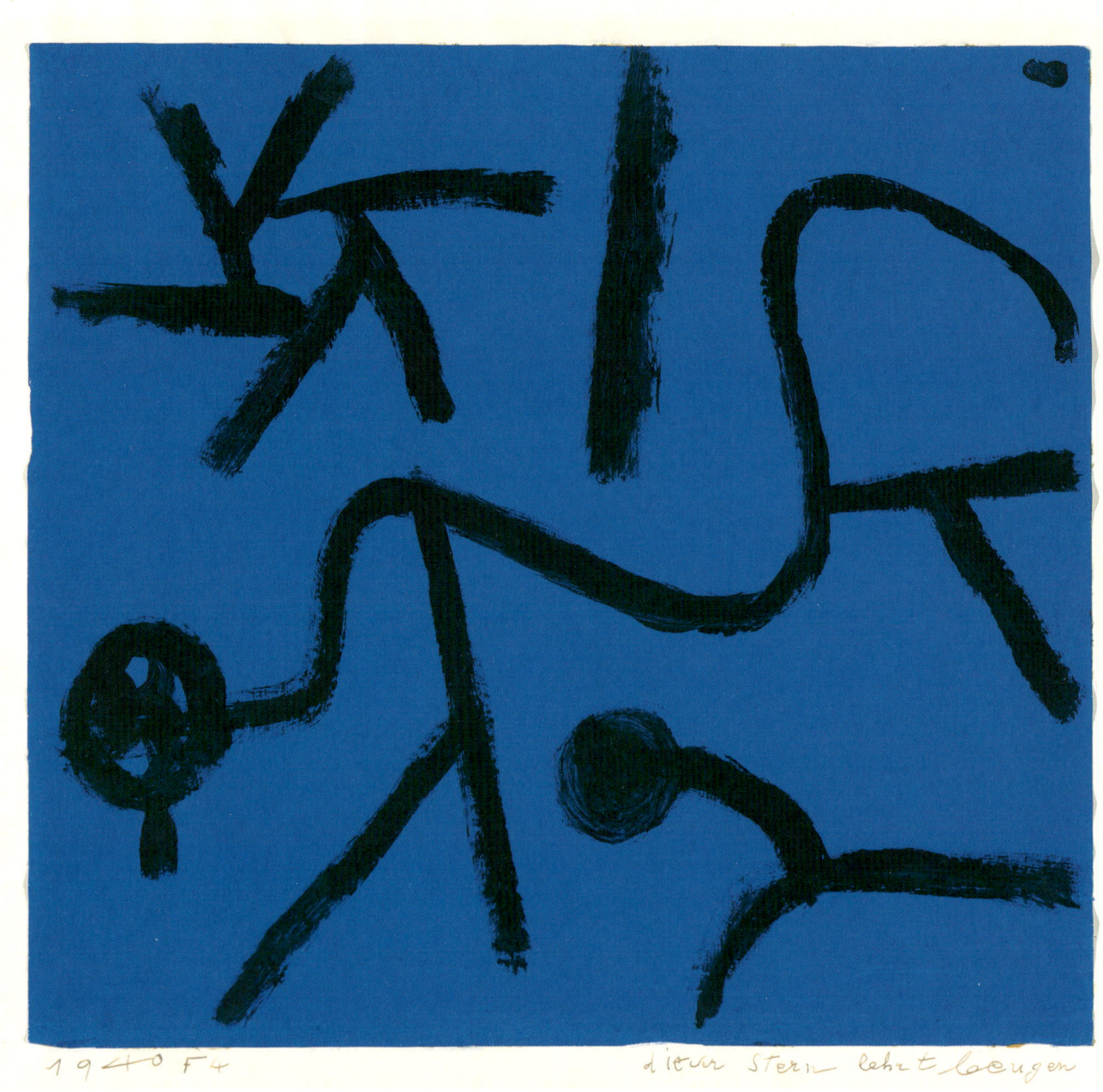

Fig. 4. This star teaches bending, 1940, 344

Introduction

'This star teaches bending' is the telling title of a work on paper which Paul Klee completed in the year of his death. This brilliant artist lived the last few years of his life in Bern, but they were years which were overshadowed by a dark star. In 1935 Klee suffered a variety of setbacks and became seriously ill. Although he never recovered from this illness, he always maintained his love of life, facing his suffering with a trenchant 'so what?' But by 1940 he had to accept that there was no hope of a cure or any improvement in his health. The star had taught him to bend to the blows of fate.

Paul Klee died in 1940 at the age of 60. He died of a mysterious disease which at the time remained undiagnosed: the symptoms included changes to the skin and problems with the internal organs. It was only 10 years after the artist's death that the illness was actually given a name in writings about Klee. The art dealer Daniel-Henry Kahnweiler wrote in a publication: 'His health was undermined for years by a terrible disease – a kind of skin sclerosis, which in the end was to carry him (Paul Klee) off'.[1] Four years later, the Klee biographer Will Grohmann wrote in his 1954 monograph: '[…] it turned out to be a malignant disease (scleroderma), a drying-out of the mucous membranes which was little known in medical circles. After five years it spread to his heart and led to his death'[2]. We still have no idea where Kahnweiler and Grohmann got this information. It is strange that the diagnosis appears in neither the correspondence between the two married couples, Paul and Lily Klee and Will and Gertrud Grohmann,[3] nor in Lily Klee's memoirs[4] which were written from 1942. The illness is also not identified in the notes published by Felix Klee, Paul and Lily's only son, on his parents.[5] Today it is no longer possible to ascer-

[1] Kahnweiler 1950, p. 23. I thank Walther Fuchs, MA, for the reference.
[2] Grohmann 1965 (4th ed.), p. 84.
[3] Will Grohmann Archive at the Stuttgart State Gallery: 103 letters, 35 postcards and 1 telegram from Lily and Paul Klee to Will and Gertrud Grohmann, for the period July 4, 1929 to September 13, 1946.
[4] Klee [from 1942] (p. 258).
[5] Notably Klee 1948 and Klee 1960/1.

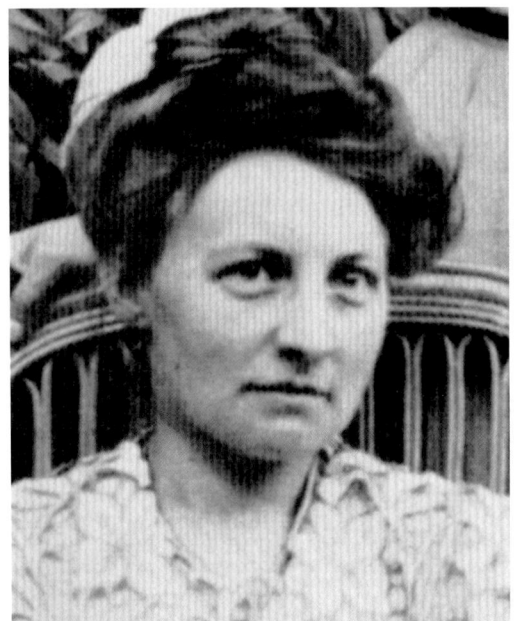

Fig. 5. Lily Klee-Stumpf, 1906

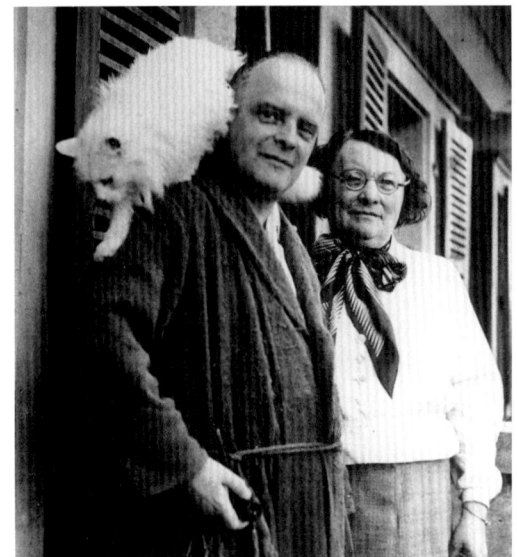

Fig. 6. Paul and Lily Klee with Bimbo the cat, Bern, 1935

tain where the diagnosis of 'scleroderma' for Paul Klee's illness originated,[6] and more recently the diagnosis has been called into question in medical circles.[7]

In 1979, Professor Alfred Krebs, who at that time was Professor of Dermatology and Venereology at the University of Bern Skin Clinic, instigated research into Paul Klee's illness. We talked to the artist's son[8] (see above) and the descendants of the now deceased doctors in Bern who treated Paul Klee or who were close to him: General Practitioner, Dr. Gerhard Schorer[9] and his locum, Dr. Max Schatzmann,[10] his boyhood friend, associate professor Dr. Fritz Lotmar,[11] and his consultant, Professor Oscar Naegeli.[12] We also spoke to Sister Virginia Bachmann, head of the Clinica Sant' Agnese in Locarno-Muralto,[13] where the artist died on June 29, 1940. As patients' records are only kept for 10 years, there was little hope that, nearly 40 years on, any trace of his medical history would remain, and unfortunately this was the case. So I had further lengthy conversations with Felix Klee[14], Max Huggler[15] and other people who knew the artist personally[16] or who could possibly contribute something with regard to his illness.[17] Professor Krebs got in touch with the management of the Tarasp sanatorium in Unterengadin,[18] where Klee went for treatment in 1936. He also checked the archives at the Bern Dermatology Clinic, where the painter consulted with Professor Oscar Naegeli in the same year.[19] We made enquiries at the Institute for Diagnostic Radiology at Bern University to find out whether Paul Klee had undergone any tests or X-rays. However, as expected, there was no evidence of any medical records, X-ray pictures or analyses.[20] I contacted both the administration and a former chief physician at the 'Centre Valaisan de Pneumologie' in Montana, as well as the local government of Montana and the canton administration in Sion to find out whether there was a patient file on Paul Klee for the year 1936 – he was recuperating at the 'Pension Cécil' in Montana at that time. I was informed that this pension was separate from the lung sanatorium, and it was not possible to track down any medical records for Paul Klee.[21] Ms. Diana Bodmer, the daughter of Dr. Hermann Bodmer, who was the last doctor to treat the artist in Locarno, was also unable to bring us any further forward.[22]

[6] Felix Klee told the author on September 20, 1983 that he did not know who had hazarded this diagnosis after the death of his father, and his mother also had no idea. The author's research to date has also failed to throw any light on this matter.
[7] Cf. Castenholz/ML 2000, pp. 144–148.
[8–20] See Appendices: Research into Paul Klee's Illness (p. 264 f).
[21–22] See Appendices: Research into Paul Klee's Illness (p. 265).

The only piece of laboratory evidence that we have is the result of a urine test carried out at the Clinica Sant' Agnese in Locarno-Muralto during Klee's final days. This was sent to Professor Alfred Krebs by Sister Virginia Bachmann in 1979.[23]

I have been fascinated by Paul Klee and his art since my adolescence, and this spurred me on to continue my research. Would I ever get a clear picture of the artist's illness? I was keen to find out whether there was any evidence to support or contradict the assumptions about his illness, so I studied notes and letters from the painter himself, from family members, friends and acquaintances, and also documents from the Paul Klee's Estate. Felix Klee gave me copies of the extensive correspondence between his parents (particularly Lily Klee) and Will and Gertrud Grohmann, much of which was previously unpublished.[24] These documents helped me to piece together an idea of the course of the illness and some of the symptoms, and Felix Klee filled me in on other important facts during our conversations.[25] I was also helped in my research by the Bern-based Klee specialists and art historians Michael Baumgartner, Stefan Frey, Jürgen Glaesemer, Josef Helfenstein, Christine Hopfengart, Max Huggler, Osamu Okuda and Hans Christoph von Tavel, the nephew of Dr. Gerhard Schorer, who all provided me with invaluable information. The administrator of the Paul Klee's Estate, Stefan Frey, was always ready to help with my research, and kindly put at my disposal an extensive, unpublished set of excerpts from letters.[26] His exhaustive work on the documents gave me a solid foundation for my work.

I also studied the extensive literature on Paul Klee,[27] particularly his diaries from 1898 to 1918 and other writings by the artist and his son Felix Klee. Other helpful literature included: Will Grohmann's seminal monograph, along with that of Carola Giedion-Welcker, Max Huggler's perceptive work, Jürgen Glaesemer's excellent texts and the collection catalogues he put together for the Paul Klee Foundation in Bern, as well as this foundation's catalogue of works, Stefan Frey's detailed chronological biography of Paul Klee, 1933–1941 (Frey 1990), 'Erinnerungen an Paul Klee' (Memories of Paul Klee), by Ludwig Grote (Grote 1959), and a perusal of many exhibition

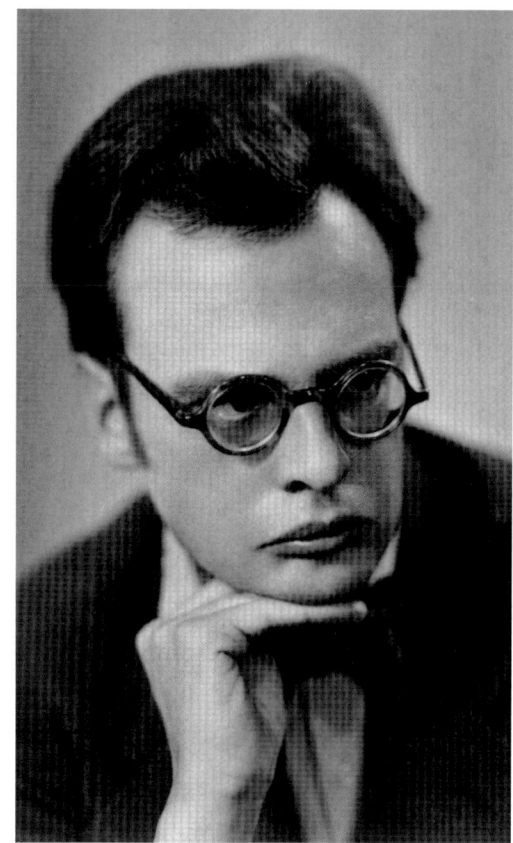

Fig. 7. Dr. h.c. Felix Klee, 1940

[23] See Appendices: Research into Paul Klee's Illness (p. 265).
[24] See note 3 (p. 11) for details of the correspondence.
[25] Conversations with Felix Klee, Bern, with Prof. Alfred Krebs and the author, Bern, November 9, 1979 and July 23, 1981, also with the author alone, Bern, September 20, 1983.
[26] Cf. Frey Zitate (quotations), pp. 1–35.
[27] See bibliography, pp. 254–258.

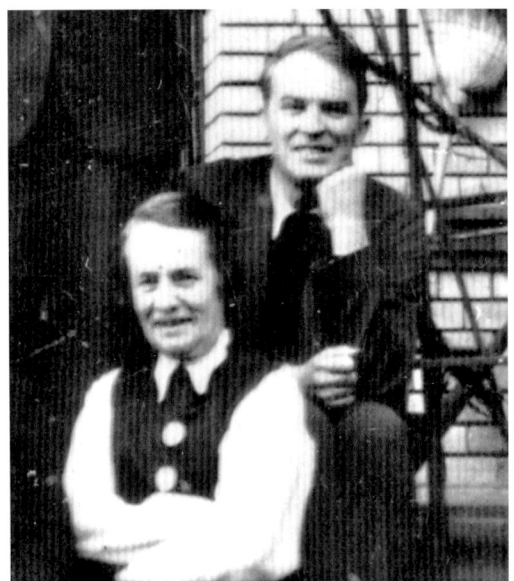

Fig. 8. Dr. Will Grohmann, PhD, and Gertrud Grohmann, 1935

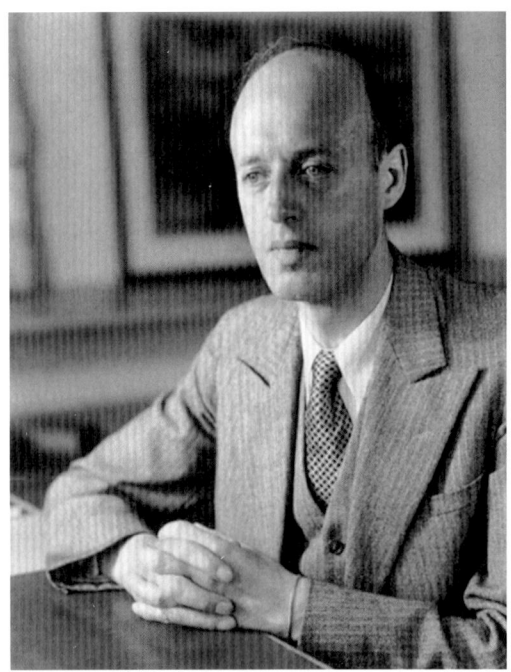

Fig. 9. Dr. Max Huggler, PhD, 1944

catalogues and press reviews. Also invaluable was the groundbreaking book 'Krankheit als Krise und Chance' (Illness as Crisis and Opportunity) by Professor Edgar Heim (Heim/ML 1980). I am also grateful for the specialist advice given to me by Professor Peter M. Villiger in his fields of rheumatology, allergology and immunology.

To date, Paul Klee's illness has been largely ignored by the medical profession, hence my desire to fill the gap in our knowledge. In all the literature on Paul Klee, there is still no extant specialist assessment by a dermatologist.

In 1978, the President of the 'Società Ticinese di Belle Arti', Sergio Grandini, asked the then chief physician of the medical department of the Clinica Sant' Agnese in Locarno-Muralto, Dr. Enrico Uehlinger, to investigate the illness and death of Paul Klee in this clinic. Unfortunately nothing came of this, as Dr. Uehlinger surmised that records were possibly handed over by the clinic to a Japanese researcher.[28] However, Osamu Okuda, art historian at the Paul Klee Foundation, Museum of Fine Arts, Bern (now research associate at the Zentrum Paul Klee, Bern), told me that this was not the case, and that the Japanese in question was called Sadao Wada.[29] He said Wada was at the Clinica Sant' Agnese in 1974 and had in fact made his own investigations, but these also turned out to be fruitless. He published his findings in 1975 in a Japanese art journal under the title 'The Last Moments of Paul Klee'.[30] It mainly contained photographs of the house where the Klees lived in Bern, Klee's tomb in the Schosshalden cemetery in Bern, the Viktoria Sanatorium in Locarno-Orselina and the Clinica Sant' Agnese in Locarno-Muralto. Wada also photographed the room where the artist died and the view from this room.

[28] Cf. letter from Dr. Enrico Uehlinger, Locarno-Minusio, to Sergio Grandini, Lugano, April 6, 1978 (ZPKB/SFK).

[29] Osamu Okuda told the author on November 1, 1998: Sadao Wada was a Japanese employee of the Berlin branch of the Bank of Japan, and was an admirer of Paul Klee and his work.

[30] Wada 1975. I thank Osamu Okuda for this information. See also Wada, Sadao, Paul Klee and his Travels, Tokyo 1979.

In my work I have the following basic objectives:
- To collect as far as possible all the information which still exists on Paul Klee's illness
- To reappraise the hypothetic diagnosis of 'scleroderma'. Could it in fact have been another disease?
- To consider whether his illness had an influence on his psyche and his creative work
- To look at Paul Klee's later works in the light of his personality, social environment, his illness and his imminent demise

In Chapter 2 I have tried to write about the medical facts in a way which is understandable to the layman, and I hope that when reading Chapters 3–6, my readers will be infected by some of the fascination that I feel for the great man and his work.

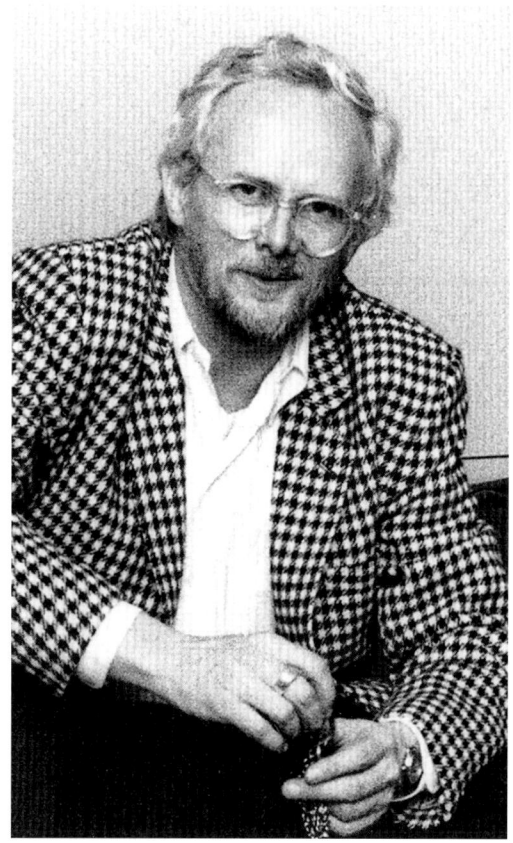

Fig. 10. Dr. Jürgen Glaesemer, PhD, 1987

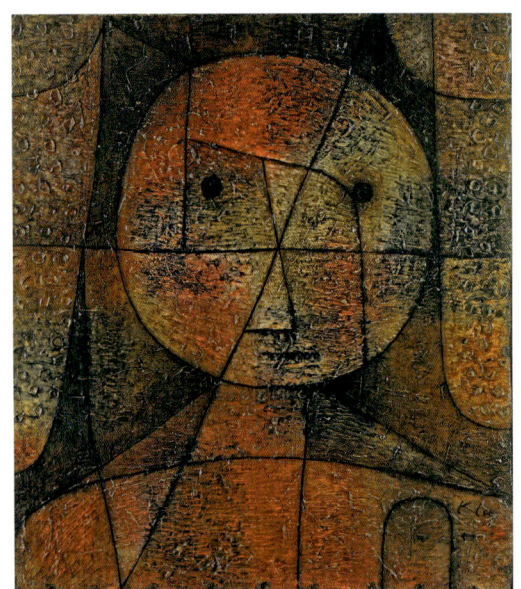

Fig. 11. Marked man, 1935, 146

Notes on Interpreting the Works of Art

Paul Klee had a very vivid imagination, and his art works and their titles in turn ignite the imagination of his viewers, adults and children alike. Upon finishing a piece of work, Klee would give it a pithy title. In the title he liked to give a pointer to help interpret his work, and at the same time he was very creative in his use of language. It is quite a feat of imagination that in around 9,800 works he very rarely repeated a title.

However, the titles still leave room for individual interpretation of the paintings and drawings. Klee was quite clear about this, saying to his viewers: 'At the end of the day [...], the signatures [by which he meant the picture titles] give a sense of my direction. But it's up to you whether you decide to go my way, whether you take your own route – or whether you just stand still and decide not to come along at all. Don't mistake the signature for an intention'[31]. In this respect, Will Grohmann was of the opinion that 'He [Klee] tended to distance himself from his work, and talked about it as if it belonged to someone else. He was rarely satisfied; sometimes he would hint that there was a mistake and would challenge us to find it with an impish grin. But he would also tell us when he was feeling proud of certain works for one reason or another. When visitors came, he liked to take the opportunity to look at his latest output, which he otherwise didn't take the time to do, and he inwardly expected his visitors to offer some objective criticism, or at least give a sign that they understood what he was trying to do. But he bemoaned the fact that most of them 'didn't add anything', they just viewed his work with silent enjoyment. He was keen to find out the effect of his works-in-progress, the feelings and ideas they aroused; he needed this as a kind of checkup, but he was not at all unhappy if the viewer's train of thought went in a totally different direction to his own. He knew this was a possibility and said 'I'm surprised, but I find your interpretation just as good as and perhaps even better than mine'[32].

Because of these comments quoted above, I have allowed myself to attempt some personal interpretation of his works. I do not in any way claim that my interpretations have any general validity, and must stress that I am not an art historian.

[31] Geist, Hans-Friedrich, in: Grote 1959, p. 87.
[32] Grohmann 1965, p. 64 f.

I wrote down my ideas spontaneously after in-depth viewing of his works. At times I may have projected too much into a picture, and I beg the reader for forgiveness if my imagination sometimes runs away with me.

Ultimately, the 'soul' of every work of art remains the artist's own secret. Klee came up with an apt metaphor in this respect: 'Art is a parable of Creation. The bond with optical reality is very elastic. The world of form is master of itself, but in itself is not art at the highest level. At the highest level there is a mystery which presides over ambiguity – and the light of intellect flickers and dies.'[33]

In this book, the illustrations showing Paul Klee's works are mostly arranged in chronological order, so that we seem to be watching scenes from a film about the last seven years of the artist's life.

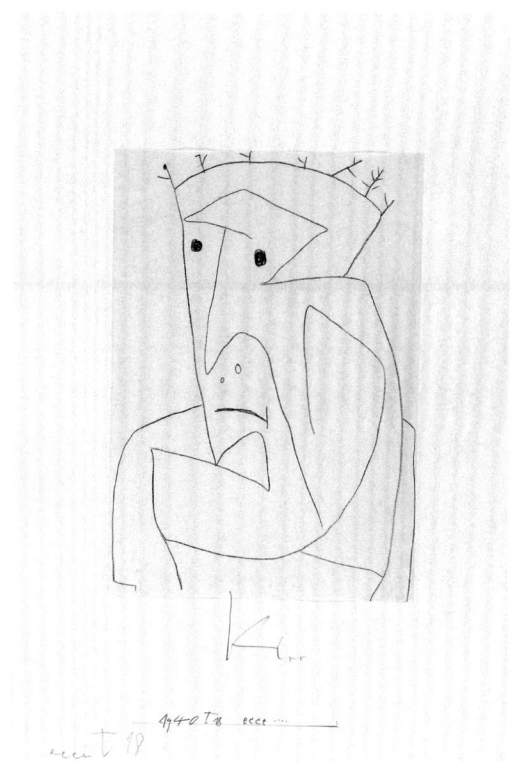

Fig. 12. Ecce ...., 1940, 138

[33] Quoted from Klee 1960/1, p. 251, and Klee 1960/2, p. 101.

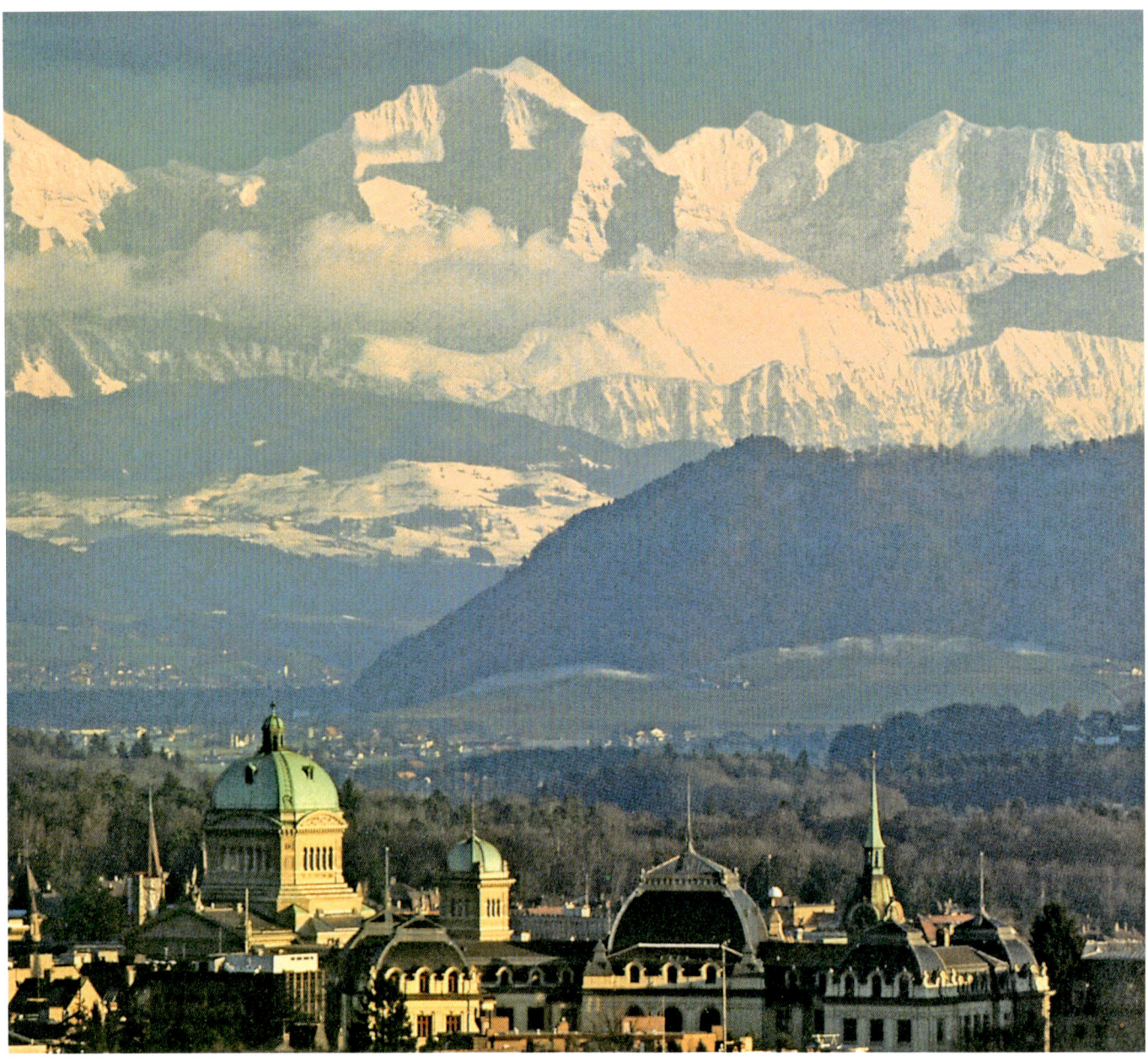

Fig. 13. Bern with the Federal Parliament Building, Belpberg and the Bernese Alps

1. Paul Klee's Life
   Major Milestones

Early Years in Bern

Paul Klee was born on December 18, 1879 in Münchenbuchsee near Bern. His father, Hans Klee, was of German nationality and worked as a music teacher at the cantonal teacher's college in Hofwil, Bern, where his students found him to be a distinctive and unusual character.[34] His mother, Ida Klee, née Frick, was from Basel and had family in the South of France. She was also musically trained. Paul Klee had a sister, Mathilde (1876–1953) who was three years older than him. In 1880 the family moved to Bern. In 1898 Paul Klee graduated from Bern Grammar School, but due to his varied talents he found it difficult to decide on a career. He was not only good at drawing, but was also a talented violinist, and he was deeply interested in literature and the theater.

Artistic Training in Munich and Italy, Sojourns in Bern and Munich

Klee finally embarked on a three-year course at the Academy of Fine Arts, Munich, followed by six months in Rome with the Swiss sculptor Hermann Haller to further expand his artistic training. Looking back he comments: 'My next task was to employ the skills I had acquired, and to make progress in my art. Bern, the home of my youth, seemed to me the ideal place for such work. [...] I had formed many ties in Munich, and one of these led to marriage with my present wife. The fact the she could practice her profession in Munich was one of the important reasons for my returning there for the second time (autumn 1906).'[35] Paul Klee's wife Lily, née Stumpf, was a pianist and supported the family by giving piano les-

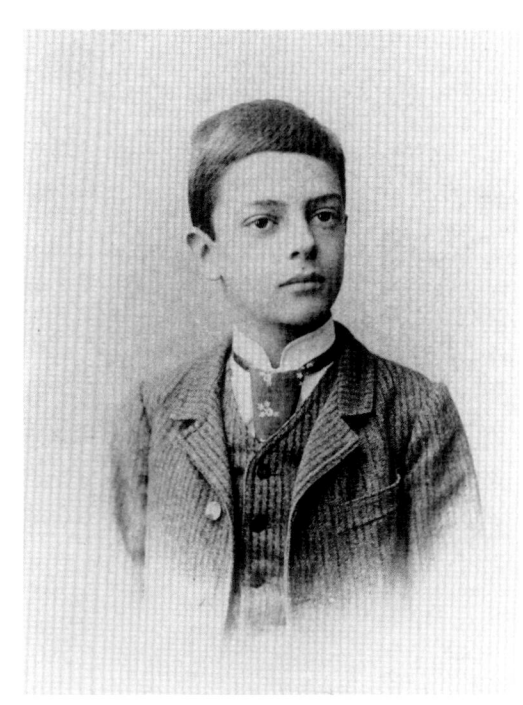

Fig. 14. Paul Klee, 1892

[34] See Appendices: Hans Klee's Personality (p. 265).
[35] Klee 1940, p. 12 (p. 258).

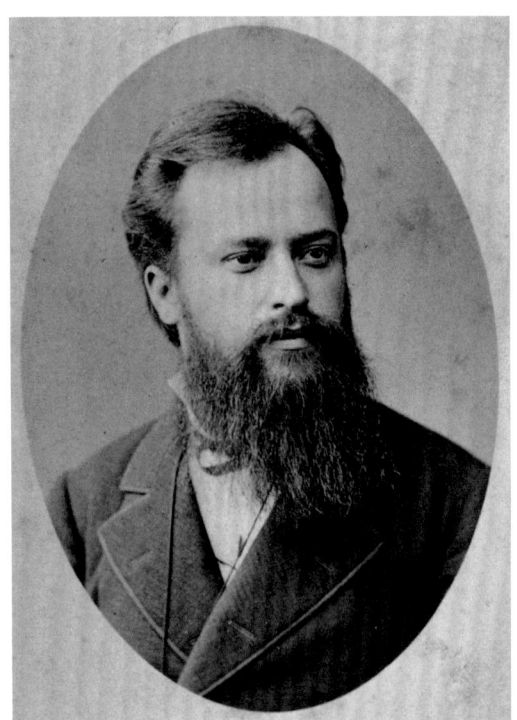

Fig. 15. Hans Klee, 1880

Schaße, schaße Rübchen,
Schwesterchen hat ein Bübchen,
Schwesterchen ist hübsch und fein,
das allerschönste Jungfräulein.
Schaße, schaße Rübchen,
Schwesterchen hat ein Bübchen.

Schaße, schaße Rübchen,
Mütterlein sitzt im Stübchen,
hat das Kindlein in dem Schoß,
ach, wie ist die Freude groß!
Schaße, schaße Rübchen,
Schwesterchen hat ein Bübchen.

Schaße, schaße Rübchen,
Bald taufen wir das Liebchen.
Da gibt's im Haus ein großes Fest
und Schmausen auf das Allerbest.
Schaße, schaße Rübchen,
Schwesterchen hat ein Bübchen.

*

Fig. 16. Poem by Hans Klee about his children, Mathilde and Paul (from the small volume of poems, 'Jugend Verse', p. 43)

[36] Klee, Diaries, no. 926 o.
[37] Klee 1940, p. 13 (p. 258).

sons. Later this was to prove a crucial factor in allowing Klee to develop himself as an artist. In 1907 their son Felix was born. In 1912 Paul Klee joined 'Der Blaue Reiter' (The Blue Rider), a group of artists including Heinrich Campendonk, August Macke, Franz Marc, Gabriele Münter and Wassily Kandinsky. In 1924 an art dealer from Braunschweig, Emmy ('Galka') Scheyer, along with Lyonel Feininger, Alexej Jawlensky, Wassily Kandinsky and Paul Klee set up a group called 'Die Blaue Vier' (The Blue Four), in order to promote the four artists in the USA.

Trip to Tunisia, Military Service during World War I, Teaching, Journey to Egypt

In 1914 Klee and two artist friends, August Macke from Bonn and Louis Moilliet from Bern, went on a two-week study trip to Tunisia. The light and color of the region made a big impression on him, and he recorded in his diary the now legendary phrase: 'Color has taken possession of me […] color and I are one.'[36] Klee's artistic evolution was hampered by three years in the army during the World War I. Fortunately, he was stationed behind the front and came through unscathed, whereas August Macke and Franz Marc were killed in action.

Klee was both matter-of-fact and modest when he looked back on his employment and the twists of fate which followed: 'In 1920 came my appointment to the staff of the Bauhaus school in Weimar. I taught there until the institution moved to Dessau in 1926. Finally, in 1930, I was asked to accept an appointment to conduct a course in painting at the Prussian Academy of Art in Düsseldorf. This offer coincided with my own desire to confine my teaching entirely to my own field. I therefore accepted and was associated with the Academy from 1931 to 1933.'[37]

A two-month trip to Egypt in 1928/29 had a similar effect on him to that of his earlier visit to North Africa: the trip to Tunisia had a strong influence on his work between 1914 and 1931; the trip to Egypt influenced his art between 1929 and 1940. Will Grohmann comments: 'Klee fed off it (the trip to Egypt) right up to his death, because here, more than in Tunis, he felt confronted by the fact that six thousand years of culture were no more than the blink of an eye in terms of world history, a fact that was reflected in the landscape, which seemed to play as big a role in it as humans. […] Klee could see creation, life and death reflected in every monument and every hill. […] Egypt gave him the courage to face ultimate simplicity, to cross the European horizon with its polarities; the Egyptian pictures are Klee's "West-East divan".'[38] Grohmann also mentions 'the oneness of life and eternity in Egypt'[39], which made a particular impression on Klee.

Dismissal, Return to Bern, Isolation
In 1933 Klee was reviled and denounced as a 'Jew' and 'foreigner' by the National Socialists, who had just come to power.[40] On March 17 his house in Dessau was searched while he and Lily were away.[41] On April 21 he was suspended from his post as Professor at the Düsseldorf Academy of Fine Arts, and a few months later he was dismissed. He did not try to defend himself against being labeled a 'Galician Jew'. He wrote to his wife: 'As far as I'm concerned, it does not seem right to do anything about this kind of crude slander. After all, if it were true that I were a Jew and that I came from Galicia, what difference would it make to my value as a person and to the value of my work? […] I would rather get into difficulties than be one of those miserable people who spend all their time trying to curry favor with the powers that be.'[42] Klee had to prove his Aryan descent and his Protestant affiliation. For many months he tried to stay in Germany, where he had an excellent reputation as an artist and art teacher, but he finally had to accept that there was no long-term future for his professional career under the Third Reich. Like other contemporary artists, his work was discredited, and in 1937 it was publicly denounced in the touring exhibition entitled 'Degenerate Art'. Looking back at that fateful year 1933, Paul Klee wrote: 'The new political climate in Germany affected the field of graphic art, both curbing academic freedom and cutting off all outlets for creative work in the arts. Since my reputation as a painter had in the course of time become international and even intercontinental, I felt that I was in a position to give up teaching and make my

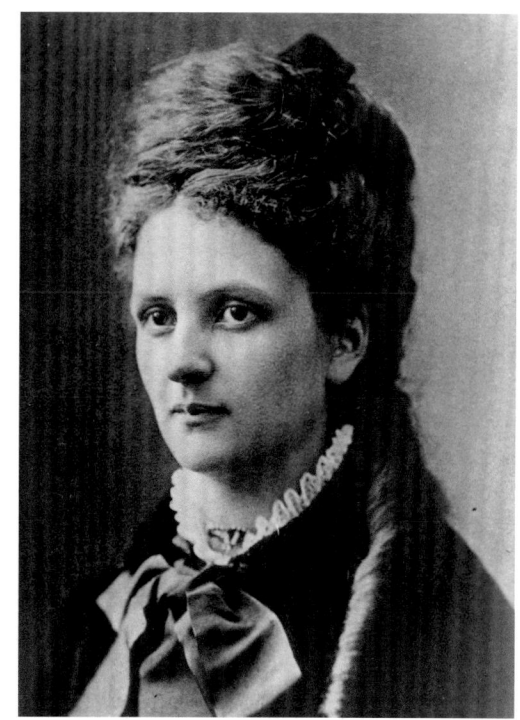

Fig. 17. Ida Klee-Frick, 1879

---

[38] Grohmann 1965, p. 72 f.
[39] Ibid., p. 73.
[40-41] See Appendices: Paul Klee and Lily Klee and the National Socialists (p. 268).
[42] Letter from Paul Klee to Lily Klee, Düsseldorf, April 6, 1933, quoted in Klee 1979, p. 1234.

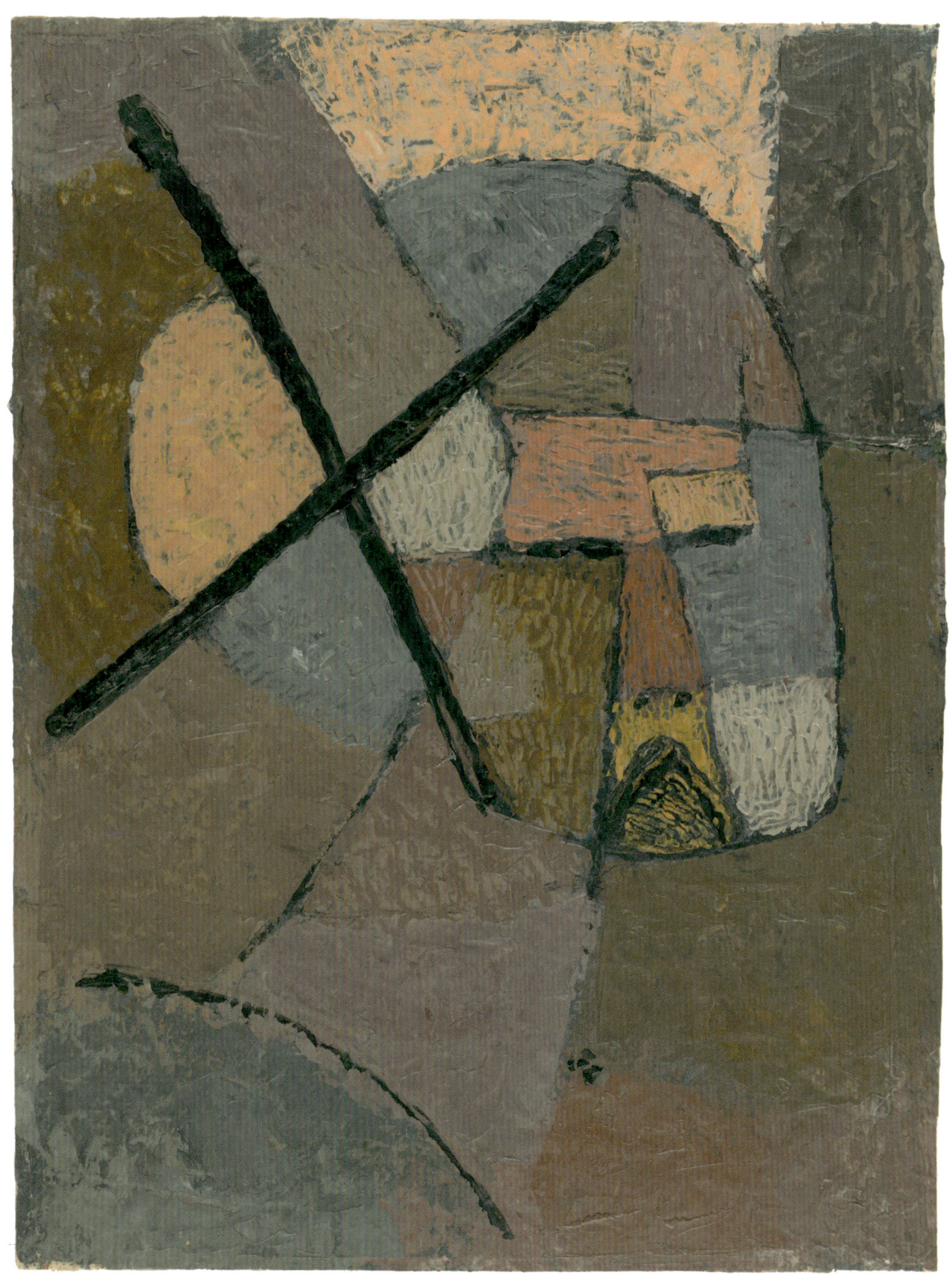

Fig. 18. Struck from the list, 1933, 424

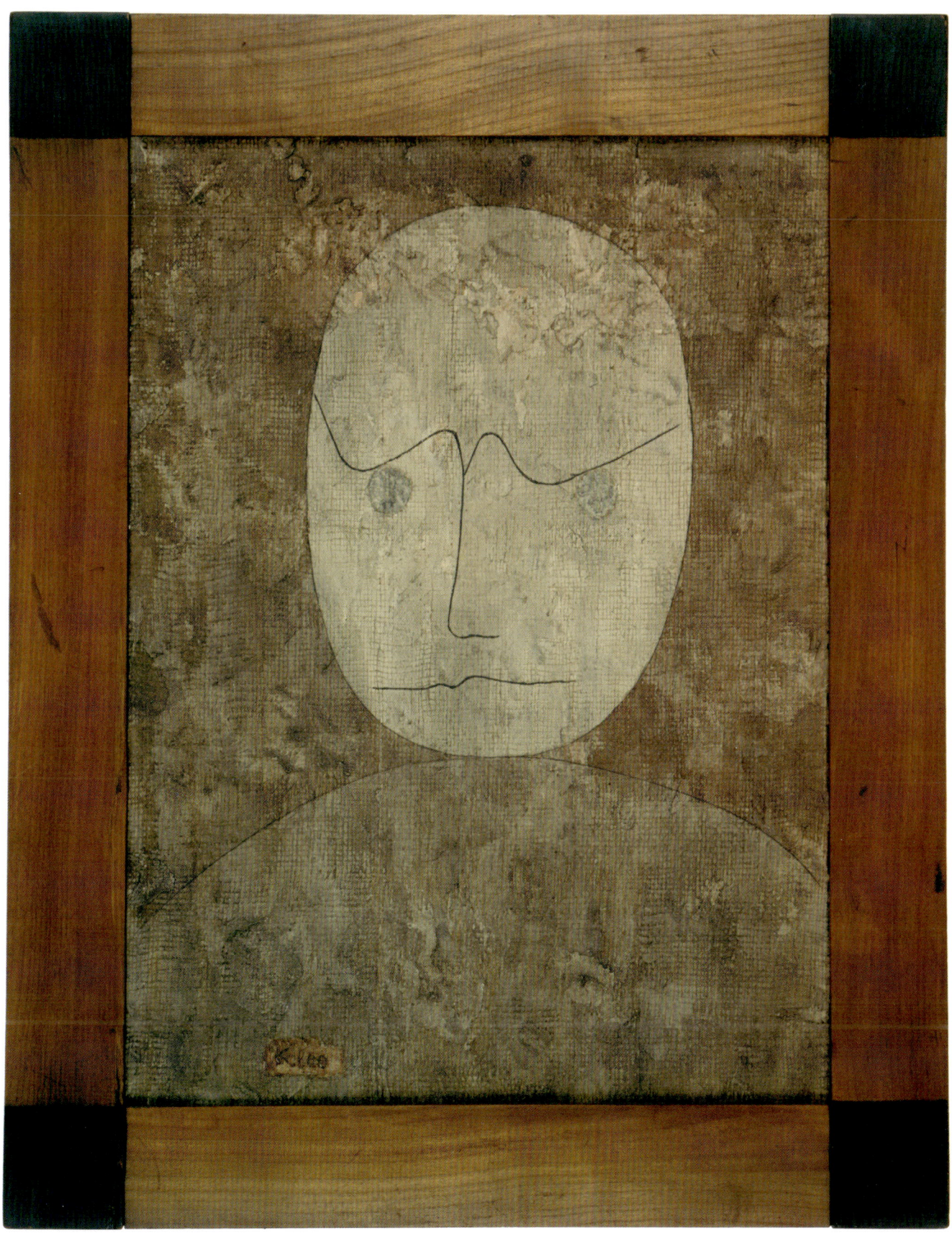

Fig. 19. Scholar, 1933, 286

Re Fig. 18. Struck from the list, 1933, 424 (p. 22)

Just three months after Hitler was elected Chancellor, Klee was suspended from his position as Distinguished Professor at the Düsseldorf Academy of Fine Arts. Eight months later (on January 1, 1934) his employment contract was terminated. Klee's art was denounced as degenerate. The artist, like many others, was 'struck from the list'. The National Socialists feared resistance, and wanted to do away with anything that smacked of intellectual superiority. The painting is a self-portrait. He is frowning angrily, and a thick, black cross is painted across his head.

Re Fig. 19. Scholar, 1933, 286 (p. 23)

This is probably also a self-portrait. Klee was an excellent teacher who loved his profession and took it very seriously. His students admired him greatly. He was very disappointed and bitter about his dismissal. This is expressed in the painting: the pensive, sad eyes, the frown, the narrow, pinched mouth. The corners of the wide, wooden frame are black. The future looks bleak.

Re Fig. 20. Rigidity, 1933, 187 (p. 25) ▷

This drawing, also from 1933, seems to show a person in a state of rigor mortis. Did Klee have a presentiment of how many soldiers would soon be lying stiffly on the battlefields? And how strange that within a few years his own body would stiffen up due to an incurable disease.

Re Fig. 21. Emigrating, 1933, 181 (p. 26)

After being dismissed from his post by the newly elected Nazis, Paul Klee and his wife had to emigrate to Switzerland. In Germany, Klee had been held in high regard as an artist and teacher, but in December 1933 he returned as an emigrant to his home town of Bern, where he felt very isolated. He felt that no one understood his brand of avant-garde art there. The drawing shows the couple's reluctance to emigrate. Lily is depicted with bowed head, and Paul with hanging arms and a skeptical, questioning expression as he faces an uncertain future.

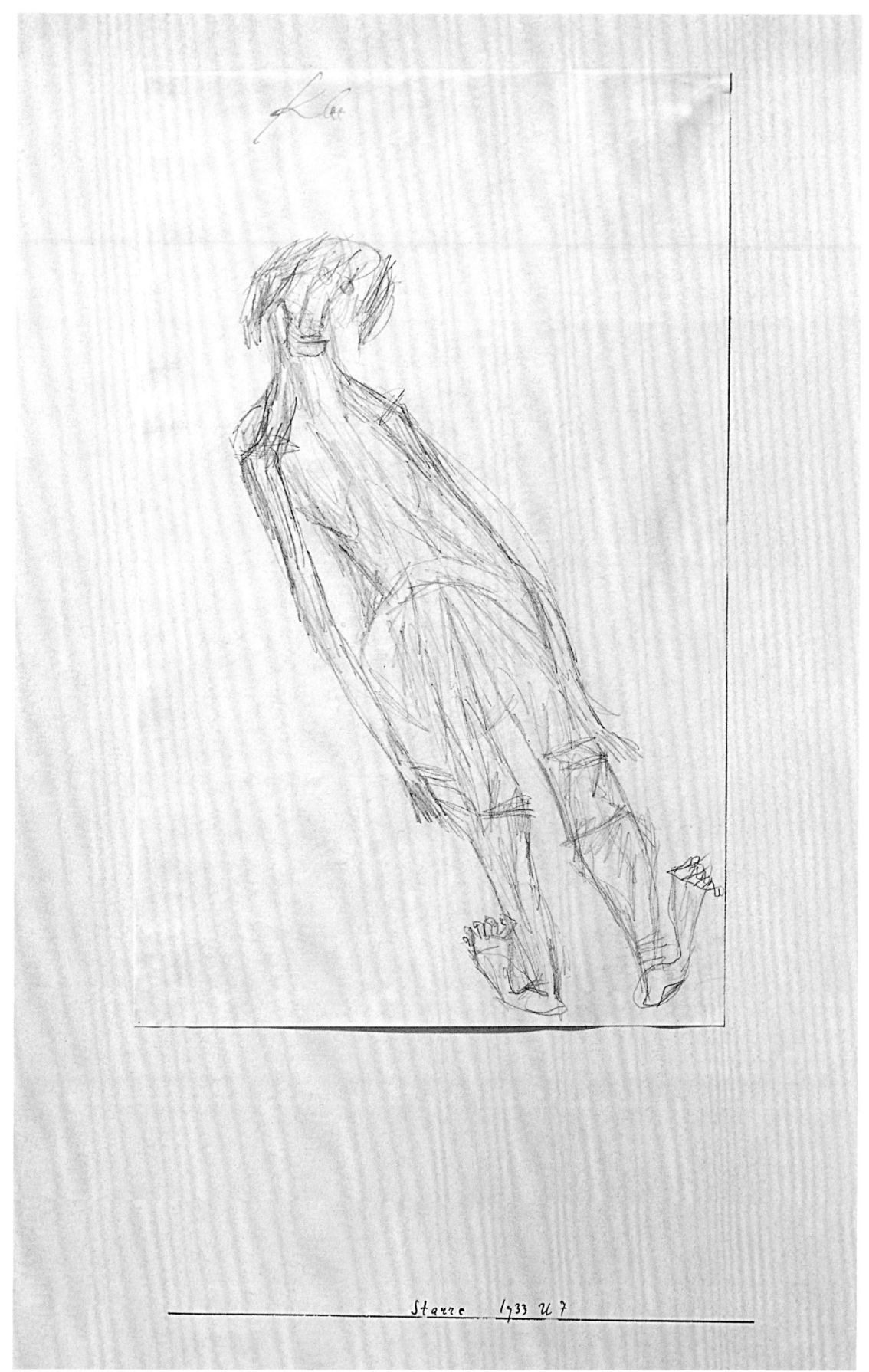

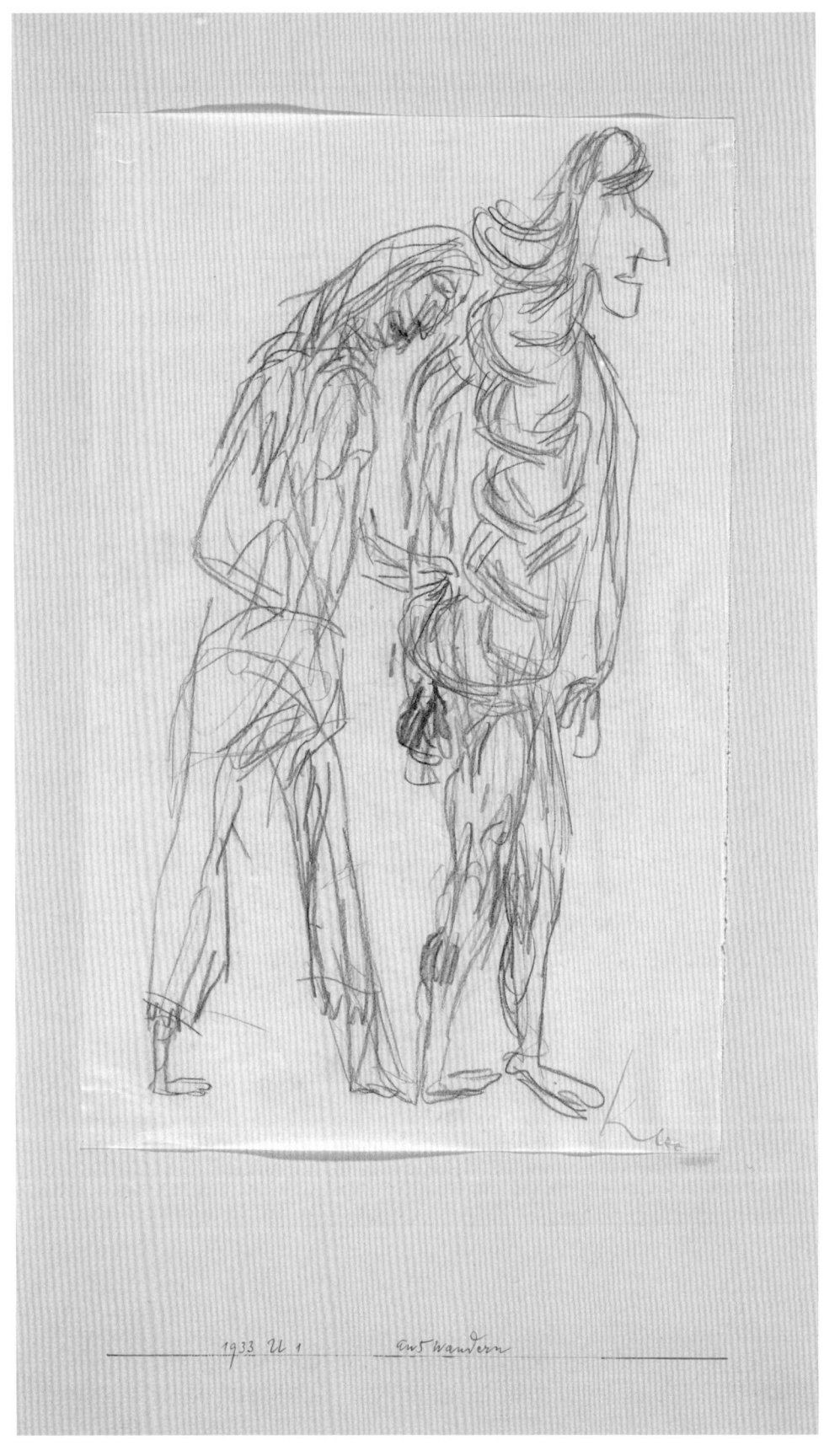

Fig. 21. Emigrating, 1933, 181

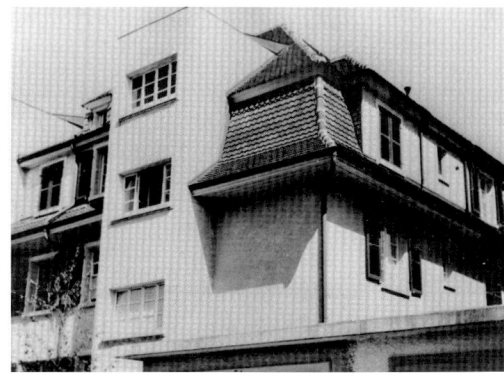

Fig. 23. Last residence of Paul and Lily Klee, Kistlerweg 6, Bern

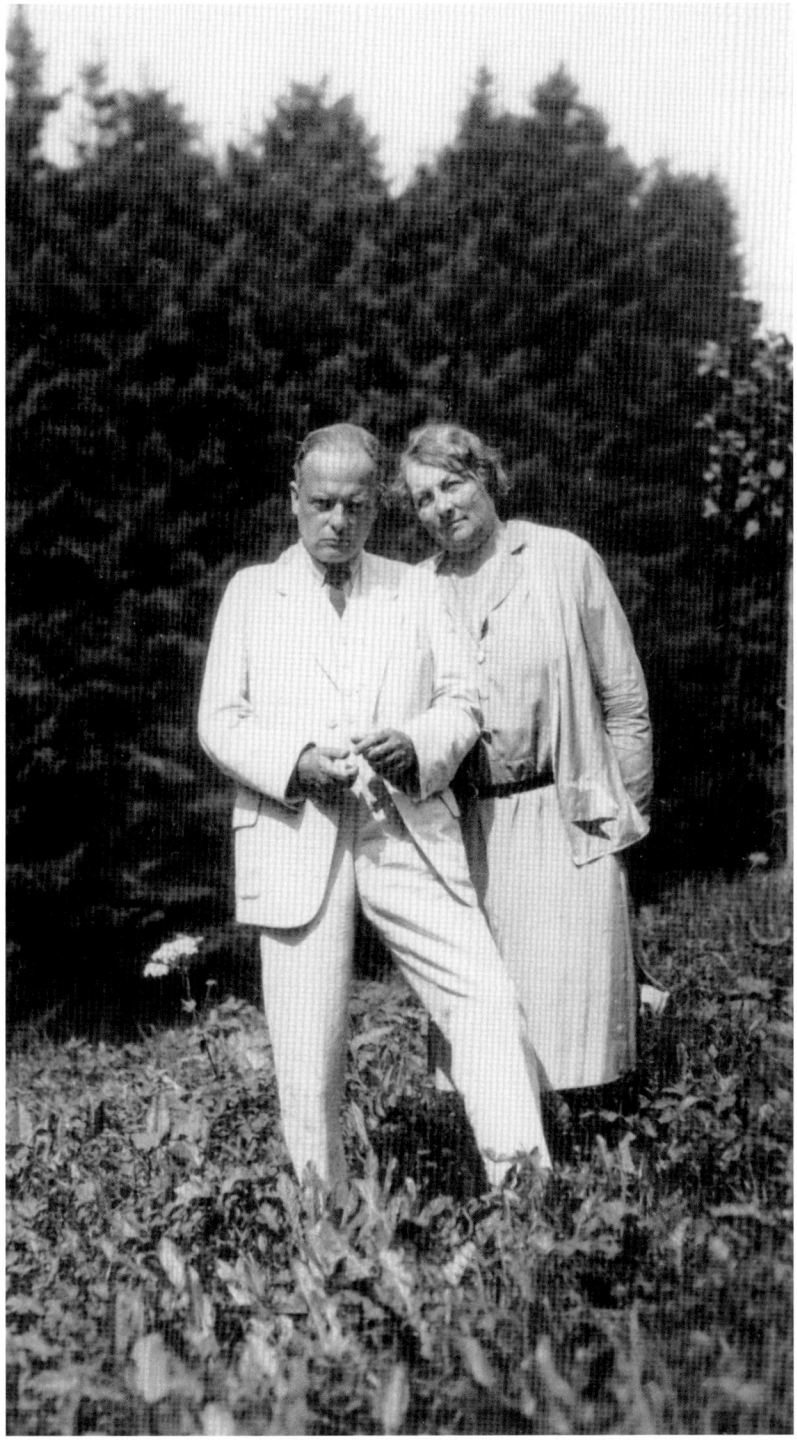

Fig. 22. Paul and Lily Klee, 1930

livelihood as an independent artist. The question of where to live henceforth was not in doubt. My close ties with Bern had never been broken; I felt keenly drawn to the city that is really my home.'[43]

[43] Klee 1940, p. 13 f (p. 258).

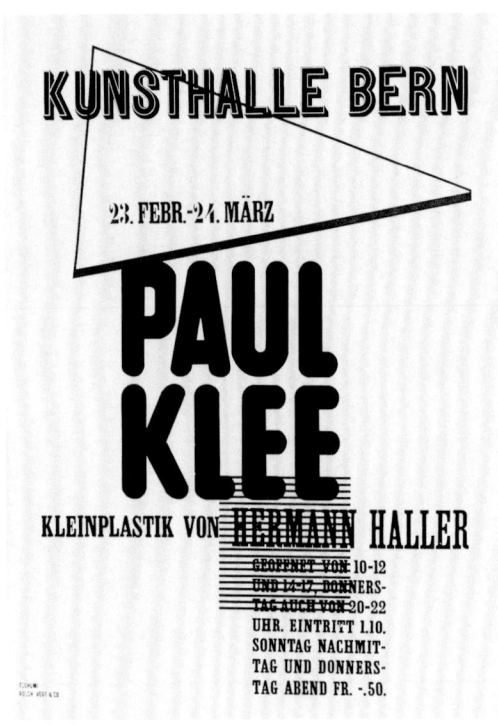

Fig. 24. Poster for the exhibition at the Kunsthalle Bern, February 23 to March 24, 1935

On December 24, 1933, Paul Klee emigrated from Düsseldorf to Bern, where Lily had arrived four days earlier. To begin with, they stayed with his father Hans and sister Mathilde at his parents' house at Obstbergweg 6, and then in early 1934, as an interim measure, they rented a furnished two-room apartment at Kollerweg 6. On June 1, 1934, they moved into a modest three-room apartment at Kistlerweg 6 in the Elfenau area of Bern. They turned the largest room into Klee's studio, the second-largest became the music room, containing the grand piano and violin, and the smallest room became their bedroom; the kitchen was also the dining room and the attic served as a guest bedroom.[44] Paul and Lily were welcomed by school friends, acquaintances and collectors such as Hans Bloesch, Dr. Fritz Lotmar, Louis Moilliet, Marie von Sinner, Hanni Bürgi-Bigler and her son Rolf, Hermann and Margrit Rupf, the artist couples Victor and Marguerite Surbek-Frey and Otto and Hildegard Nebel, and the professor of German language and literature, Fritz Strich. The Klees also soon made new friends, such as the art historians Bernard Geiser, Max Huggler and Georg Schmidt, the collectors Hans and Erika Meyer-Benteli, the German musicologist Hans Kayser and the sculptor Max Fueter.[45] But despite this, the artist felt unexpectedly isolated. Their son Felix was working as an opera director in Germany: from 1933 to 1938 in Ulm and then until 1944 in Wilhelmshafen.

Klee's break with the past had an effect on his productivity: in the year of his dismissal he produced his highest total of works to date, 482, but in the first year of his emigration he only produced 219.[46] Paul Klee became very quiet, as he concentrated more and more on his work. In February 1935 he wrote to Wassily Kandinsky: 'Our health and a few basic material needs are all we require to do our work. We really need nothing more. My work is my main source of optimism, and if it is to be in silence, then that is not necessarily a bad thing.'[47] Klee's words reflect his isolation, but also his unassuming, unpretentious and adaptable nature. They also tell us how much his work meant to him. During his Swiss exile, Klee largely retreated into his shell, hiding away in his little studio which was also a vast and beautiful world of art. Max Huggler refers to this as his 'inner emigration'.[48]

44 Cf. Frey 1990, p. 112.
45 Cf. ibid.
46 Cf. Glaesemer 1976, p. 308
47 Letter from Paul Klee to Wassily Kandinsky, Bern, February 1935, quoted in Kuthy 1984, p. 15.
48 Huggler 1969, p. 156.

Klee Exhibitions in Switzerland: Attracting Little Interest

As early as 1910, the Bern Museum of Fine Arts put on an exhibition of 56 graphic works by Paul Klee.[49] Klee's friend from schooldays, the editor and critic Hans Bloesch, was one of the few who championed the talented artist in public. On the occasion of a second small exhibition of Klee's work at the Bern Museum of Fine Arts in 1911, Bloesch put together 'the first ever full review of Paul Klee's work'.[50] The Bern public found the artist too avant-garde. Despite Ferdinand Hodler, Bern was still very much wedded to the traditional naturalistic style of art. There was plenty of culture on offer in the city,[51] but very little could be described as progressive. There were no internationally renowned groups of like-minded artists trying to push the boundaries, such as 'Die Brücke'[52] ('The Bridge') in Dresden and 'Der Blaue Reiter'[53] ('The Blue Rider') in Munich. With only a few exceptions, Klee could not find any connection with the artists working in Bern. It's easy to understand his disappointment when he writes of the 'bland illusion of the Bernese milieu.'[54]

In February 1935, 14 months after Klee's return to Bern, Max Huggler welcomed the artist by putting on a major exhibition of 273 works at the Bern Kunsthalle.[55] Looking back on this event, Huggler wrote: 'The exhibition […] attracted little interest: we put together treasured items from Klee's own portfolio covering his various creative periods, but this remarkable show had absolutely no effect on the local art scene, in the same way as the art associations, artists' groups and other cultural institutions had ignored his presence in Bern. […] His work had no connection with the Swiss artistic tradition, and no one was prepared for the direction he was taking: his work was just there, like an erratic boulder.'[56] The 'Welcome Exhibition' in Bern was subsequently taken over by the Basel Kunsthalle,[57] where some of the works were lambasted by local art critics. An editor of the 'National-Zeitung' wrote: 'It seems to us that Klee is a uniquely subtle and very sensitive artist, but he is an artist with limited creative powers. We just cannot find artistic value in every one of his ideas and in every variation of his favourite motifs. A lot of his work seems quite insignificant. Some of it has an Arts and

[49] Cf. von Tavel 1988, p. 13.
[50] Ibid., p. 14. The text from Hans Bloesch, Ein moderner Graphiker, in: Die Alpen, vol. VI, issue 5, January 1912, pp. 264–272, is reproduced in excerpts in Du 1948, p. 61.
[51] Cf. von Tavel 1988, p. 13.
[52] 'Die Brücke', a group of German Expressionist artists, was founded in 1905 in Dresden by E. L. Kirchner, E. Heckel, F. Bleyl, K. Schmitt-Rottluff. In 1906 they were joined by E. Nolde and M. Pechstein. Also affiliated at times were Kees van Dongen, Otto Müller, the Finnish artist Axel Gallén and the Swiss Cuno Amiet. The group broke up in 1913. (From: Darmstaedter 1979, p. 105).
[53] 'Der Blaue Reiter' was an artistic movement founded in 1912 in Munich (named after a painting by W. Kandinsky). The group included W. Kandinsky, F. Marc, A. Macke, P. Klee and E. Campendonk. Alongside 'Die Brücke' (see note 52), 'Der Blaue Reiter' was the most important group of Expressionist artists in Germany. (From: Darmstaedter 1979, p. 84).
[54] Cf. von Tavel 1988, p. 9. This title comes from Paul Klee's diaries, in: Klee Tgb., no. 963. Thanks to Josef Helfenstein for this reference. And von Tavel 1988, p. 20: 'When Klee targets the "bland illusion of the Bernese milieu", particularly the unperturbed everyday life which was barely affected by the war, we get a real feel for his relationship to the city where he grew up and spent large parts of his life. For him, Bern was both impalpable and uninteresting. After the promising start at the Museum of Fine Arts, Bern offered him nothing as an avant-garde artist. He thought the cultural events were nothing more than idle socializing. And although there were many interesting people who lived there, he never got to know them, their thinking or their work because there was no focal point where intellectuals and artists could rub shoulders.'
[55] Paul Klee, Bern Kunsthalle, from February 23 to March 24, 1935 (catalogue: 273 works).
[56] Huggler 1969, p. 156.
[57] Paul Klee, Basel Kunsthalle, from October 27 to November 24, 1935 (catalogue: 191 works).

Crafts influence and could be used as a design for carpets or textiles. And to the uninitiated, much of his work looks like hieroglyphics, totally incomprehensible. What heightens our skepticism is the similarity of his work to children's drawings and the like. We don't see it as a very positive sign when a man in his fifties finds inspiration in such things.'[58]

In 1936 Paul Klee was not accepted for the major 'National Art Exhibition' in Bern.[59] However, in the same year he was shown at the Zurich Kunsthaus as part of the 'Time Problems in Swiss Painting and Sculpture' exhibition. Indeed, together with Jean Arp and Le Corbusier, he was hailed as one of the three leading international proponents of Swiss avant-garde art.[60] But the 'Luzerner Nachrichten' published a review which showed little understanding of the artists exhibiting in Zurich: 'It [the "National Art Exhibition" in Bern] cold-shouldered dreamers like the Surrealists and design engineers like the abstract artists. These "outsiders", these art revolutionaries, have now been gathered together in a kind of front by the Zurich exhibition.'[61]

In 1938 the Association of Modern Swiss Artists, known as the 'Allianz' group, honoured Klee with a special place at their exhibition in Basel entitled 'New Art in Switzerland'.[62]

In 1940 the Kunsthaus Zurich organized a major exhibition to coincide with Klee's 60th birthday. His later works from 1935 to 1940 were shown, but they also aroused controversy. After the exhibition, Jakob Welti, cultural editor of the 'Neue Zürcher Zeitung', went as far as to say he thought Klee's art was the work of someone mentally ill![63] Two days later the Bernese lawyer, Fritz Trüssel, president of the museum committee at the Bern Museum of Fine Arts, complained in a letter to the chief editor of the 'Neue Zürcher Zeitung', 'that a publication like yours [...] should attempt to dispatch an artist of such range and international standing as Klee with such a hackneyed play on words.' He stressed that Klee was 'mentally in good health' and 'in no way mentally ill'.[64]

---

[58] Published by an editor with initials 'hgr.' in the 'National-Zeitung', no. 2018, Basel, November 19, 1935, reproduced in: Du 1948, p. 72.

[59] Cf. Werckmeister 1987, p. 52.

[60] Cf. ibid.

[61] 'Luzerner Nachrichten', no. 140, June 16, 1936, quoted in Werckmeister 1987, p. 52.

[62] New Art in Switzerland, Basel Kunsthalle, from January 9 to February 2, 1938 (catalogue: 7 works by Paul Klee). Cf. Geelhaar 1979, p. 6 f.

[63] Cf. Welti, Jakob, Aus dem Zürcher Kunsthaus, in: Neue Zürcher Zeitung, March 30, 1940, morning edition: 'This Saturday afternoon at 3.00 pm sees the opening of the April exhibition at the Kunsthaus. After our interesting excursion to the strange "schizophrenic garden", which proved to be too elevated for many visitors, we are now climatically and visually back in the more familiar realms of Swiss Mittelland art. The exhibition space has been given to eight artists from the Aargau.' Quoted in Frey 1990, p. 123. Jakob Welti was referring to the main peak of the 2,910 metres high Glärnisch massif (Canton Glarus), which was known as 'Vrenelisgärtli', and linking it to the idea of schizophrenia and Klee's art, which often used a kind of garden landscape as a central theme. Thanks to the art historian Walther Fuchs for the geographical reference. Documented in detail by Walther Fuchs in: 'Paul Klee and Medicine', exhibition at the Medical History Museum, University of Zurich, Zurich, March 31 to October 9, 2005.

[64] Letter from Dr. iur. Fritz Trüssel to Willy Bretscher, Bern, April 1, 1940, typewritten, 21 x 30 cm, Bern Museum of Fine Arts. Thanks to Walther Fuchs for this reference.

'And My Sole Remaining Wish Is to Be a Citizen of This City'

In 1934, a few months after moving from Düsseldorf to Bern, Paul Klee enquired about becoming a Swiss citizen. He was informed that he would need a permanent residence permit and '[...] that citizens of the German Reich are only eligible for this when they have lived in Switzerland continuously and legally for a period of 5 years'.[65] To begin with, he and his wife were only given a restricted residence permit, which had to be extended every year. In 1934 no allowance was made for the fact that Klee had lived in Bern for the first 19 years of his life and had later spent extended periods of time there.

Once the mandatory five years had passed, on the very same day that he received his permanent residence permit – April 24, 1939 – the artist applied for Swiss citizenship through his lawyer, Fritz Trüssel (Swiss Federal Archive). He was actively supported in this by his friend Conrad von Mandach, curator of the Bern Museum of Fine Arts, and by the director of the Bern Kunsthalle, Max Huggler.[66] After Klee had been repeatedly subjected to police questioning, on November 13, 1939, the Canton and Municipality of Bern recommended to the Federal Justice and Police Department that Klee should be granted his federal permit. He received it on December 19, 1939, despite the embarrassing and humiliating reports which were made.[67] However, in order for the permit to be legally valid, he still had to apply for the so-called 'Landrecht' – the right to live in the canton – and for municipal citizenship of the city of Bern. He submitted this application on January 15, 1940, along with a short biography dated January 7, 1940 (see pages 32–35), which finished with the sentence: 'I have been living here [in Bern] ever since [his emigration from Germany], and my sole remaining wish is to be a citizen of this city.'[68] On March 12, 1940, Klee provided another piece of required information, and then on March 15, 1940, the Bern Municipal Police Department requested the Municipal Council to grant him citizenship of the city of Bern. Two weeks later, the cultural editor of the 'Neue Zürcher Zeitung' branded him as mentally ill (as previously mentioned). Klee decided not to take legal action in this respect, for fear of jeopardizing his ongoing naturalization process.[69]

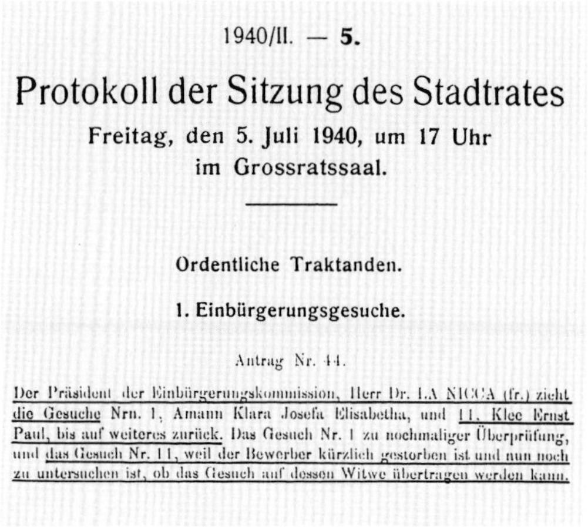
1940/II. — **5.**

Protokoll der Sitzung des Stadtrates

Freitag, den 5. Juli 1940, um 17 Uhr im Grossratssaal.

Ordentliche Traktanden.

1. Einbürgerungsgesuche.

Antrag Nr. 44.

Der Präsident der Einbürgerungskommission, Herr Dr. LA NICCA (fr.) zieht die Gesuche Nrn. 1, Amann Klara Josefa Elisabetha, und 11, Klee Ernst Paul, bis auf weiteres zurück. Das Gesuch Nr. 1 zu nochmaliger Überprüfung, und das Gesuch Nr. 11, weil der Bewerber kürzlich gestorben ist und nun noch zu untersuchen ist, ob das Gesuch auf dessen Witwe übertragen werden kann.

Fig. 25. Extract from the minutes of the Bern Municipal Council meeting on July 5, 1940 (Bern Municipal Archive)

Fig. 26. (pp. 32–35): Paul Klee's biography, Bern January 7, 1940 (Bern Police Department) ▷

[65] See Appendices: Paul Klee's Efforts to Gain Swiss Citizenship (p. 265).

[66–69] See Appendices: Paul Klee's Efforts to Gain Swiss Citizenship (p. 266).

Lebenslauf

Ich bin am 18 Dezember 1879 in München=
=buchsee geboren. Mein Vater war Musik=
lehrer am Kantonalen Lehrerseminar Hofwyl,
und meine Mutter war Schweizerin. Als ich im Frühjahr
1886 in die Schule kam, wohnten wir in der
Länggasse in Bern. Ich besuchte die ersten vier
Klassen der dortigen Primarschule. Dann
schickten mich meine Eltern ans Städtische
Progymnasium, dessen vier Klassen ich absolvierte,
um dann in die Literarschule derselben Anstalt
einzutreten. Den Abschluss meiner allgemeinen
Bildung bildete das Kantonale Maturitätsexamen,
das ich im Herbst 1898 bestand.

Die Berufswahl ging äusserlich glatt
von Statten. Obwohl mir durch das Maturitäts-
zeugnis alles offen stand, wollte ich es wagen,
mich in der Malerei auszubilden und die Kunst=
=malerei als Lebensaufgabe zu wählen. Die
Realisierung führte damals — wie teilweise auch
heute noch — auf den Weg ins Ausland.
Man musste sich nur entscheiden zwischen Paris
oder Deutschland. Mir kam Deutschland

Gefühlsmässig mehr entgegen.

Und so begab ich mich auf den Weg nach der bayrischen Metropole, wo mich die Kunstakademie zunächst an die private Vorschule Knirr verwies. Hier übte ich Zeichnen und Malen, um dann in die Klasse Franz Stuck der Kunstakademie einzutreten

Die drei Jahre meines Münchner Studiums erweiterte ich dann durch eine einjährige Studien= =reise nach Italien (hauptsächlich Rom)

Und nun galt es, in stiller Arbeit das Gewonnene zu verwerten und zu fördern. Dazu eignete sich die Stadt meiner Jugend, Bern, auf das beste, und ich kann heute noch als Frucht dieses Aufenthaltes eine Reihe von Radierungen aus den Jahren 1903 bis 1906 nachweisen, die schon damals nicht unbeachtet blieben.

Mannigfache Beziehungen, die ich in München angeknüpft hatte, führten auch zur ehelichen Verbindung mit meiner jetzigen Frau. Dass sie in München beruflich tätig war, war für uns ein wichtiger Grund, ein zweites Mal dorthin zu übersiedeln (Herbst 1906) Nach aussen setzte ich mich als Künstler langsam durch und jeder Schritt vorwärts war

war an diesem damals kunstzentralen Platz von Bedeutung.

Mit einer Unterbrechung von drei Jahren während des Weltkriegs durch Garnisonsdienst in Landshut, Schleissheim und Gersthofen, blieb ich in München niedergelassen bis zum Jahr 1920. Die Beziehungen zu Bern brachen schon äusserlich nicht ab, weil ich alljährlich die Ferienzeit von 2-3 Monaten daselbst im Elternhaus verbrachte.

Das Jahr 1920 brachte mir die Berufung als Lehrer an das staatliche Bauhaus zu Weimar. Hier wirkte ich bis zur Übersiedelung dieser Kunsthochschule nach Dessau im Jahre 1926. Endlich erreichte mich im Jahr 1930 ein Ruf zum Leiter einer Malklasse an der preussischen Kunstakademie zu Düsseldorf. Dieses kam meinem Wunsch entgegen, die Lehrtätigkeit ganz auf das mir eigentümlichen Gebiet zu beschränken, und so lehrte ich denn an dieser Kunsthochschule während der Jahre 1931 bis 1933.

Die neuen politischen Verhältnisse Deutschlands erstreckten ihre Wirkung auch auf das Gebiet der bildenden Kunst und hemmen nicht nur die Lehrfreiheit, sondern auch die Auswirkung des privaten künstlerischen Schaffens. Mein Ruf als Maler hatte im Laufe der Zeit sich über die staatlichen, ja auch über die continentalen Grenzen hinaus ausgebreitet, so dass ich mich stark genug fühlte, ohne Amt im freien Beruf zu existieren.

Die Frage von welchem Orte aus das geschehn würde, beantwortete sich eigentlich ganz von selber. Dadurch, dass die guten Beziehungen zu Bern nie abgebrochen waren, spürte ich zu deutlich und zu stark die Anziehung dieses eigentlichen Heimatortes. Seitdem lebe ich wieder hier und es bleibt nur noch ein Wunsch offen, Bürger dieser Stadt zu sein

Bern den 7 Jänner 1940

Paul Klee

Biography

I was born on December 18, 1879, in Münchenbuchsee. My father was a music teacher at the cantonal teacher's college in Hofwil; my mother was Swiss. When I started school in the spring of 1886, we lived on Länggasse in Bern. I attended the first four classes of primary school in that city. Then my parents sent me to the municipal grammar school; I stayed there through the fourth and last class and then attended the school of literature in the same institution. My general education was concluded with the cantonal examination, which I passed in the autumn of 1898.

It seemed that my choice of career should be easy. I was now qualified, thanks to my cantonal certificate, to enter any profession. However I decided to study painting and devote my life to art, however hazardous such a career might be. Such studies were best undertaken in those days – as to some extent they still are today – abroad. The choice lay only between Paris and Germany. I felt more emotionally drawn to Germany. And so I set out for the Bavarian metropolis. At the Academy of Fine Arts they recommended that I first attend Knirr's preparatory school. There I practiced drawing and painting, and subsequently entered Franz Stuck's class at the Academy.

After three years studying in Munich, I spent a further year of study and travel in Italy, chiefly in Rome. My next task was to employ the skills I had acquired, and to make progress in my art. Bern, the home of my youth, seemed to me the ideal place for such work, and I still can point to the fruits of this stay: the etchings I did from 1903 to 1906, which even at that time attracted a certain amount of attention.

I had formed many ties in Munich, and one of these led to marriage with my present wife. The fact that she could practice her profession in Munich was one of the important reasons for my returning there for the second time (autumn 1906). As an artist I was slowly achieving recognition, and every step forward in Munich was of importance, for the city was then a center of the art world.

I remained a resident of Munich until 1920, except for an interruption of three years during the World War, when I served on garrison duty in Landshut, Schleissheim and Gersthofen. All through this period my ties with Bern remained unbroken; every year I holidayed for two or three weeks at my parents' home there.

In 1920 came my appointment to the staff of the Bauhaus school in Weimar. I taught there until the institution moved to Dessau in 1926. Finally, in 1930, I was asked to accept an appointment to conduct a course in painting at the Prussian Academy of Art in Düsseldorf. This offer coincided with my own desire to confine my teaching entirely to my own field. I therefore accepted and was associated with the Academy from 1931 to 1933.

The new political climate in Germany affected the field of graphic art, both curbing academic freedom and cutting off all outlets for creative work in the arts. Since my reputation as a painter had in the course of time become international and even intercontinental, I felt that I was in a position to give up teaching and make my livelihood as an independent artist. The question of where to live henceforth was not in doubt. My close ties with Bern had never been broken; I felt keenly drawn to the city that is really my home. I have been living here ever since, and my sole remaining wish is to be a citizen of this city.

Bern, January 7, 1940
Paul Klee

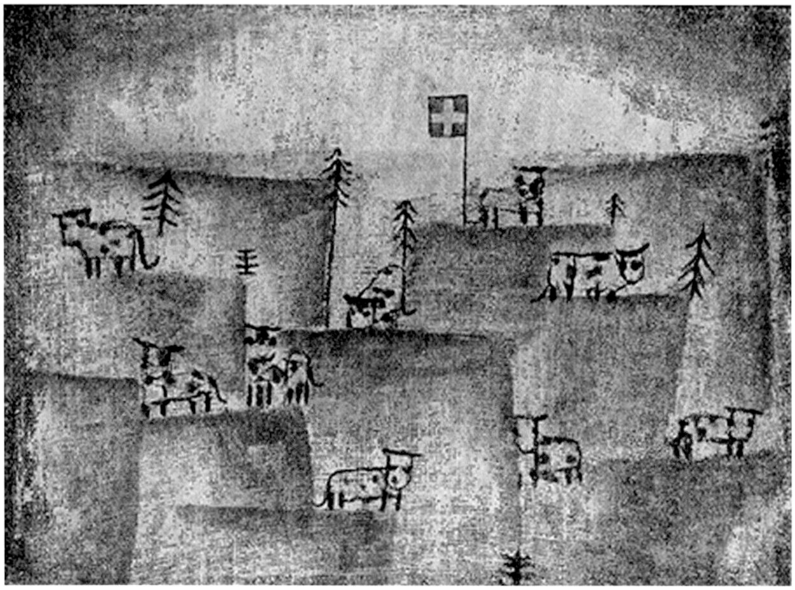

Fig. 27. Swiss landscape, 1919, 46

On their return to Switzerland in 1934, as Germans, Paul and Lily Klee applied for Swiss citizenship. Klee had to submit to embarrassing questioning by the naturalization authorities. After a visit to Klee, a police official remarked in his report – referring to this painting – that the cows 'looked stupid', and 'Isn't this painting a direct attack on what some people call "Kuhschweizer" (Swiss cow herders, a pejorative term for the Swiss)?' Despite such fatuousness, the artist, who had spent more than half his life in Bern, would probably have been granted Swiss citizenship in the end, but he died six days before the meeting of the Bern Citizenship Commission where his case was to be decided.

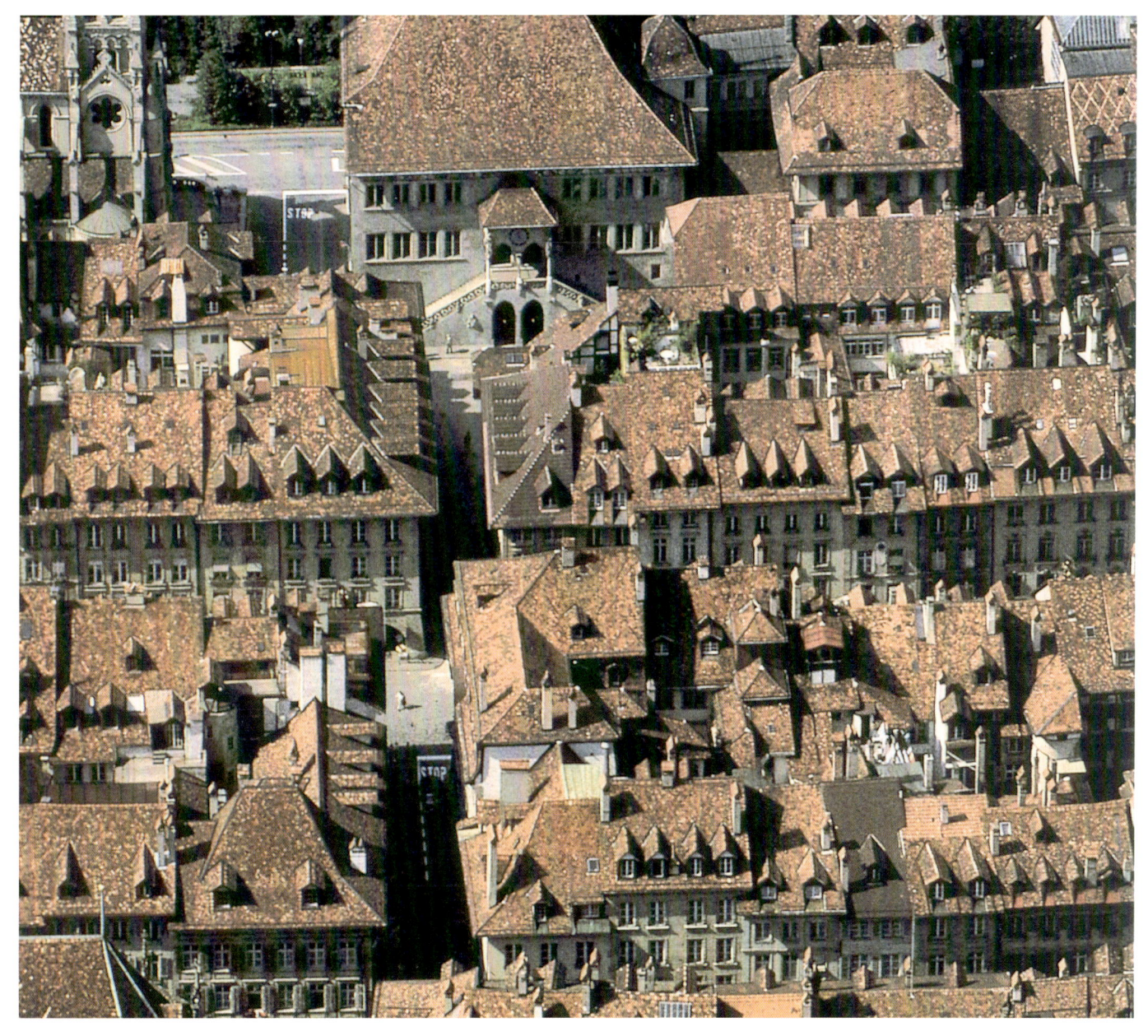

Fig. 28. Bern old town with the town hall (top)

On June 19, 1940, ten days before his death, he still had to deal with questions from the Bern Citizenship Commission while he was seriously ill in the Clinica Sant' Agnese in Locarno.[70] His application for citizenship was then finally put on the agenda for the meeting of the Bern Municipal Council to be held on July 5, 1940 (fig. 25).[71] Paul Klee died six days before this meeting took place. His final wish was never granted – to be a citizen of the city in which he had lived half his life.

[70-71] See Appendices: Paul Klee's Efforts to Gain Swiss Citizenship (p. 265 f).

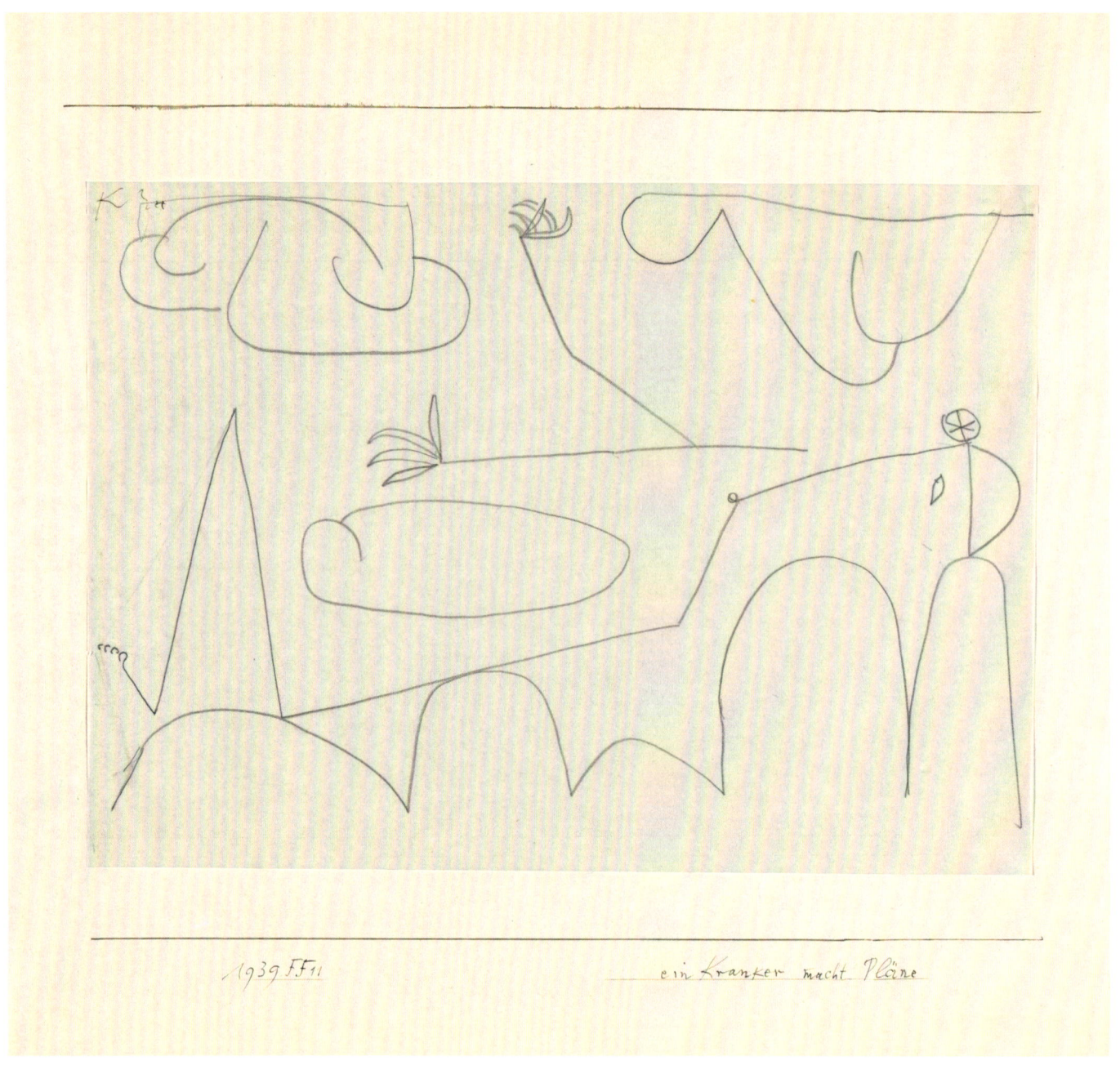

Fig. 29. A sick man makes plans, 1939, 611

2. Paul Klee's Illness

First Symptoms – Persistent Bronchitis, Pneumonia, Pleurisy and Permanent Fatigue

Paul Klee's illness first reared its head in the summer of 1935. The artist had never before suffered ill-health 'apart from a few childhood illnesses'[72], but at the end of August he caught 'a bad cold'[73]. Lily Klee reported that he had suffered badly from persistent and deep-rooted bronchial catarrh.[74] Paul Klee felt constantly tired.[75] But he didn't seek medical help until later, when he noticed that his body temperature was slightly elevated in the evenings. On October 21, 1935,[76] thanks to the intervention of his school friend, the Bern neurologist Dr. Fritz Lotmar, he visited the internist Dr. Gerhard Schorer.[77] The latter observed that 'the heart was not functioning properly',[78] and ordered complete physical rest.[79] But Klee's condition continued to deteriorate, and from October 25 he was confined to his bed.[80] From November 15 to 17 he had a high fever (over 39°C); Dr. Schorer suspected lung complications[81] – probably pneumonia and pleurisy. There were no antibiotics, so Paul Klee had to rally his powers of resistance and try to beat the illness on his own. But he was in a very weak state.[82] It was also not yet possible to take an X-ray of his lungs and heart.[83]

[72] Letter from Lily Klee to Daniel-Henry Kahnweiler, Bern, November 30, 1935 (location unknown): 'My husband was never ill, apart from in his early childhood, and this is why the disease affected him so badly. He was unlike other people who often have something wrong with them, and who as a result build immunity against such attacks.' And letter from Lily Klee to Gertrud Grote, Bern, January 12, 1936 (ZPKB): 'My husband had never been seriously ill, so when the illness came, it felled him like a tree.'

[73] Letter from Lily Klee to Gertrud Grohmann, Bern, October 11, 1935 (AWG).

[74] Cf. letter from Lily Klee to Will Grohmann, Bern, October 23, 1935 (AWG).

[75] Cf. letter from Lily Klee to Dr. Gerhard Schorer, Bern, March 8, 1936 (photocopy ZPKB/SFK).

[76] Klee 1935/1936 (p. 258), p. 1: '21. X. evening 37.6 (at the doctor's)'.

[77] Cf. letter from Lily Klee to Will Grohmann, Bern, October 23, 1935 (AWG), and cf. letter from Lily Klee to Gertrud Grohmann, Bern, November 23, 1935 (AWG).

[78] Letter from Lily Klee to Will Grohmann, Bern, October 23, 1935 (AWG).

[79] Cf. ibid.

[80] Klee 1935/1936 (p. 258), p. 2: '26. X. in bed', cf. letter from Lily Klee to Nina Kandinsky, Bern, November 3, 1935 (BK/CGPP), cf. letter from Lily Klee to Rudolf Probst, Bern, November 10, 1935 (PBD), and cf. letter from Lily Klee to Daniel-Henry Kahnweiler, Bern, November 22, 1935 (location unknown).

[81] Cf. Klee 1935/1936 (p. 258), p. 4, cf. letter from Lily Klee to Gertrud Grohmann, Bern, November 23, 1935 (AWG), and cf. letter from Lily Klee to Rudolf Probst, Bern, November 26, 1935 (PBD).

[82] Cf. letter from Lily Klee to Daniel-Henry Kahnweiler, Bern, January 4, 1936 (location unknown).

[83] Cf. letters from Lily Klee to Will Grohmann, Bern, December 2, 1935, and December 29, 1935 (AWG), and cf. letter from Lily Klee to Gertrud Grohmann, Bern, March 29, 1936 (AWG).

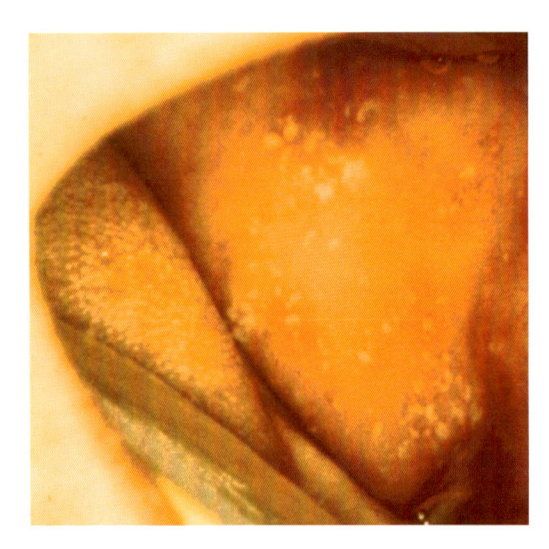

Fig. 30. Measles: 'Koplik's spots', small white spots on the inside of the mouth. I thank Prof. Christoph Aebi for the photo.

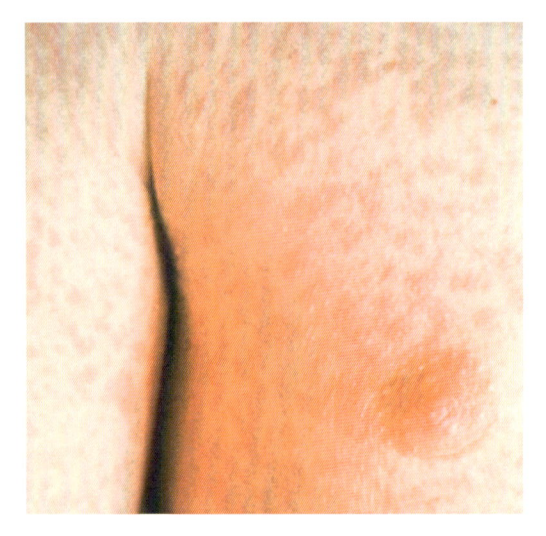

Fig. 31. Measles: rash with red spots over the whole body, including the face. I thank Prof. Christoph Aebi for the photo.

84   Letter from Otto Nebel to Lily Klee, Bern, November 20, 1935 (ZPKB/SFK).
85   Letter from Lily Klee to Nina Kandinsky, Bern, February 13, 1936 (BK/CGPP).
86   Cf. letter from Lily Klee to Emmy Scheyer, Bern, March 8, 1936 (NSMP).
87   Letter from Lily Klee to Will Grohmann, Bern, April 9, 1936 (AWG).
88   Letter from Lily Klee to Nina Kandinsky, Bern, April 14, 1936 (AWG).
89   Letter from Lily Klee to Will Grohmann, Bern, October 29, 1936 (AWG).
90   Personal communication, Felix Klee to the author, Bern, September 20, 1983.
91   Klee 1989, p. 47.

Measles?

Coinciding with the high fever in mid-November 1935, Paul Klee apparently came out in a short-lived rash all over his body. The German artist Otto Nebel (who also lived in Bern) writes in a letter to Lily Klee on November 20, 1935: 'Thank goodness the doctor is such an excellent diagnostician. It is very odd that he should catch the measles – and even stranger that we can't work out how he got infected.'[84] It is not clear from the letter how Nebel came by this information. The skin rash was not described in any more detail. It's curious that Lily Klee doesn't mention the 'measles' until three months later in a letter to Nina Kandinsky, the wife of Wassily Kandinsky: 'I don't know whether I told you that he [Paul Klee] has had the measles really badly. In older age, measles is a very serious complaint and can lead to severe complications – this is what has happened to my husband. He has been ill for four months (!).'[85] In March 1936 she tells Emmy Scheyer the same thing.[86] In April 1936 it was possible to have an X-ray examination, and eight days later she writes to Will Grohmann: '[…] it was chronic double pneumonia caused by the measles (!). The doctor made this diagnosis earlier.'[87] We can assume that Lily is referring to the diagnosis of 'chronic double pneumonia' and not to the measles. She tells Nina Kandinsky: 'He has had prolonged chronic double pneumonia (caused by the measles).'[88] However, in 1936 Paul Klee started to experience other changes to his skin, so Dr. Schorer referred him to Professor Naegeli, a specialist in dermatology. Immediately after this consultation, Lily told Will Grohmann: 'The doctors now think it wasn't the measles!! So what was it?'[89] Felix Klee could not tell us anything concrete about his father's 'measles', as he was working as an opera director in Germany at the time.[90] In an interview with Sabine Rewald he could only add: 'We always thought it [the illness] was a result of the measles, but the dermatologists disputed this.'[91]

So did Paul Klee actually have measles in the middle of November 1935, or was there some other reason for his skin rash?

Measles has characteristic symptoms which are normally easy to diagnose: initially these include sore throat, catarrh, runny nose, conjunctivitis, light sensitivity, tiny white spots on the inside of the mouth ('Koplik's spots', fig. 30), mild fever which after three to five days suddenly develops into a high fever up to 40°C, and the characteristic measles rash, where the entire body and face are covered in red spots (fig. 31). After three or four days the fever subsides and the rash disappears. In the recovery phase which follows, the skin starts to peel very finely, except on the hands and feet (fig. 32).[92] Lily Klee asked a friend, Ju (Juliane) Aichinger-Grosch, to stay with them to help nurse Klee through his illness. She spent several months with the Klees from the end of November 1935 and made the following comment: 'Klee's whole body was peeling like in a bad case of scarlet fever.'[93] This is an interesting observation, as in cases of scarlet fever, large pieces of skin tend to peel off the trunk and particularly the palms of the hands and soles of the feet six days to six weeks after other symptoms have subsided.[94] Lily Klee doesn't mention anything about peeling from the hands and feet. Besides, scarlet fever can easily be distinguished from measles: in scarlet fever the fever is generally very high, with tonsillitis, inflamed pharynx and 'strawberry tongue', and the rash consists of very fine, tiny, red spots which do not run together as in measles.[95] We have to qualify the remark that Ju Aichinger-Grosch made in 1959; it seems highly unlikely that Klee was suffering from scarlet fever in 1935.

In terms of differential diagnosis, a drug-induced exanthema should be considered, i.e. a rash covering a large area caused by an adverse reaction to a drug which has been ingested or injected. These eruptions often look like measles, scarlet fever or rubella (fig. 33). They can also cause fever and subsequent skin peeling. Professor Alfred Krebs, an internationally renowned specialist in drug-induced exanthema, thinks this is the most likely cause of Paul Klee's rash in November 1935.[96] It is interesting to note that one year later, in November 1936, Paul Klee had a feverish reaction to injections. His wife wrote about this to Hermann and Margrit Rupf: 'It has now been definitely confirmed that the fever was a result of the injections. […] The fever lasted 3 days until Sunday morning, and it was a really high fever.'[97] It is also interesting to note that a few weeks before his death, the artist was afflicted by a rash similar to the one he had in 1935. Lily told

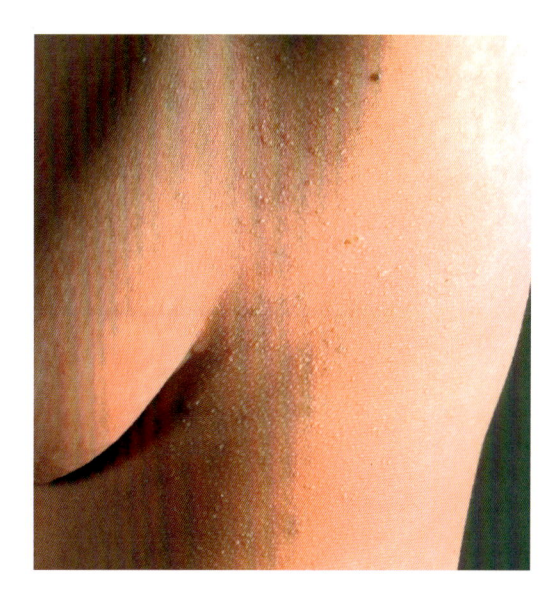

Fig. 32. Fine flaking of the rash as it starts to fade, associated both with measles and drug-induced exanthema

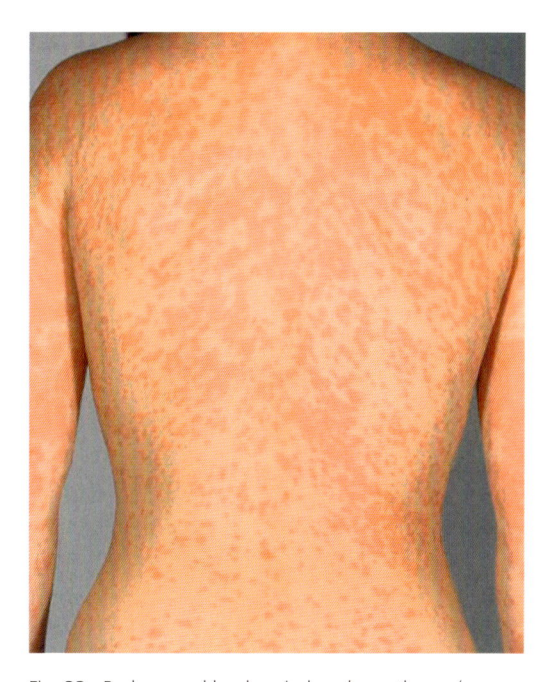

Fig. 33. Rash caused by drug-induced exanthema (as a result of oversensitivity to a drug)

[92] Cf. Pschyrembel/ML 1998, p. 987 f.
[93] Aichinger-Grosch 1959, p. 52 f.
[94] Cf. Pschyrembel/ML 1998, p. 1412.
[95] Cf. ibid., p. 1411 f.
[96] Verbal communication, Prof. Alfred Krebs, specialist in skin diseases, venereology and internal medicine, Bern, to the author, Bern, June 1, 2003, after thorough study of all relevant data.
[97] Letter from Lily Klee to Hermann and Margrit Rupf, Bern, November 25, 1936 (HMRS).

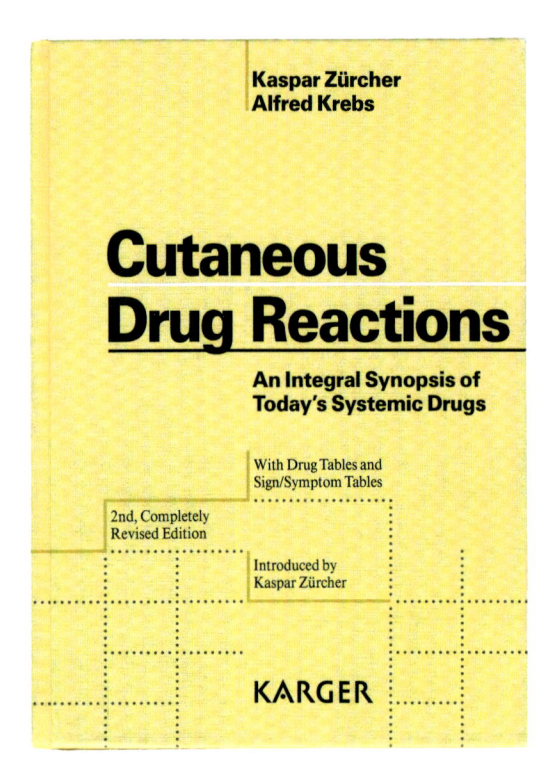

Fig. 34. Handbook by Dr. Kaspar Zürcher and Prof. Alfred Krebs on skin reactions to internal drugs (English edition 1992)

Will Grohmann in July 1940: 'The skin rash appeared again, a little less severe but basically the same as the one he had 5 years ago, right at the start of this terrible illness.'[98] Was it another drug-induced exanthema? Was it perhaps caused by the same drug as in 1935, or at least by another chemically related drug with similar allergenic properties?

We can perhaps throw some light on this by studying three entries in Paul Klee's temperature chart which Lily Klee kept from October 1935 until April 1936. On November 5, 1935, Lily noted his morning temperature as 'morning 36.7' and next to it 'doctor' (fig. 35) – probably a visit by Dr. Schorer during the morning – and his evening temperature as 'eve. 37.5', adding next to it 'Theominal' (fig. 35).[99] She noted another doctor's visit on November 8 and the remark 'new medication' (fig. 35).[100] She recorded the next doctor's visit on November 12, along with a prescription for the evening: '2 x powder and Theominal'.[101] The 'powder' probably refers to the 'new medication' mentioned on November 8. Another doctor's visit is noted in the temperature chart on November 14, 1935.[102]

The drug 'Theominal' is no longer available. It was produced by Bayer and consisted of a mixture of theobromine and luminal in a ratio of 10:1. It was used in the treatment of cardiovascular disease. The theobromine is no longer in common use; however luminal (a barbiturate, active ingredient phenobarbital) is still used as a sedative/hypnotic and in the treatment of febrile seizures and epilepsy.[103] It is now known that bromines (which also occur in sedatives/hypnotics and cough medicine) sometimes cause adverse reactions in the form of acne, papules, ulcers and rashes with tiny spots of blood.[104] Barbiturates can also cause drug-induced exanthema, particularly maculopapular rashes and urticaria.[105] So it is quite possible that the luminal contained in the Theominal triggered an allergic reaction in Paul Klee in the form of a measles-like rash. An allergic reaction could also have been caused by the unknown 'new medication' in powder form which Klee took for the first time on November 8, 1935. Apparently, the rash first appeared ten days after the first dose of Theominal and seven days after first

[98] Letter from Lily Klee to Will Grohmann, Bern, July 7, 1940 (AWG), quoted in Frey 1990, p. 124.
[99] Klee 1935/1936 (p. 258), p. 3.
[100] Ibid.
[101] Ibid., p. 4.
[102] Ibid.
[103] See Appendices: Composition of and Medical Indicators for the Drug 'Theominal' (p. 267).
[104] Cf. Zürcher and Krebs/ML 1992, p. 268 f.
[105] Cf. Zürcher and Krebs/ML 1992, p. 164 f.

taking the 'powder'. This is a typical incubation period for allergies.

It is still not clear whether Dr. Schorer actually saw Klee's rash. Lily's notes in the temperature chart indicate that Paul Klee visited Dr. Schorer on October 21 and 25, 1935 ('at the doctor's') and that Dr. Schorer visited his patient on October 29 and on November 1, 5, 8, 12 and 14 ('doctor').[106] Other possible visits are not recorded. We can pinpoint the rash as occurring during his high fever between November 15 and 17. Dr. Schorer would surely have noticed the typical measles symptoms during the three-to-five day preliminary phase of the rash (see pages 40 and 41) when he made his visit on November 12. He was, after all, a very experienced and distinguished physician. So it seems highly likely that he in fact never saw the short-lived rash, but only saw his patient after it had disappeared. And, as previously mentioned, the high fever could have been linked to the pneumonia and pleurisy.

There is little evidence to suggest that measles is an accurate diagnosis. The artist Otto Nebel mentions in a letter that Paul Klee had measles, but without specifying further (see note 84), and Lily does not mention it in her letters until three months later – also without any medical verification. What is more, Lily wrote almost a year later that the doctors had discounted measles.

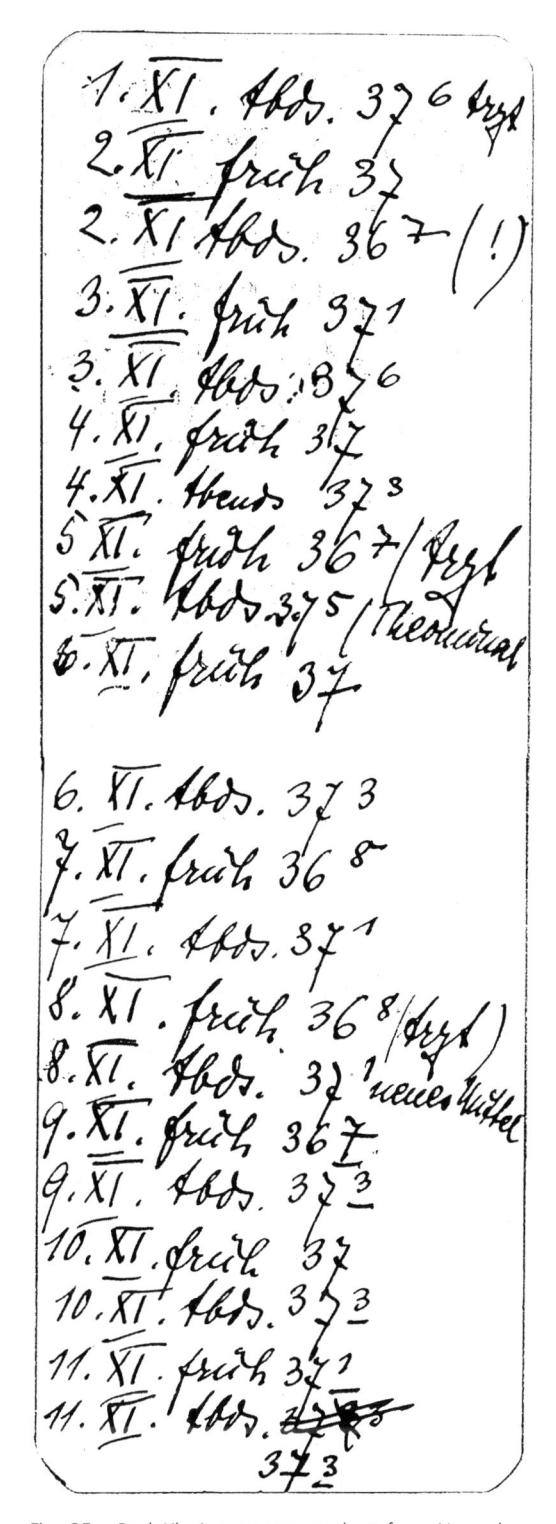

Fig. 35. Paul Klee's temperature chart from November 1–11, 1935, recorded by Lily Klee

[106] Klee 1935/1936 (p. 258), p. 1–4.

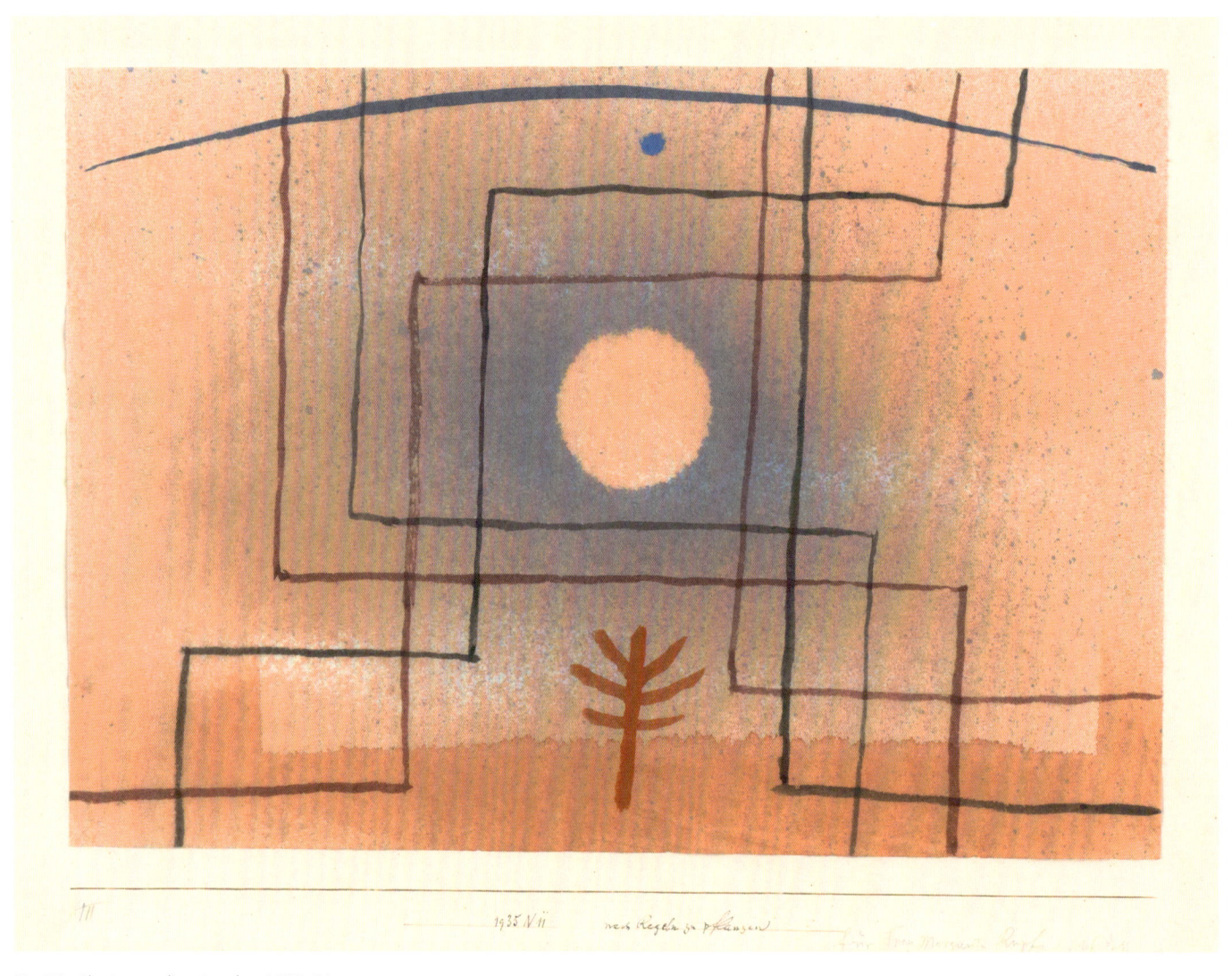

Fig. 36. Plant according to rules, 1935, 91

This watercolor was a Christmas present from Paul Klee to the ailing art patron, Margrit Rupf, in 1935. At the same time, it provides us with the first written evidence from the artist that he was also unwell. He added to the dedication 'in the hope we'll both soon be feeling better'. In the middle foreground a newly set plant is growing from the earth. It does not yet bear flowers or fruit. Above it, the sun is shining through a blue haze. The plant and the sun are contained within a regular, geometric structure. A plant needs just the right conditions to grow, flower and mature, and when planting, certain rules have to be followed: it is necessary 'to plant according to rules'.

Long Convalescence, Debility, Heart and Lung Complications

Klee's health deteriorated further after the high fever phase of his illness in mid-November 1935. He needed a lot of time to recuperate and was totally bedridden for six weeks.[107] In December 1935 he was allowed to get up for two and a half hours a day.[108] At Christmas in 1935 he gave his friends, the collectors Margrit and Hermann Rupf, a watercolor entitled 'Plant according to rules' (fig. 36). He dedicated it 'to Mrs. Marguerite Rupf, in the hope that we'll both soon be feeling better.'[109] This is the first time Paul Klee mentioned in writing that he was ill. In January 1936 Klee was getting up for three to four hours every day[110], in February this had stretched to afternoons[111] and in March he was up for almost the whole day.[112] Lily thought it was a good sign that her husband began working again at the beginning of April 1936: '[…] and today is a special day, because he has painted again for the first time (!), and a few days ago he did a drawing.'[113]

From October 18, 1935 to April 18, 1936 Lily Klee kept a detailed and regular record of her husband's body temperature. This shows that, apart from during the fever attack in mid-November 1935, his temperature was generally steady, with slightly elevated evening temperatures between 36.6 and 37.9°C (average 37.3°C) before the fever attack and between 36.5 and 37.7°C (average 37.2°C) after the attack.[114]

On April 1, 1936, Klee finally had the heart/lung X-ray which was planned in October 1935. Lily Klee reports the result of the examination: '[…] it was chronic double pneumonia […]'[115] and 'his heart is back to normal'.[116] In May 1936 she declares delightedly, 'He [Paul Klee] is doing very well, even though he is still very weak, and still looks thin and ill. […] But it is a miracle that he has come this far after such a terrible illness, we feel like he has been given back to us. He really was at death's door, and even though he is starting to get better, I feel as though I have had a black cloud hanging over me for months.'[117] At the end of June 1936 she adds that further serious complications – pleurisy and cardiac dilation – had arisen alongside the pneumonia and measles (fig. 37).[118]

[107] Klee 1935/36 (p.258), p. 2: '26 X [Oct.] morning 36.8 in bed' marks the beginning of his bed confinement, and a letter from Lily Klee to Lucas Lichtenhan, Bern, December 6, 1935 (photocopy: ZPKB/SFK): 'After being bedridden for six weeks, he [Paul Klee] briefly got up for the first time' marks the end of his total bed confinement.

[108] Cf. letter from Lily Klee to Will Grohmann, Bern, December 29, 1935 (AWG).

[109] Glaesemer 1976, p. 318.

[110] Cf. letter from Lily Klee to Daniel-Henry Kahnweiler, Bern, January 4, 1936 (location unknown).

[111] Cf. letter from Lily Klee to Nina Kandinsky, Bern, February 13, 1936 (BK/CGPP).

[112] Cf. letter from Lily Klee to Daniel-Henry Kahnweiler, Bern, March 10, 1936 (location unknown), and cf. letter from Lily Klee to Gertrud Grohmann, Bern, March 29, 1936 (AWG).

[113] Letter from Lily Klee to Will Grohmann, Bern, April 9, 1936 (AWG).

[114] Cf. Klee 1935/1936 (p.258), pp. 1–4: 26 evening temperature readings from October 18, 1935 to November 12, 1935; pp. 5–17: 146 evening temperature readings from November 22, 1935 to April 18, 1936.

[115] Letter from Lily Klee to Will Grohmann, Bern, April 9, 1936 (AWG).

[116] Letter from Lily Klee to Nina Kandinsky, Bern, April 14, 1936 (BK/CGPP).

[117] Letter from Lily Klee to Gertrud Grohmann, Bern, May 16, 1936 (AWG).

[118] Cf. letter from Lily Klee to Emmy Scheyer, Bern, June 28, 1936 (NSMP).

In June 1936 Paul Klee took a break to convalesce in Tarasp in the Unterengadin with Hermann and Margrit Rupf. He felt good while he was there, apart from some shortness of breath when walking uphill, when the Föhn wind was blowing and after meals.[119] In August and September 1936 Klee stayed at the 'Pension Cécil' in Montana, a high-altitude health resort in Valais, and felt a further improvement in his health.[120] According to Lily Klee, he also had an electrocardiogram in 1936[121], but we have no details about where it was carried out or what the findings were.

It is interesting to note how Klee himself felt about his illness at the end of 1936, compared to the view of certain people who were close to him:

Paul Klee writes to Will Grohmann: 'I am certainly glad to receive your good wishes [for his birthday on December 18, and for the New Year] and I am sure some of them will come true. It will be a step forward for me if I can just shake off some of the worries which are holding me back in my work. I mean by this, that I am still much too conscious of the changes in my body and spend too much time thinking about them'.[122] Klee seems to be saying that he still feels weak and has to consciously avoid too much physical activity.

Lily Klee states: 'Paul is doing very well, thank goodness. He has produced one or two nice pieces of work, which is really wonderful. And he is definitely looking a little better.'[123]

Dr. Gerhard Schorer replies to Lily Klee: 'Thank you very much for the two reports on your husband's condition. I am very pleased that he seems to be making a sustained recovery. He is coming to see me in the next few days and we can decide what we need to do next. In the meantime, please accept my very best wishes for you and Mr. Klee for the coming year.'[124]

Hermann Rupf confides to Wassily and Nina Kandinsky: 'We were at the Klee's on Friday evening and today they came to us for lunch. It is very distressing to see such a unique and wonderful man in such bad health. Mrs. Klee seems to think he is doing well, but he is very resigned and serious, although

---

[119] Cf. letter from Paul Klee to Lily Klee, Tarasp, June 17, 1936, quoted in Klee 1979, p. 1272.

[120] Cf. letters from Lily Klee to Will Grohmann, Bern, August 24, 1936, August 18, 1936 and October 13, 1936 (AWG), also cf. letters from Lily Klee to Emmy Scheyer, August 26, 1936 and November 3, 1936 (NSMP). From this we can gather that Paul Klee stayed at the 'Pension Cécil' in Montana between August 17, 1936 and October 1, 1936. It was not initially clear whether this pension was an annexe of the Valais Pneumology Sanatorium, which mainly treated TB patients, or whether it was a private establishment. My research shows that it was in fact a privately-run hotel (see note 21, p. 12, and p. 265).

[121] Cf. letter from Lily Klee to Nina Kandinsky, Bern, September 5, 1936 (BK/CGPP).

[122] Letter from Paul Klee to Will Grohmann, Bern, December 31, 1936 (AWG).

[123] Letter from Lily Klee to Will Grohmann, Bern, December 31, 1936 (AWG).

[124] Letter from Dr. Gerhard Schorer to Lily Klee, Bern, January 2, 1937 (ZPKB/SFK).

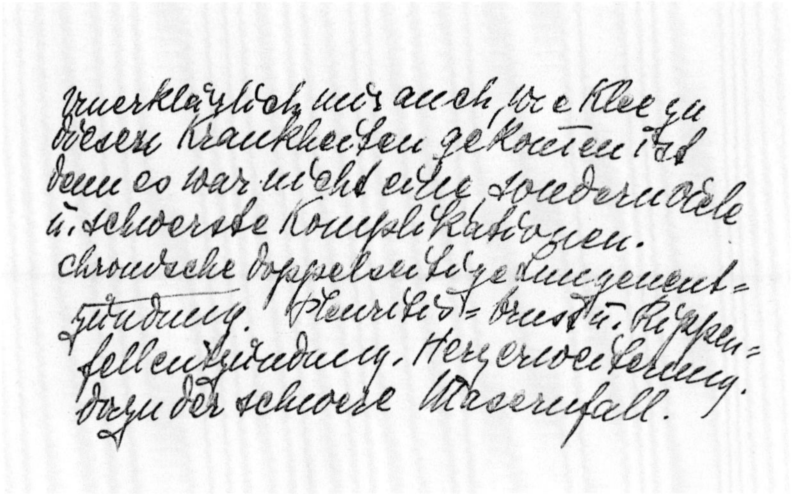
Unerklärlich ist mir auch, wie Klee zu
diesen Krankheiten gekommen ist
denn es war nicht eine sondern viele
u. schwerste Komplikationen.
chronische doppelseitige Lungenentzündung. Pleuritis = Brust u. Rippenfellentzündung. Herzerweiterung.
dazu der schwere Masernfall.

I also have no idea how Klee came to have these illnesses, because it wasn't just one complication, it was several serious ones. <u>Chronic</u> double pneumonia. Pleurisy = inflammation of the pleura. Cardiac dilation. And a serious case of measles.

Fig. 37. Extract from a letter from Lily Klee to Emmy Scheyer, Bern, June 28, 1936 (Norton Simon Museum, Pasadena – The Blue Four Galka Scheyer Collection)

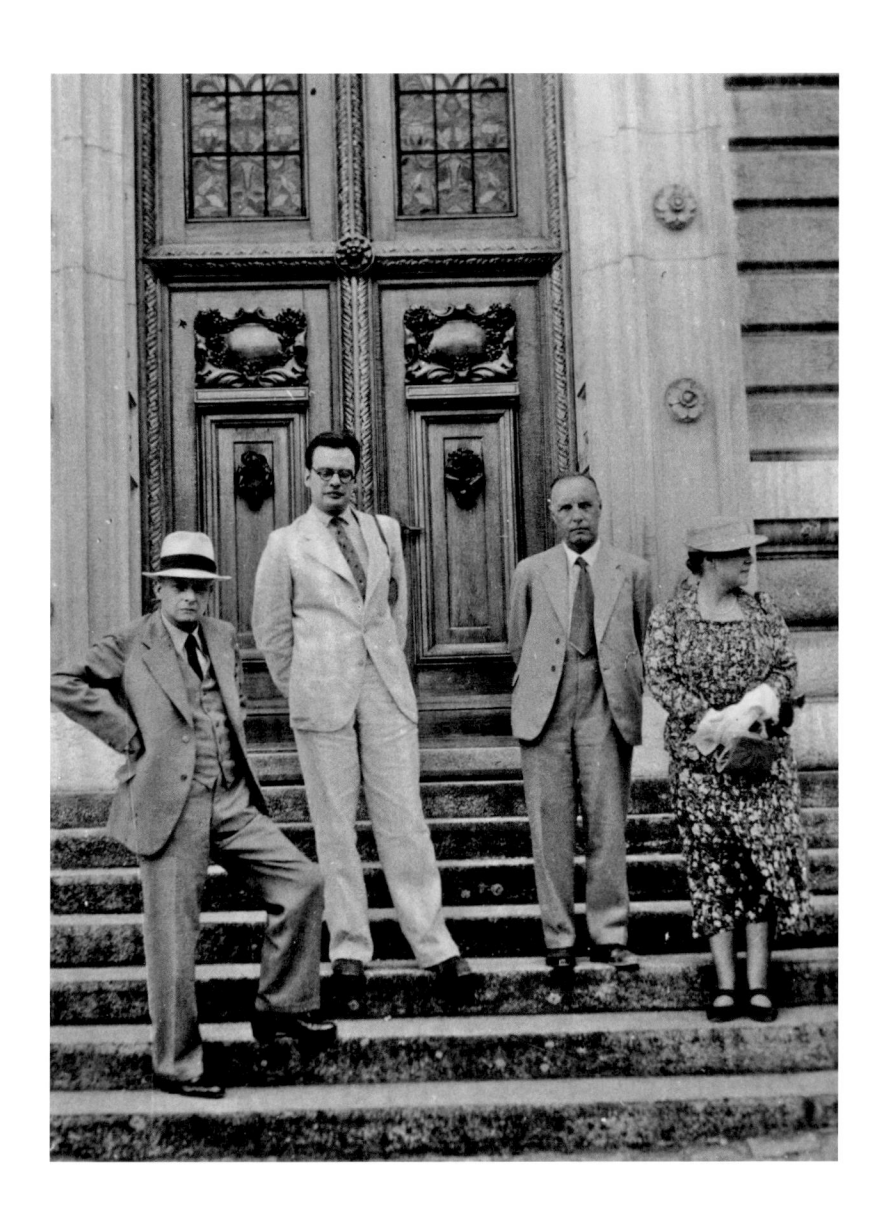

Fig. 38. Paul Klee and Felix Klee with Hermann and Margrit Rupf-Wirz in front of St. Ursus cathedral in Solothurn, 1937

he still has his old traits of intellectual superiority and calmness, mixed in with a hint of mockery.'[125]

A Possible Diagnosis: Scleroderma

In autumn 1936 Paul Klee once again suffered some kind of changes to his skin, but his wife did not pinpoint them or describe them in detail. We assume that Dr. Schorer was the first to notice them. Along with Dr. Lotmar, he suggested that Paul Klee should visit Professor Oscar Naegeli, chief physician at the University Dermatology Clinic for a specialist examination (fig. 39).[126] The examination was carried out in the outpatients department at the University Dermatology Clinic at the Inselspital in Bern (fig. 40) on October 28 and 29[127], but unfortunately we don't have the results. Did Professor Naegeli diagnose the skin changes as 'scleroderma'? We can't say for sure, but we can probably make that assumption. But why weren't Paul Klee and his family informed? Perhaps it was because at that time it was not common practice to pass on the diagnosis of a serious, terminal disease to the patient and his close relatives. This was done to protect the patient, and because it was thought that knowledge of the disease and the prognosis would only depress the patient and lead to an exacerbation of the illness. The patient's hopes of recovery or cure would also be dashed.[128]

Scleroderma is a very rare, chronic, inflammatory disease which affects the connective tissue of the skin, blood vessels and internal organs.[129] Connective tissue diseases are also known as 'collagenoses' and can lead to changes in the connective tissue, with outer tissue cells attaching themselves to inner cells, for example, the epidermis to the subcutis. The term 'connective tissue disease' encompasses a range of diseases which cause similar changes to the connective tissues: scleroderma, systemic Lupus erythematosus, dermatomyositis/polymyositis, mixed forms (= mixed collagenoses, mixed connective tissue diseases MCTD, where the symptoms of two or more collagenoses combine, and rheumatoid arthritis), overlap syndrome (where two collagenoses occur in parallel) and undefined connective tissue diseases UCTD.[130]

---

[125] Letter from Hermann Rupf to Wassily and Nina Kandinsky, Bern, December 20, 1936 (BK/CGPP).

[126] Letter from Dr. Gerhard Schorer to Paul Klee, Bern, October 23, 1936 (ZPKB/SFK): 'Dear Mr. Klee, Dr. Lotmar and I both feel that you should visit Prof. Naegeli for an examination. He is a dermatologist and we would like to get a second opinion from him. If I do not hear from you otherwise, I will contact Mr. Naegeli and advise him of your symptoms. With best wishes to you and your wife, Yours sincerely, G. Schorer'. (fig. 39).

[127] Letter from Dr. Gerhard Schorer to Paul Klee, Bern, October 26, 1936 (ZPKB/SFK): '[…] Many thanks for your note. Prof. Naegeli looks forward to seeing you on Wednesday, October 28 at 4.00 pm at the dermatology clinic, Inselspital […]' and letter from Lily Klee to Hilde Nebel, Bern, October 29, 1936 (SLB/SLA): 'My husband had a skin examination yesterday, carried out by Prof. Naegeli at the dermatological clinic […].'

[128] From a letter from Hermann Rupf to Wassily and Nina Kandinsky, Bern, December 9, 1936 (BK/CGPP): 'It is very difficult to do anything about Klee's choice of doctor, because he is being treated by his old friend Dr. Lotmar and also by Dr. Schorrer, and he has every confidence in them. They are both very competent and they have tried all the latest procedures, but unfortunately Klee has not responded to them. He has been given other advice, but he refuses to take it because he feels that Schorrer is doing everything humanly possible, and he trusts him totally. As a result he has ignored all other advice. But his doctors are offering little hope; they say it is lung cancer. We are the only ones they have told, as they do not want him to find out. They want to make this last part of his life as easy and comfortable as they can, and also want to shield Mrs. Klee from the truth, otherwise she will be very distressed and will not be help him or herself. The doctors want to give them hope and spare them too much worry in their lives until the end comes. We know some other people who were in this situation, and looking back we can see that it was the right thing to do.' [I'd like to comment on two points in this letter: (1) Dr. Lotmar was not personally treating Klee, but was in constant contact with the doctor who was treating him, Dr. Gerhard Schorer, and (2) I find it hard to believe that Dr. Lotmar or Dr. Schorer diagnosed 'lung cancer'. It seems more likely that Hermann and Margrit Rupf heard from Lily Klee that Paul Klee had lung problems, which they then took to mean 'lung cancer'.]

[129] Cf. Mehlhorn/ML 1994, p. 8.

[130] Cf. Gadola and Villiger/ML 2006, pp. 74–94.

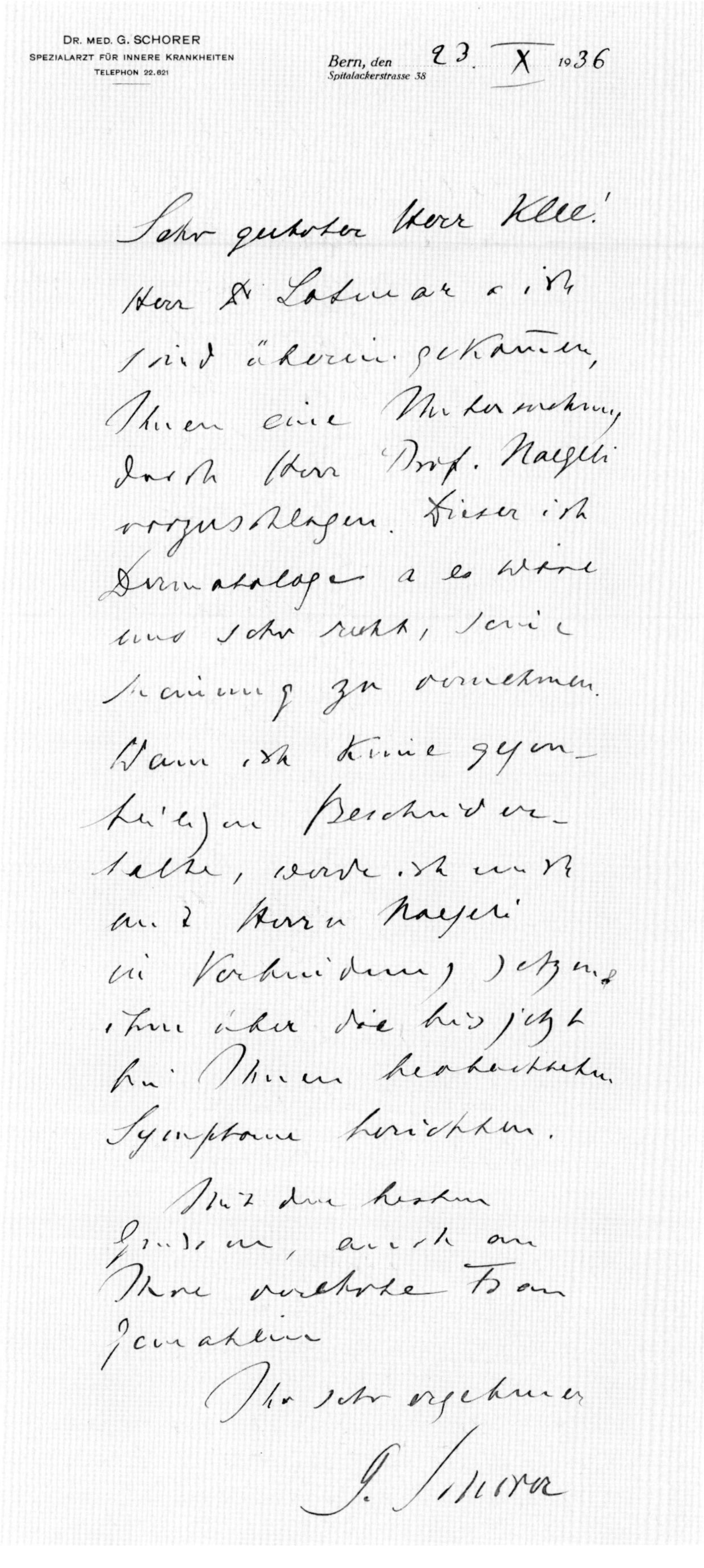

Dr. med. G. Schorer
Spezialarzt für innere Krankheiten
Telephon 22.621

Bern, den 23. X 1936
Spitalackerstrasse 38

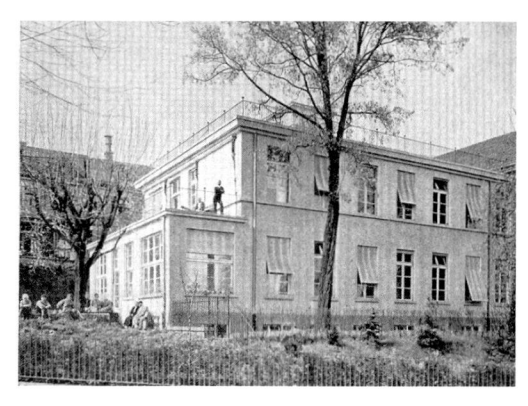

Sehr geehrter Herr Klee!

Herr D. Lotmar u. ich sind überein gekommen, Ihnen eine Untersuchung durch Herrn Prof. Naegeli vorzuschlagen. Dieser ist Dermatologe u. es wäre uns sehr recht, seine Meinung zu vernehmen. Wann ich keine gegenteiligen Bescheid erhalte, werde ich mich mit Herrn Naegeli in Verbindung setzen u. ihm über die bis jetzt bei Ihnen beobachteten Symptome berichten.

Mit den besten Grüssen, auch an Ihre verehrte Frau Gemahlin

Ihr sehr ergebener

G. Schorer

Fig. 40. University Dermatology Clinic, Inselspital, Bern, ca. 1930

Fig. 39. Letter from Dr. Gerhard Schorer to Paul Klee, Bern, October 23, 1936 (see note 126).

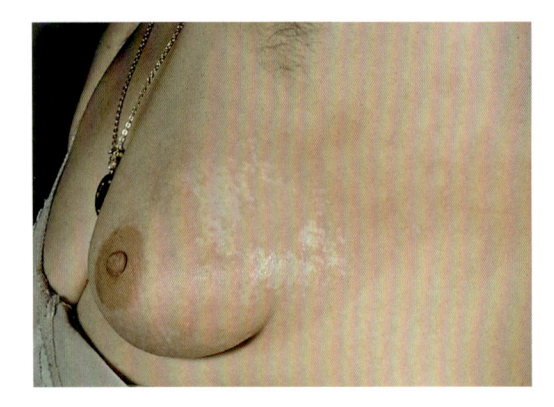

Fig. 41. Morphea, inflammation stage with reddening

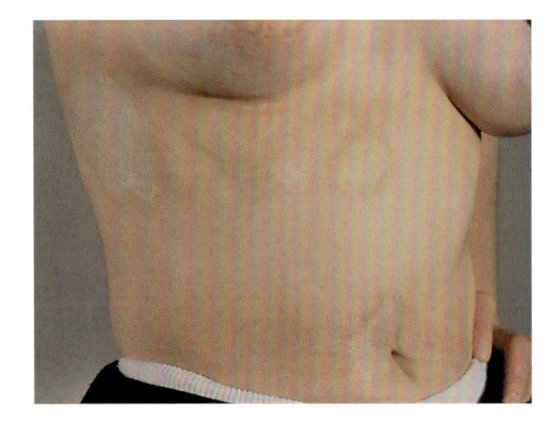

Fig. 42. Morphea, with lilac ring

Scleroderma is classified as a rheumatic disease, and these days it is generally regarded as an autoimmune disease. For mostly unknown reasons the immune system loses control. The body's defences turn against themselves, so instead of attacking external bacteria or viruses, they attack the body's own cells and organs. As a result the antibodies mistakenly attack other cells within the body, as though these cells were suddenly harmful to the organism. In scleroderma, the immune system attacks the body's own connective tissue, triggering an inflammatory reaction which leads to thickening and hardening of these tissues. The skin can become hard and immobile, otherwise known as 'armor-like'; it also becomes very dry and in some cases itchy. Gradually the epidermis begins to thin (atrophy), brown and white patches of pigmentation appear on the skin, and tiny blood vessels (telangiectasia) start to show through. These changes restrict certain functions, for example, they can affect elasticity and mobility, particularly in the hands. Sufferers often experience difficulty swallowing and mild joint pain, particularly in the smaller joints.[131] If the major internal organs are affected, then sooner or later the disease becomes terminal.

The name scleroderma comes from the Greek and means 'hard skin' (scleros = hard, derma = skin). Even in ancient times, Hippocrates and other doctors mentioned instances of skin hardening.[132] In 1753 Carlo Curzio, a Neapolitan doctor, reported on a patient who had skin hardening on her face and in the lining of her mouth, along with difficulties in swallowing and speaking.[133] In Bordeaux in 1847, the French doctor Elie Gintrac (1791–1877) described for the first time four cases of these skin changes in women and coined the term 'sclérodermie'.[134] In 1889 the Viennese dermatologist Moritz Kaposi (1837–1902) gave an excellent description of the typical facial changes caused by scleroderma: 'When the face is afflicted, the features appear set, totally immobile, and incapable of any expression. The countenance seems made of stone, as if sculpted from marble, and evinces neither pain nor joy.' Professor Ernst G. Jung provides us with another interesting angle from the realms of mythology. He describes the 'armor-like skin' of Achilles in the Greek sagas and Siegfried in the Germanic sagas, which makes us think of generalized sclero-

[131] Cf. Gadola and Villiger/ML 2006, p. 86 f.
[132] Cf. Castenholz/ML 2000, p. 16 f.
[133] Cf. Castenholz/ML 2000, p. 34.
[134] Cf. ibid., p. 52 f.

derma. But it is well known that both these heroes met their fate because they had one small, unhardened spot. Ernst G. Jung draws a kind of parallel between these ancient myths and the 20th century in his allusion to Paul Klee's presumed progressive systemic scleroderma.[135] Around 1900 it was discovered that not just the skin but also the inner organs could be affected.[136] In 1942, the term 'collagenoses' was first used.[137] Before that, scleroderma was also known in German as 'Darrsucht',[138] stemming from the archaic word 'darr', meaning dry. The word 'Darrsucht' conveys the idea of a 'dry consumption', a 'wasting disease, where the body effectively consumes itself and dries out'.[139]

Overview of the Forms of Scleroderma
There is a 'circumscribed' or localized form of scleroderma called **'morphea'**. This only affects the skin, and initially manifests as a slowly spreading red patch (fig. 41) which develops into a shiny, whitish hardened plaque with a 'lilac ring' at the border (fig. 42). The ring also gradually whitens and the surface becomes thinner. The white patches which remain can measure several centimeters in diameter, but they are generally harmless and are only a problem from a cosmetic point of view (fig. 43).[140]

There are other forms of the disease which affect the skin to various extents and which can attack internal organs such as the esophagus, stomach, gastrointestinal tract, lungs, heart and kidneys. The blood vessels, joints and muscles can also be affected. This is therefore known as a 'systemic disease', nowadays commonly called **'systemic sclerosis'** or 'progressive systemic sclerosis' ('progressive' because new symptoms arise and the disease gets worse). It develops in patients between the ages of 35 and 65,[141] and women contract it three to four times more often than men.[142]

Systemic sclerosis manifests in two forms: 'limited' and 'diffuse'. The **'limited form'** represents 95% of cases and affects the face, hands and forearms, and occasionally the feet and lower legs. The internal organs are only attacked much later, normally after many years.[143] This form of systemic scle-

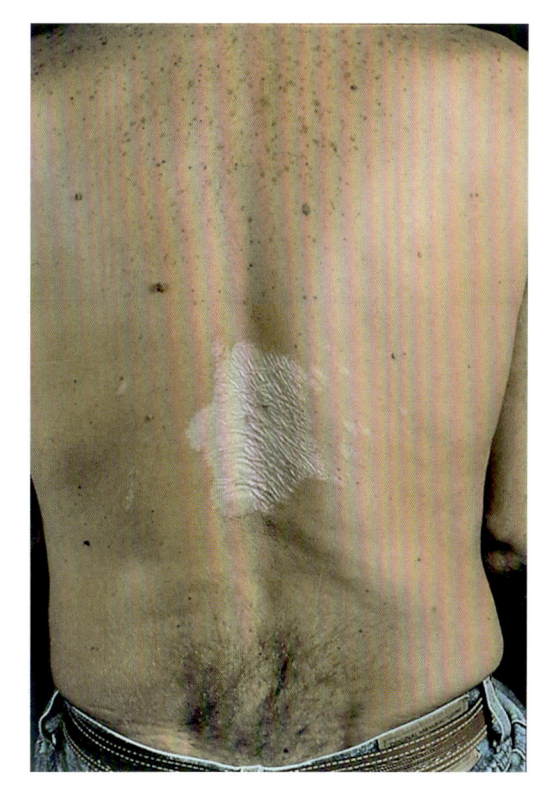

Fig. 43. Morphea, final stage

[135] Cf. Jung/ML 2005, p. 573 f.
[136] I thank Prof. Urs Boschung, Director of the Institute of Medical History, Bern University, for providing this reference and also the previous quotation from Moritz Kaposi.
[137] Cf. Castenholz/ML 2000, p. 70.
[138] Cf. Kumer/ML 1944, p. 313.
[139] Cf. Brockhaus 1894–1897, vol. 4, p. 816.
[140] Cf. Krieg/ML 1996, pp. 724–728. Only the rare variety of localized scleroderma, known as 'disseminated localized scleroderma', with widespread lesions, can occasionally develop into 'progressive scleroderma' [systemic sclerosis] (cf. ibid., p. 725).
[141] Cf. Gadola and Villiger/ML 2006, p. 86.
[142] Cf. ibid., p. 86, and cf. Röther and Peter/ML 1996, p. 381.
[143] Cf. Moll/ML 1991, p. 93.

rosis does not normally improve on its own, but often stays the same for years.[144] Pulmonary arterial hypertension can gradually develop, which has a poor prognosis.[145] There are normally few other general symptoms, but the hands can be badly affected and, in both forms, swallowing can become difficult and painful. The **'diffuse form'**, which represents the other 5% of cases, afflicts the face and large areas of the skin and in some cases the whole skin.[146] However, hands and feet are normally not affected. The internal organs are often attacked early on, sometimes after only a few months, and in the past this serious form of the disease resulted in death within three to five years.[147] Nowadays, drugs can slow the progression of the disease, with women tending to live longer than men.[148] The incidence of the limited form is on average 10–20 cases per million population per year, for the diffuse form it is only one case per million.[149]

The table on page 53 summarizes the main differences between the different forms of scleroderma.

Skin Disorders

In order to verify whether the hypothetical diagnosis of 'scleroderma' fits in with the skin disorders and other symptoms which Paul Klee experienced in autumn 1936, we now need to take an in-depth look at the disease.

There is no evidence of morphea, so straight away we can remove this from the equation.

In both forms of systemic sclerosis, there are characteristic changes to the facial skin. The skin becomes stiff and taut, the facial features stiffen, facial expression is lost, and the nose becomes pointed.[150] The lips become thinner, the mouth shrinks, and it becomes difficult to open the mouth and look after the teeth.[151] Radial wrinkles appear around the mouth ('tobacco pouch mouth').[152] This is known as **'mask face'**.[153] Paul Klee certainly had a mask-like face in the last years of his life, though it was not so pronounced. We can see this if we compare a photo from 1939 (fig. 46)[154] with one from 1925 (fig. 45).[155] Felix Klee says his father's skin 'tightened' and his

---

[144] Cf. Krieg/ML 1996, p. 732, and cf. Gadola and Villiger/ML 2006, p. 87.
[145] Cf. Gadola and Villiger/ML 2006, p. 87.
[146] Cf. Moll/ML 1991, p. 93, and cf. Gadola and Villiger/ML 2006, p. 87.
[147] Cf. Krieg/ML 1996, p. 730.
[148] Cf. Mittag and Haustein/ML 1998, p. 550.
[149] Cf. Moll/ML 1991, p. 93, cf. Mittag and Haustein/ML 1998, p. 545, and cf. Gadola and Villiger/ML 2006, p. 86.
[150] Cf. Röther and Peter/ML 1996, p. 384.
[151] Cf. Krieg/ML 1996, p. 731.
[152] Cf. Röther and Peter/ML 1996, p. 384.
[153] Cf. ibid.
[154] In this photo, Paul Klee's facial skin looks stiff and taut.
[155] Here Paul Klee's facial skin looks softer, smoother, and more elastic than in the 1939 photo (fig. 46).

Morphea	**Systemic sclerosis**	
	Limited form (95%)	Diffuse form (5%)
Patches appear on the skin, predominantly on the trunk. Internal organs are not affected. Harmless, purely cosmetic problem.	Skin affected locally, particularly the face ('mask face'), hands ('sclerodactyly') and forearms, occasionally the feet and lower legs. Mucous membranes can often also be affected. Internal organs are afflicted later (after many years). Death usually results from pulmonary hypertension as a late effect or from another illness.	Large areas of the skin affected, particularly the face ('mask face'), the neck, upper chest and back. Whole skin surface can be affected, but rarely the hands and legs. Mucous membranes can also be affected. Internal organs afflicted early on (after a few years). Can lead to death within five to ten years.

Table 1. Summary of the different forms of scleroderma

appearance changed.[156] More precisely, he told me that his father's skin became noticeably tighter on his face and neck.[157] Max Huggler also confirmed this.[158] Even the eyelids can be affected[159], which throws light on Paul Klee's comment in 1939 that he could no longer hold a monocle between his eyebrow and cheek, '[…] as I can no longer wear a monocle on my youthful countenance'.[160] This is clear evidence of loss of mobility in the eyelid.

On July 11, 1990 Stefan Frey had a telephone conversation in Bern with Dr. Jean Charlet, the last dentist to treat Paul Klee. From this he gleaned the following: in the last years of Paul Klee's life it was always difficult to give him dental treatment, and the patient could no longer open his mouth very wide. The mouth opening had become small; the lips and surrounding tissues had lost their elasticity. Dr. Charlet did not notice any cracking of the lips, but was always afraid that forcible opening of the mouth would cause them to crack. Klee was grateful to him for treating him gently. (This also emerges in a letter from Paul Klee to Lily Klee: 'I have been spending a lot of time at the dentist's, and this state of affairs is going to continue, but I am becoming accustomed to it. He really is very skilful.'[161]) Dr. Charlet also reported that he observed 'early-stage periodontosis' (shrink-

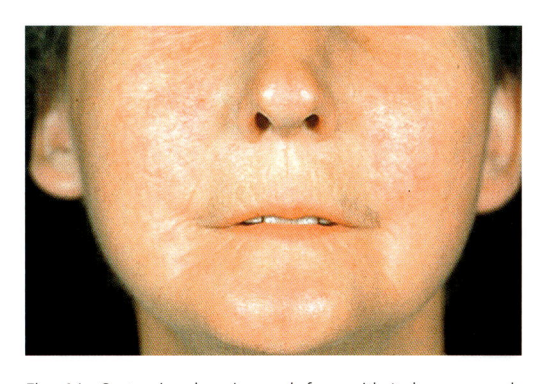

Fig. 44. Systemic sclerosis: mask face with 'tobacco pouch mouth'

[156] Cf. Klee 1989, p. 46.
[157] Personal communication, Felix Klee to the author, Bern, September 20, 1983.
[158] Telephone conversation between Max Huggler and the author, CH–7554 Sent, August 15, 1981.
[159] Cf. Krieg/ML 1996, p. 730.
[160] Letter from Paul Klee to Lily Klee, Bern, April 25, 1939, quoted in Klee 1979, p. 1286.
[161] Letter from Paul Klee to Lily Klee, Bern, June 10, 1939; Briefe II, p. 1294.

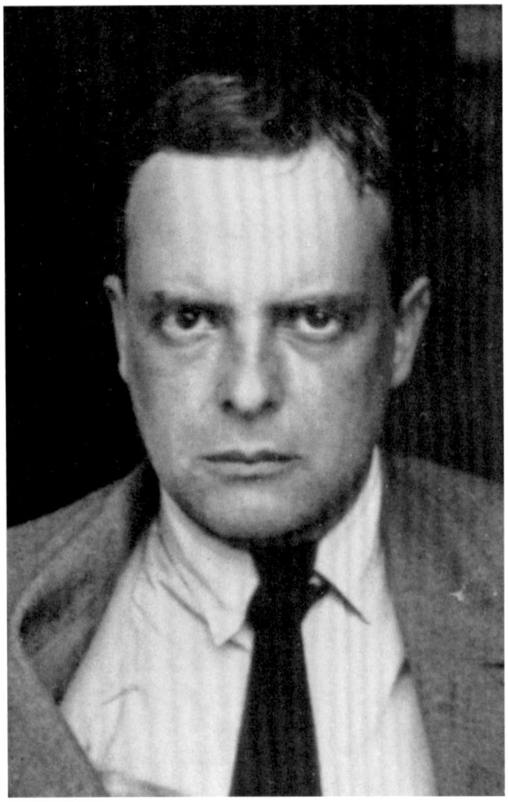

Fig. 45. Paul Klee, 1925

Fig. 46. Paul Klee, 1939 ▷

age of the gums) and that he had to carry out a few fillings. His patient's facial expression had become stiffer, but he did not notice a shortening or hardening of the tongue frenulum. He said Klee could speak quite normally.[162] The dentist's observations closely match the symptoms of systemic sclerosis.

In May 1938 Lily Klee writes: 'He [Paul Klee] has had really bad pains again, which seem to be connected to his gland and skin problems'.[163] We can assume from this that his skin changes were getting worse rather than better. With respect to the 'gland problems' mentioned, see my explanation on page 61.

In July 1940 Lily Klee writes: 'On May 10 (1940) my husband traveled to [Locarno] Orselina to the Viktoria Sanatorium, as he had been unwell for some time. I followed him a week later (though I had not planned to), because I felt very worried. His condition was fair for the first two weeks, but then he suddenly became very ill. The skin rash appeared again, a little less severe but basically the same as the one he had 5 years ago, right at the start of this terrible illness.'[164] It seems this rash only lasted a short while, so it does not have any particular bearing on the progression of the illness and should not really be considered typical of systemic sclerosis. In all likelihood it was once again a 'drug-induced exanthema' caused by intolerance to pills or injections. It is possible the rash was triggered by the same drug which caused it in 1935, or by a chemically related drug (see pages 41 and 42).

In addition to the facial changes, systemic sclerosis afflicts other parts of the skin. As previously mentioned, the hands are particularly affected in the limited form, as opposed to the diffuse form which rarely affects the hands. The skin of the hands becomes hard, waxy and immobile. The fingers become thick and stiff and feel difficult to bend (**'sclerodactyly'**, figs. 49–51, pages 58 and 59). The fingers lose their sensitivity (responsiveness) and the sense of touch is impaired. In serious cases the fingers curl stiffly inwards (fig. 50, page 58) and finger mobility can be severely limited. For some patients this can lead to a loss of independence.

[162] Cf. recording of telephone conversation between Stefan Frey and Dr. Jean Charlet (1906–1990), Bern, July 11, 1990 (SFB).
[163] Letter from Lily Kee to Curt Valentin, Bern, May 15, 1938 (MoMAANY/VP).
[164] Letter from Lily Klee to Will Grohmann, Bern, July 7, 1940 (AWG), excerpts quoted in Frey 1990, p. 124.

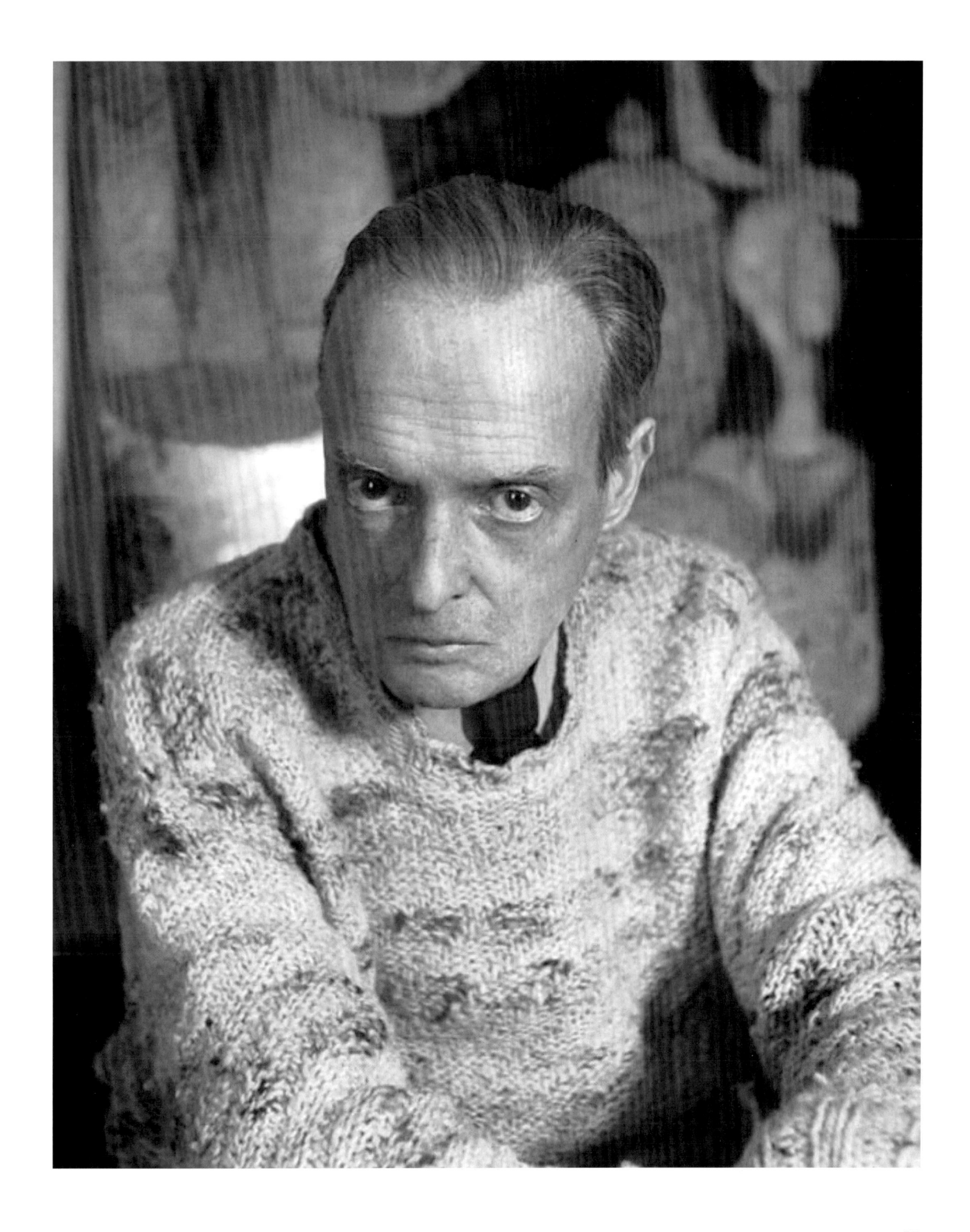

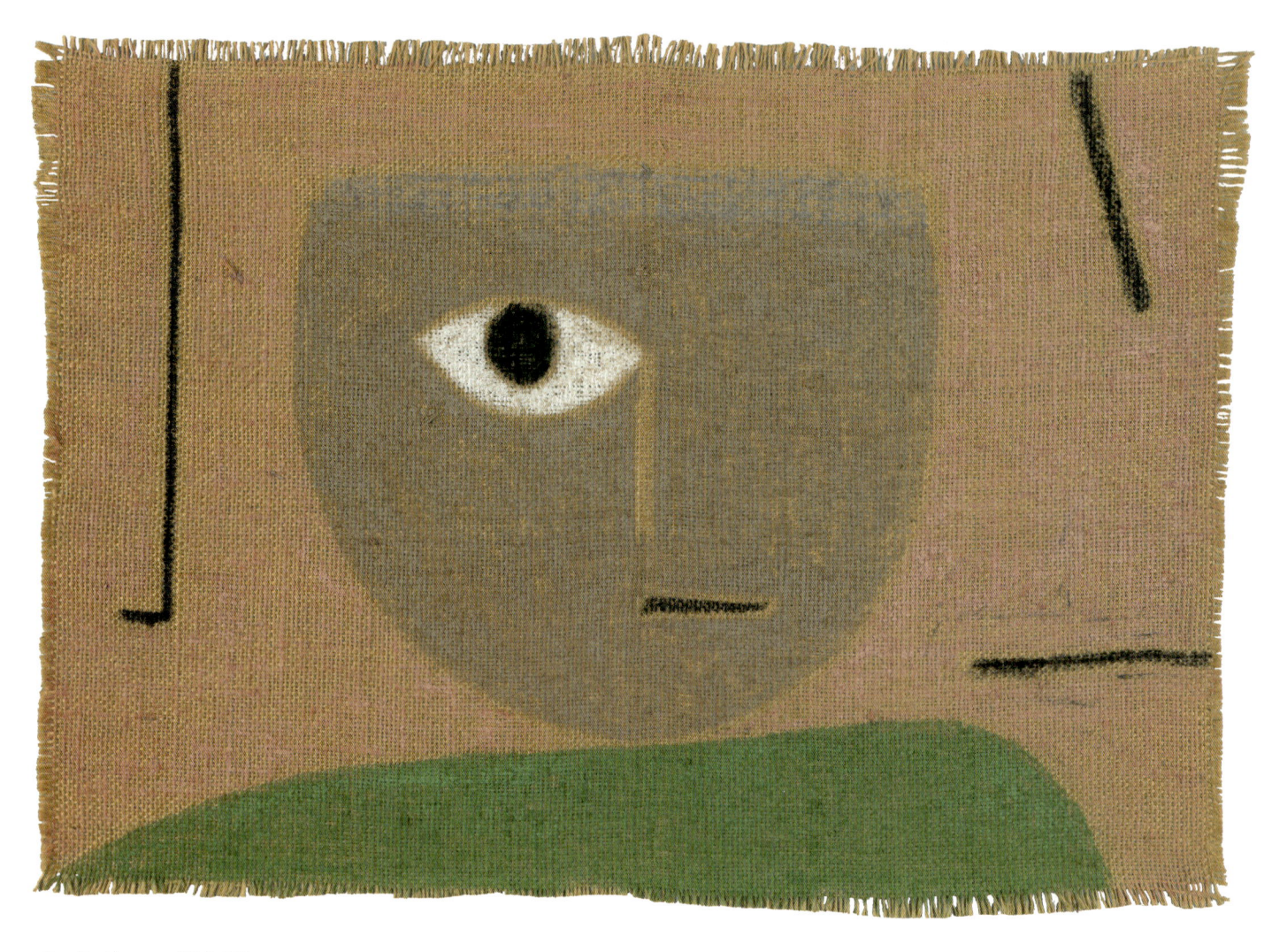

Fig. 47. The eye, 1938, 315

The artist depicts himself in a moss-green pullover. The head is mask-like, as in scleroderma, with taut skin, a pointed nose and narrow mouth. One eye is closed, the other is wide open. It gazes at us solemnly: contemplative, melancholy, questioning. This painting in pastels is stripped down to basics, with just three unconnected black lines on an orange background. The composition is balanced, but the person in the painting is not. His condition is unstable.

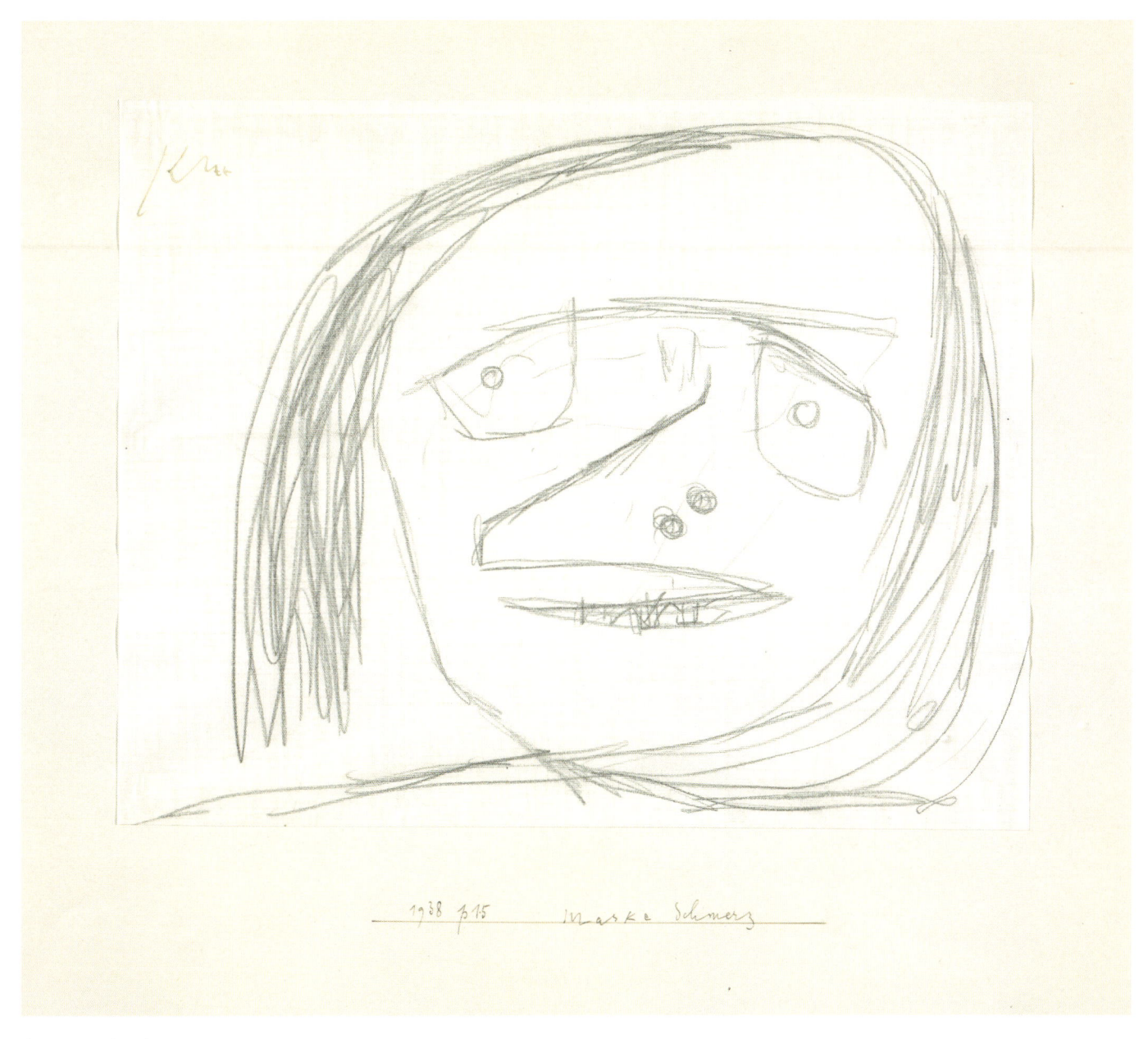

Fig. 48. Mask: pain, 1938, 235

When Paul Klee drew this mask-like face, he was already suffering from the mask-like skin changes which are typical of his illness. He calls the drawing 'Mask: pain' and emphasizes 'recurring pain'. His chronic disease means that he has serious discomfort when swallowing, shortness of breath when physically exerting himself and general debility, but above all he is suffering psychologically and emotionally. He bears his pain and suffering with great fortitude.

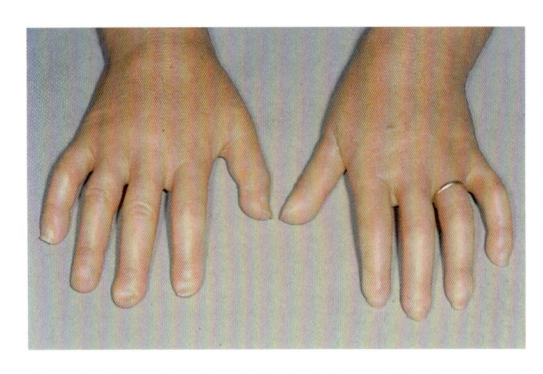

Fig. 49. Systemic sclerosis: limited form with sclerodactyly (see p. 54)

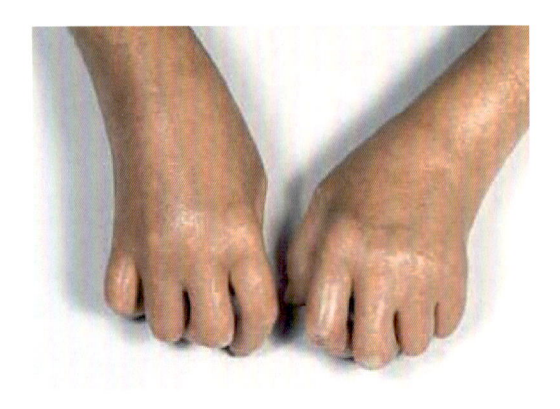

Fig. 50. Systemic sclerosis: limited form with sclerodactyly and finger contracture (see p. 54)

[165] Cf. Röther and Peter/ML 1996, p. 383, cf. Krieg/ML 1996, p. 730, and cf. Gadola and Villiger/ML 2006, p. 88.

[166] Cf. Moll/ML 1991, p. 96, cf. Krieg/ML 1996, p. 730, and cf. Ruzicka/ML 1996, p. 1201: In systemic sclerosis, especially the limited form, calcium deposits can build up on the fingers, knuckles, elbows and knees, also in muscles and tendons (known as 'Thibierge-Weissenbach syndrome'). These symptoms were never noted in Paul Klee.

[167] Cf. Krieg/ML 1996, p. 730.

[168] Personal communication, Felix Klee to the author, Bern, September 20, 1983.

[169] Telephone conversation between Max Huggler and the author, CH–7554 Sent, August 15, 1981.

[170] Note from Kathi Zollinger-Streiff (daughter of Bruno Streiff) to the author, CH–8044 Gockhausen, June 20, 2005, after a conversation with her father in November 2004. Bruno Streiff (1905–2005) visited Paul Klee in August or September 1939 in Bern.

[171] Personal communication, Felix Klee to Prof. Alfred Krebs and the author, Bern, November 9, 1979.

[172] Klee 1989, p. 46 f. Felix Klee had some knowledge of scleroderma in 1989. He knew that the disease can affect the hands, but confused the stiffness and restricted mobility of the fingers with paralysis.

The finger ends become tapered ('Madonna fingers'). Circulatory disorders gradually develop in the fingers due to the thickening and hardening of the vascular walls (fig. 56, page 63). This restricted circulation leads to a lack of oxygen in the tissues and parts of the tissue can die off ('rat-bite necrosis', fig. 51, page 59).[165] Minor injuries can result in ulcers on the fingertips and finger joints, and calcium excretion.[166] Ridges and lumps can appear on the fingernails; sometimes small blood spots appear on the cuticles and enlarged blood vessels in the nail-fold (see fig. 54, page 62).[167]

It can no longer be determined whether Klee had problems with other areas of his skin other than on his face and neck. But judging by Felix Klee's remarks, it is clear that he did not suffer from sclerodactyly. His fingers did not thicken and their mobility was in no way impaired.[168] This was also confirmed by Max Huggler[169] and Bruno Streiff, one of the artist's Bauhaus students, who visited Paul Klee in Bern in 1939.[170] According to his son, Klee was still able to do fine, detailed work right to the end.[171] Felix Klee also noted in 1989: 'This illness (scleroderma) has a lot of different symptoms. A lot of sufferers have paralyzed hands. This didn't happen to my father, otherwise he would not have been able to continue drawing and painting.'[172] The fact that the hands remained unaffected is significant in terms of differential diagnosis (see pages 78 f and 106).

Mucous Membrane Disorders

Mucous membrane disorders can also lead to a variety of problems, particularly when they occur in the mouth and in the esophagus (see pages 62 f).

When the tongue is affected by systemic sclerosis, it initially thickens up, then later the surface of the tongue starts to thin, becoming smooth, dry and fissured (fig. 52).[173] The tongue can also become smaller and less mobile.[174] Sometimes the band of tissue that attaches the tongue to the floor of the mouth can become thick, hard and shortened ('frenulum sclerosis').[175] The oral and genital mucous membranes can be affected in a similar way to the tongue.[176] If the salivary glands are also affected it can lead to an unpleasantly dry mouth ('Sicca syndrome') and if the vocal cords harden, it can result in hoarseness.[177] Early on in the disease there can be signs of widening of the 'periodontal space', the space between the teeth and the gums, particularly around the molars. This presents without inflammation, loculation and mostly without loosening of the teeth ('Stafne sign'=early form of 'periodontosis'=gum recession).[178] There is an increased likelihood of caries. Furthermore, tear secretion is reduced and the conjunctiva dries out. These changes to the mucous membranes occur in both forms of systemic sclerosis.[179]

Paul Klee did not show any of these symptoms, apart from periodontosis in the early stages. This was confirmed by his son[180], and also by his dentist, Dr. Jean Charlet.[181]

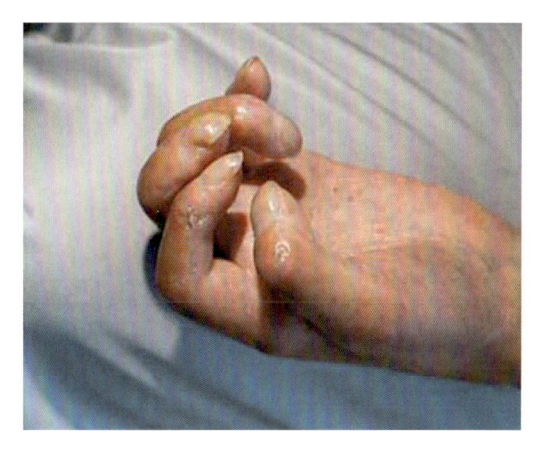

Fig. 51. Systemic sclerosis: sclerodactyly with dead tissue ('rat-bite necrosis') and ulceration (see p. 58)

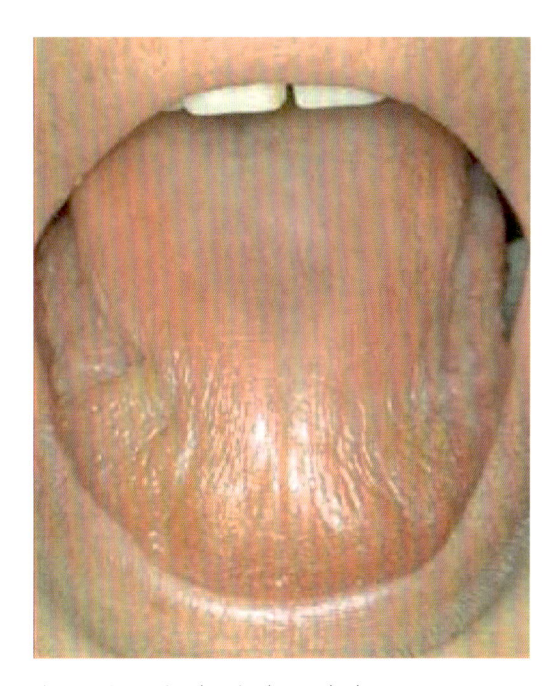

Fig. 52. Systemic sclerosis: dry, cracked tongue

[173] Cf. Krieg/ML 1996, p. 730.
[174] Cf. Moll/ML 1991, p. 96.
[175] Cf. ibid.
[176] Cf. ibid., and cf. Krieg/ML 1996, p. 730.
[177] Cf. ibid.
[178] See Appendices: Early Signs of Systemic Sclerosis on the Gums (p. 267).
[179] Cf. Moll/ML 1991, p. 96 f.
[180] Personal communication, Felix Klee to the author, Bern, September 20, 1983.
[181] Cf. recording of telephone conversation between Stefan Frey and Dr. Jean Charlet, Bern, July 11, 1990.

Raynaud's Syndrome

'Raynaud's syndrome'[182] presents in around 75% (60–90%) of cases of systemic sclerosis, especially in the limited form. It is a characteristic vascular disorder which affects the blood flow to the fingers, and it normally appears months or even years before the onset of the disease in the limited form.[183] In the diffuse form, Raynaud's syndrome presents shortly before or at the onset of the disease[184] or much later.[185] Emotional stress and cold are classic triggers of the phenomenon, causing a sudden narrowing of the arteries supplying blood to the fingers, which then turn pale or white ('dead finger', fig. 53). The blood vessels are depleted of oxygen and contain too much carbonic acid, causing the fingers to gradually turn blue ('cyanosis'). Finally as the blood vessels dilate, blood rushes back to the fingers, causing them to become red and painful.[186] In cold weather the pains can even start while the fingers are turning white. Young women in particular are often diagnosed with a harmless form of this circulatory disorder which is not linked with an underlying disease.[187] These days, other characteristic changes in the small blood vessels in the nail-fold have been identified: in the nail-fold capillaroscopy the capillaries have a corkscrew appearance and have wide ends ('giant capillaries', fig. 55, page 62).[188] Neither Paul Klee himself nor his wife or friends ever mentioned or described these very obvious symptoms of Raynaud's syndrome, and Felix Klee also assured me that his father did not suffer from it.[189]

In December 1938 Lily Klee remarks that Dr. Schorer had 'finally given us a diagnosis: vasomotor neurosis. This is a disorder of the nerves of the blood vessels and glands and this is causing all the problems. So it is an organic neuropathic disease.'[190] The term 'vasomotor neurosis' is misleading and indeed is no longer used in medical circles. It could wrongly lead to the assumption that it is identical to Raynaud's syndrome, but this is in fact not the case. In his interesting historical retrospective of scleroderma,[191] Gabriele Castenholz observes that the medical textbooks of the 1920s and 1930s stated that scleroderma resulted from changes to the blood vessels and nerves. The disease was therefore designated a 'vasomotor trophic neurosis'[192] ('vasomotor'=pertaining to

[182] Cf. Krieg/ML 1996, p. 729 f.
[183] Cf. ibid., p. 730, cf. Röther and Peter/ML 1996, p. 383, cf. Moll/ML 1991, p. 97, and cf. Gadola and Villiger/ML 2006, p. 87.
[184] Cf. Gadola and Villiger/ML 2006, p. 87.
[185] Cf. Moll/ML 1991, p. 96.
[186] Cf. Haustein/ML 1996, p. 336.
[187] Cf. ibid.
[188] Communication by Prof. Peter M. Villiger, Director and Chief Physician of the University Clinic and the Polyclinics of the Department of Rheumatology and Immunology/Allergology, Inselspital, Bern, to the author, Bern, September 16, 2005.
[189] Personal communication, Felix Klee to the author, Bern, September 20, 1983.
[190] Letter from Lily Klee to Gertrud Grote, Bern, December 17, 1938 (ZPKB).
[191] Cf. Castenholz/ML 2000, pp. 13–80 and 94–130.
[192] Ibid., p. 54: 'Various terms are used to describe scleroderma as a result of the changes to the nerves: "angiotropho neurosis" (Lewin and Heller 1895) and "vasomotor trophic neurosis" (Cassirer and Hirschfeld 1912/1924 and Curschmann 1926).' And p. 60: 'In 1924 R. Cassirer and E. Hirschfeld also published an article on scleroderma in "Spezielle Pathologie und Therapie innerer Krankheiten", vol. 10 (Nervenkrankheiten III), chapter entitled "Vasomotorische Neurosen" [ed. Kraus, F., and Brugsch, Th., Wien 1924, pp. 622–665]'.

blood vessels; 'trophic'=pertaining to the nourishment of tissues and organs; 'neurosis' here refers only to 'nerve changes' and not to the modern psychiatric use of the term to mean a mental disorder). At that time, according to Gabriele Castenholz's study, ductless gland disorders were also considered to be a cause of scleroderma.[193] Lily Klee's comments after Professor Naegeli's examination seem to support this: 'He [Paul Klee] is having treatment again because he has internal secretion problems (his glands), resulting from his long and serious illness.'[194] And: 'As his skin is still bad, he has had his blood and metabolism checked for calcium and phosphorus.'[195] (At that time it was thought that scleroderma was caused by changes to calcium metabolism as a result of thyroid disorders.[196]) This could have provided the doctors with additional evidence to support their diagnosis of 'scleroderma', but we do not know the results of the examination. Lily Klee does not mention any particular treatment as a result of the examination, so we can assume that the results were normal. Nowadays, scleroderma is not thought to be linked to endocrine disorders.

As a result of the thickening and hardening of the blood vessel walls in the connective tissues (see fig. 56, page 63), collateral vessels can form on the skin, known as 'teleangiectasia' (see also page 50).[197]

It is hard to establish when Paul Klee's underlying illness really began. But the first phase, with the persistent, feverish bronchitis, pneumonia and pleurisy, the long confinement to bed and the extreme fatigue before the ostensible measles outbreak in 1935, would seem to indicate the start of the autoimmune disease. These symptoms (as described on page 39) are typical signs of systemic sclerosis.

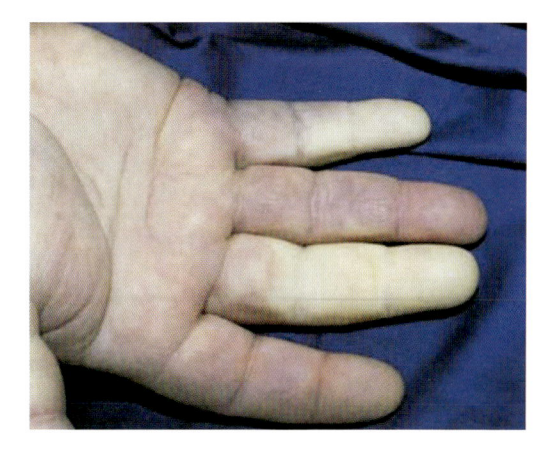

Fig. 53. Raynaud's syndrome: 'dead finger'

[193] Cf. Castenholz/ML 2000, pp. 63–66. Besides the thyroid gland, the parathyroid glands were thought to be a possible root cause of scleroderma. And Mayr/ML 1935, p. 70: 'Some cases seem to be linked to thyroid activity or to other ductless glands.'
[194] Letter from Lily Klee to Emmy Scheyer, Bern, November 3, 1936 (NSMP).
[195] Letter from Lily Klee to Will Grohmann, Bern, October 29, 1936 (AWG).
[196] Castenholz/ML 2000, p. 64: 'Ehrmann and Brünauer (1931) report that it is widely believed that scleroderma is caused by changes to calcium metabolism as a result of parathyroid disorders. It is supported by clinical findings such as calcification of the connective tissue and osteoporosis. Neuber (1935) and Thies and Misgeld (1975) also consider this to be the most widely held theory in the 1930s.' Then as now, it was important to determine the levels of calcium and phosphates in the serum when parathyroid disorders were suspected (particularly 'hyperparathyroidism' as a result of an overactive thyroid). These days other examinations may also be carried out, e.g. to determine parathormone levels in the serum.
[197] Cf. Röther and Peter/ML 1996, p. 383, and cf. Gadola and Villiger/ML 2006, p. 86.

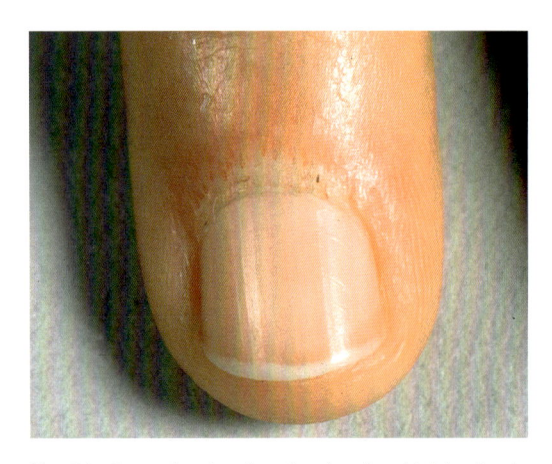

Fig. 54. Systemic sclerosis: sclerodactyly with bleeding in the cuticles and enlarged micro blood vessels in the nail-fold (see p. 58). Similar changes occur with systemic Lupus erythematosus (see p. 102).

nail   nail-fold   capillaries   giant capillary

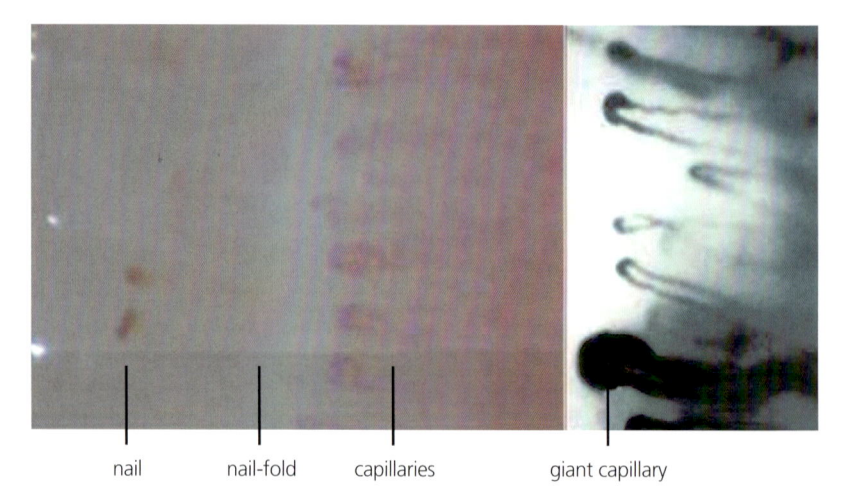

Fig. 55. Raynaud's syndrome: nail-fold capillaroscopy with giant capillaries (see p. 60)

Internal Organ Disorders

Clinical evidence demonstrates that the following internal organs are affected: the digestive tract (in up to 85% of cases), the lungs (40–90%), the heart (20–25%) and the kidneys (10–40%).[198] Autopsies have shown that in 30–80% of patients the disease causes changes in the connective tissues of the heart (fibrotic changes), and that in up to 80% of sufferers the kidneys show similar signs of the disease.[199]

Digestive Tract Disorders

In over 75% of systemic sclerosis cases – including both forms of the disease – patients have difficulty swallowing, due to a hardening of the connective tissues and a narrowing of the lower third of the esophagus ('esophageal stenosis').[200] Combined with this, the patient also produces less saliva, and this makes it difficult, or even impossible, to swallow solid foods. The muscles of the esophagus no longer force the food quickly down into the stomach (fig. 58, page 64). Solid foods get stuck in the esophagus, with resulting pain, and as a result, the patient can only take in small portions of liquid foods. The stomach contents then wash back into the esophagus ('reflux') and the lower portion of the esophagus becomes inflamed. This is experienced as heartburn, a burning sensation behind the lower part of the breastbone.[201]

---

[198] Cf. Mittag and Haustein/ML 1998, pp. 546–549.
[199] Cf. ibid., p. 548 f.
[200] Cf. Röther and Peter/ML 1996, p. 385, and cf. Mittag and Haustein/ML 1998, p. 546.
[201] Cf. ibid., p. 384 f, and p. 546.

In the summer of 1938, Paul Klee was described for the first time as having 'swelling in the esophagus'.[202] Later on, Felix Klee wrote: 'My father often had difficulty eating; his esophagus had lost its elasticity and would no longer pass solid food down to his stomach. Although this condition had its ups and downs, my father must have suffered unspeakably for almost five years, from the beginning of the disease to his death.'[203] And: 'He [Paul Klee] couldn't even swallow a grain of rice. For months he could only eat a liquid diet. No bread, nothing! Because of his swallowing difficulties, he always ate alone.'[204] Felix Klee also told me that his father was a good cook and generally prepared his own meals. He could only eat small portions of liquid foods and often disappeared into the kitchen to get them ready.[205] The art historian Carola Giedion-Welcker also confirms this eating pattern. She visited the invalid four months before his death and records the event in her monograph on Klee: 'While we were talking, he was constantly running into the little kitchen next door; he joked that women didn't like cooking so much these days, so he had to do it himself. But he was hiding something much more tragic, the fact that at that time he could only eat specially prepared liquid foods [...].'[206] In March 1939 Herman Rupf also comments on Paul Klee's eating problems: 'He looks a little better, but a trip to Paris is out of the question because he is still having problems with a stomach blockage, which forces him to eat at home as he feels unable to visit a hotel or restaurant.'[207] As a layman, Hermann Rupf wrongly describes the probable narrowing of the esophagus as a 'stomach blockage'. Paul Klee himself twice mentions his swallowing difficulties to his wife; on May 26, 1939, when Lily was staying at a spa near Lucerne, he says: 'Overall I am feeling a little better; it is easier than before to swallow my food.'[208] And one day after arriving at the Sanatorium Viktoria in Locarno-Orselina on May 11, 1940, he tells Lily: 'The diet, I imagine, is going to do me some good; the difficulty is more one of the mechanism of swallowing [...].'[209] (fig. 59, page 65).

The comments made by Paul and Felix Klee, and also by Carola Giedion-Welcker, clearly indicate a narrowing of the esophagus. There is also a telling drawing done by Klee in

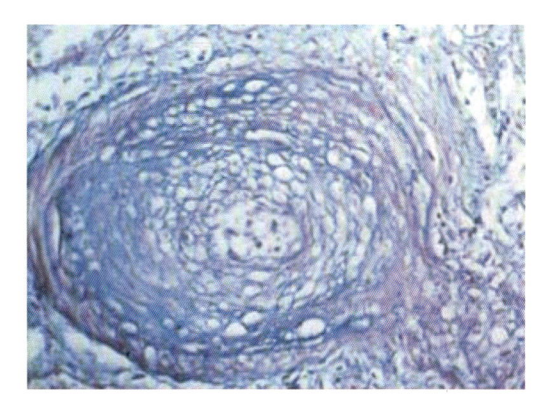

Fig. 56. Systemic sclerosis: blood vessel with 'onion skin' thickening and hardening of the wall tissue (see pp. 58 and 70)

[202] Letter from Dr. W. von Bremer, PhD, Berlin, to Paula Aichinger, Berlin, July 12, 1938 (ZPKB/SFK).
[203] Klee, 1960/1, p. 110.
[204] Klee 1989, p. 46 f.
[205] Personal communication, Felix Klee to Prof. Alfred Krebs and the author, Bern, November 9, 1979.
[206] Giedion/Welcker 2000, p. 101.
[207] Letter from Hermann Rupf to Wassily and Nina Kandinsky, Bern, March 12, 1939 (BK/CGPP).
[208] Letter from Paul Klee to Lily Klee, Bern, May 26, 1939, quoted in Klee 1979, p. 1292.
[209] Postcard from Paul Klee to Lily Klee, Locarno-Orselina, May 11, 1940, quoted in ibid., p. 1298.

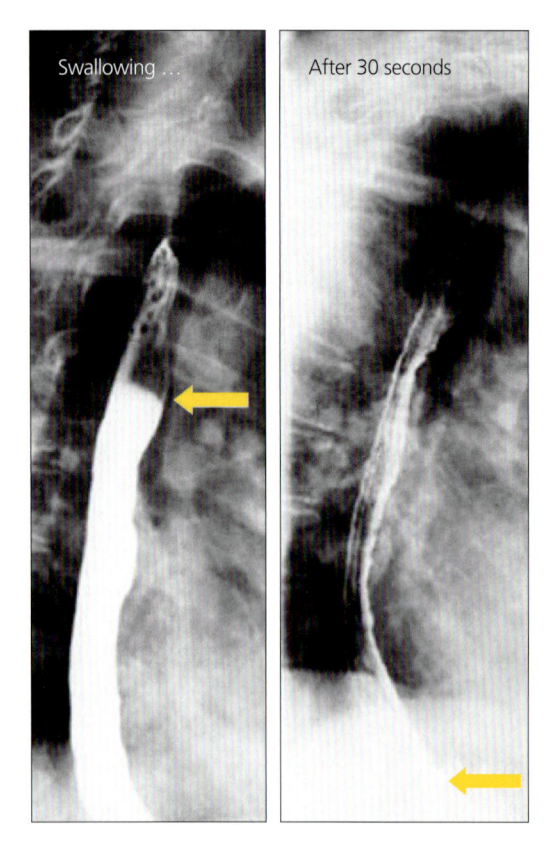

Fig. 57. X-ray of a normal esophagus: The food (represented by barium sulfate, shown here in white) travels through the esophagus to the stomach.

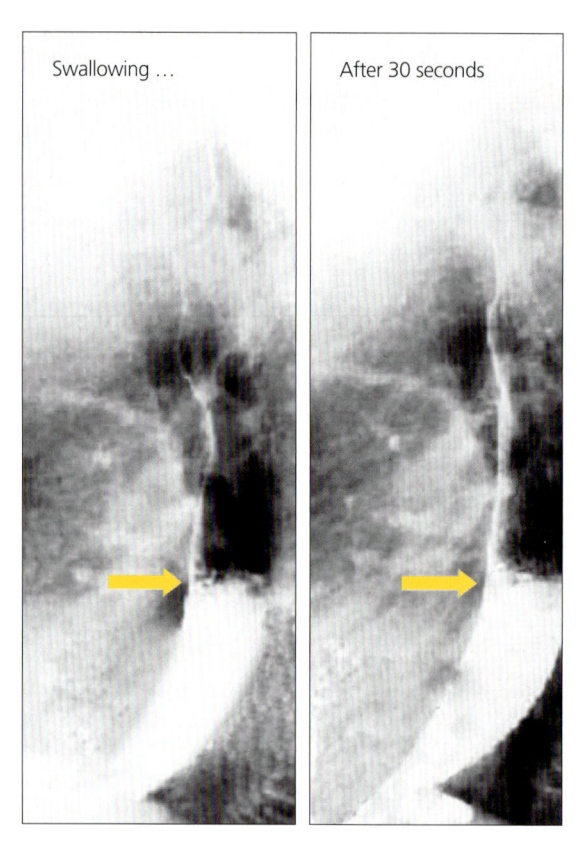

Fig. 58. Systemic sclerosis: X-ray of a rigid esophagus with narrowing in the lower part.

The swallowed barium meal remains longer in the esophagus.

1939 with the title 'Never again that dish!' (fig. 61, page 66). I thanks Hans Christoph von Tavel for this reference,[210] and also Michael Baumgartner for pointing out a mention of this drawing and its immediate predecessor entitled 'Herring, for me?!' (fig. 60, page 66) in a paper by Christina Kröll, a doctoral student. She writes: 'Sometimes within a title [by Paul Klee] there is a real little dialogue [...] or one title follows another to create a short story: mir Hering?! ['Herring, for me?!'] nie mehr jene Speise! ['Never again that dish!'] (both from 1939).'[211]

Sometimes other portions of the digestive tract are affected by the disease. In certain cases the stomach ceases to produce gastric acid.[212] In a diet plan, probably prepared by Lily Klee for her husband, covering the period December 28, 1935 to January 17, 1936, it is noted that six drops of hydrochloride were given on nine occasions with lunchtime meals (fig. 62, page 68).[213] This could indicate a lack of gastric acid.

[210] Cf. Letter from Hans Christoph von Tavel, to the author, CH–1169 Yens, February 16, 2000.
[211] Kröll 1968, p. 40. I thank Michael Baumgartner for the reference, Bern, February 12, 2002.
[212] Cf. Krieg/ML 1996, p. 731.
[213] Cf. diet plan for the period December 28 [1935] to January 17 [1936], probably prepared by Lily Klee (ZPKB/SFK). Note: the years are not written in the diet plan, simply 'Saturday, 28.12.'. By checking a table in 'Helveticus 5', Hallwag-Verlag, Bern 1945, p. 86, it can be determined that between 1930 and 1939 the only time that December 28 fell on a Saturday was in 1935.

We can safely assume that this diet plan was put together for the artist, as in the margins there is a note of the number of hours of rest required each day. We know that at this time he had to spend a lot of time lying down.

Changes in the stomach: the stomach lining becomes smooth. Hardening of the sphincter at the entrance to the stomach can lead to spasms in the upper abdomen. Sometimes benign gastric ulcers develop with bleeding and perforation.[214] According to his wife's report on January 31, 1937, Klee did in fact suffer 'stomach bleeding due to a gastric ulcer'.[215] The treatment consisted of a 'strict diet' for six weeks, made up of

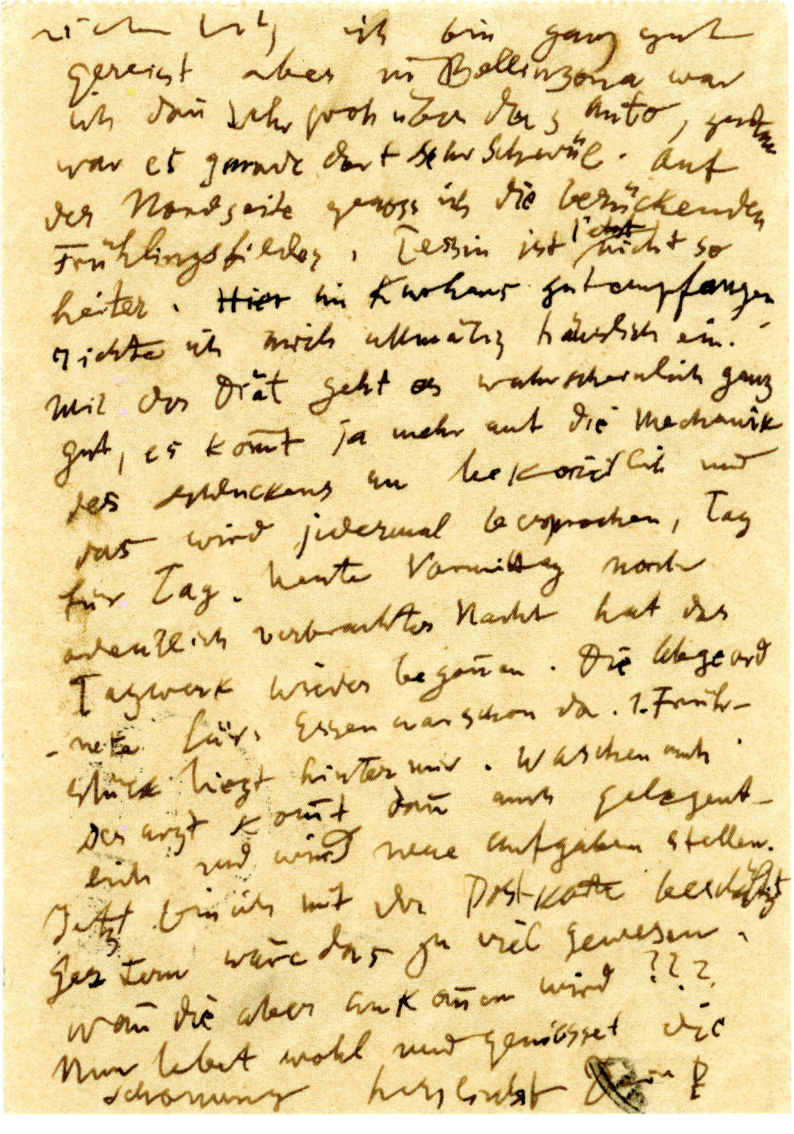
Liebe Lily, ich bin ganz gut gereist aber in Bellinzona war ich dann sehr froh über das Auto, gestern war es gerade dort sehr schwül. Auf der Nordseite genoss ich die berückenden Frühlingsbilder. Tessin ist jetzt nicht so heiter. Hier im Kurhaus gut empfangen richte ich mich allmälig häuslich ein. Mit der Diät geht es wahrscheinlich ganz gut, es kommt ja mehr auf die Mechanik des Schluckens an. Bekömmliches wird jedesmal besprochen, Tag für Tag. Heute Vormittag nach ordentlich verbrachter Nacht hat das Tagwerk wieder begonnen. Die Wägerin … Essen war schon da. 1. Frühstück liegt hinter mir. Waschen auch. Der Arzt kommt dann auch gelegentlich und wird neue Aufgaben stellen. Jetzt bin ich mit der Postkarte beschäftigt. Gestern wäre das zu viel gewesen. Wann die aber ankommen wird ??? Nun lebt wohl und geniesset die Schonung. herzl Grüsst Euer P

Fig. 59. Postcard from Paul Klee to Lily Klee, Locarno-Orselina, May 11, 1940

Dear Lily, The trip was quite tolerable, but by the time I reached Bellinzona I was very glad of the car, it was very sultry there yesterday. I enjoyed the enchanting succession of spring scenes on the northern side. Ticino is not so bright at the moment. I was well received here at the sanatorium and am gradually making myself at home. The diet, I imagine, is going to do me some good; the difficulty is more one of the mechanism of swallowing, and what will suit me is to be discussed each day before every meal. This morning, after a fairly good night, the day's routine has begun again. The nurse has been with the food. My first breakfast is already behind me. Washing too. The doctor will come by occasionally to prescribe some new treatment routines. Now I am busy writing this postcard. Yesterday that would have been too much for me. But I wonder when it will arrive??? Anyway, goodbye for now and enjoy your rest. Love, Paul

214 Cf. Krieg/ML 1996, p. 731.

215 Letter from Lily Klee to Will Grohmann, Bern, February 11, 1937 (AWG).

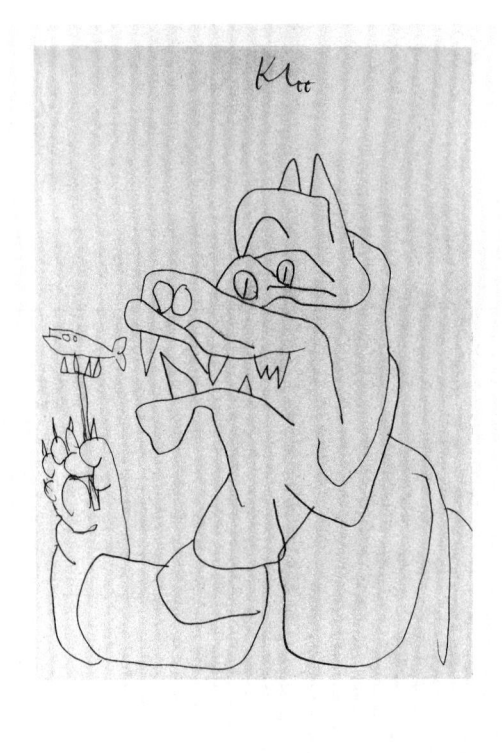

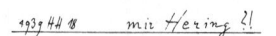

Fig. 60. Herring, for me?!, 1939, 658

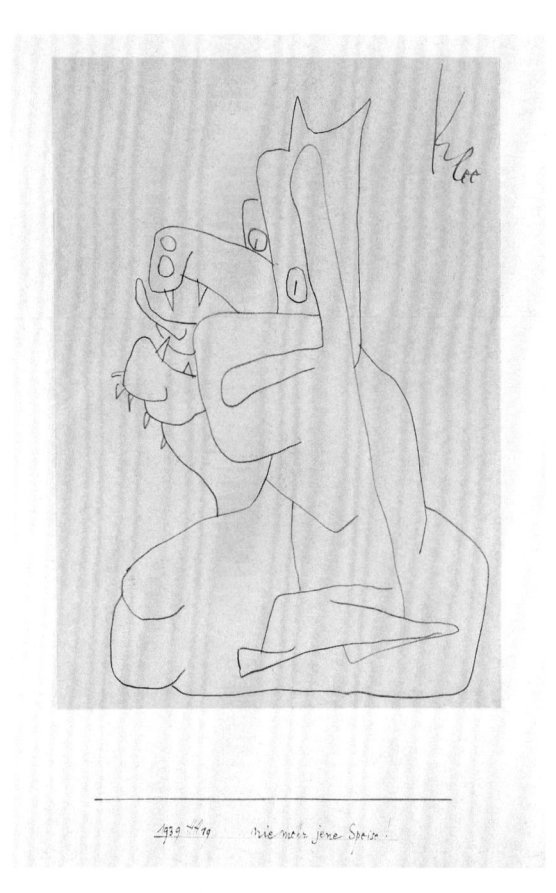

Fig. 61. Never again that dish!, 1939, 659

The illustrations show a monstrous beast, which in the first drawing 'Herring, for me?!' is holding a herring on a fork in front of its open mouth. Its eyes show its anticipation of the food. The exclamation mark in the title emphasizes this. But the question mark next to it raises a doubt as to whether this 'food' is really edible. The second drawing confirms this suspicion: the beast seems to be choking on it. Has the fish got stuck in its throat? The beast's eyes are terrified. It is holding up its left paw, its index finger raised in warning: 'Never again that dish!'

Paul Klee suffered a lot of pain due to the narrowing of his esophagus. Solid foods caused discomfort by getting stuck in the esophagus, and he could only consume more liquid foods. As so often, the artist associates a physical or mental condition, a discovery, a feeling or a sense of outrage with an imaginative and often comical drawing.

a mixture of 'milk, eggs, a little Nestle whole milk, glucose, etc.'[216] Lily Klee then very carefully and cleverly worked out a 'transition diet'[217] for a six-week period. Included are '[…] (light meat dishes, young chicken, trout), porridge, noodles, eggs, spinach, asparagus. He [Paul Klee] is tolerating everything very well. (Orange juice, apple sauce.) And still plenty of milk […]'[218] The diet helped to strengthen the invalid.[219] He put on weight, was able to go for short walks when the weather was good and on Easter Monday 1937 he even visited the exhibition 'Wassily Kandinsky/French Masters of our Time', Bern Kunsthalle, February 21 to March 29, 1937.[220] In July 1937 Lily Klee writes to Will Grohmann: 'He is working hard and producing a lot of new and interesting things. He is in one of his very creative periods again. He is in a drawing phase. He sits until 11 o'clock every evening letting sheet after sheet fall to the floor, just like he used to. Strange! But he is still not totally well and is constantly under the doctor's supervision.'[221] Hermann Rupf is a little more restrained in evaluating his friend's condition: 'Paul Klee is in reasonable health, but his cough has not disappeared and he is physically very broken down compared to before.'[222]

Paul and Lily Klee took trips to recuperate in the mild climate of Ticino (in the 'Casa Adula' in Ascona in September and October 1937)[223] and at altitude (in Beatenberg above Lake Thun in late summer 1938).[224] These holidays had a beneficial effect. Lily reported from Ascona on September 22, 1937: 'My husband feels very well here and has started to work (very colorful pastels.)'[225]

In spring 1939 Paul Klee mentions intestinal problems. He tells his wife, who is staying at the Sonnmatt spa hotel near Lucerne: 'Your suggestion that I come to lunch is tempting, but I have qualms about traveling in the mornings because of my physical condition. It is absolute hell for me if I have an episode of diarrhea in the car. It does not happen every day, but I have to anticipate that it might.'[226] This fits in with the symptoms of systemic sclerosis. If the small or large intestine is affected by the disease, both dilation and contraction can occur. It can lead to a bacterial overgrowth of the intestine, to a disruption in the absorption of nutrients into the blood

[216] Letter from Lily Klee to Will Grohmann, Bern, March 20, 1937 (AWG).
[217] Letter from Lily Klee to Nina Kandinsky, Bern, March 23, 1937 (BK/CGPP).
[218] Letter from Lily Klee to Nina Kandinsky, Bern, March 23, 1937 (BK/CGPP).
[219] Cf. ibid.
[220] Cf. letter from Lily Klee to Nina Kandinsky, Bern, April 13, 1937 (BK/CGPP).
[221] Letter from Lily Klee to Will Grohmann, Bern, July 8, 1937 (AWG).
[222] Letter from Hermann Rupf to Wassily and Nina Kandinsky, Bern, August 9, 1937 (BK/CGPP).
[223] Cf. letters from Lily Klee to Will Grohmann, Ascona, September 15, 1937, September 27, 1937, and October 13, 1937 (AWG), and cf. letter from Lily Klee to Curt Valentin, Ascona, October 17, 1937 (MoMAANY/VP).
[224] Cf. letter from Lily Klee to Gertrud Grote, Bern, December 17, 1938 (ZPKB).
[225] Letter from Lily Klee to Hermann and Margrit Rupf, Ascona, September 22, 1937 (HMRS), cf. letter from Lily Klee to Will Grohmann, Ascona, September 27, 1937 (AWG), and cf. letter from Lily Klee to Curt Valentin, Ascona, October 17, 1937 (MoMAANY/VP).
[226] Letter from Paul Klee to Lily Klee, Bern, May 6, 1939, quoted in Klee 1979, p. 1287 f.

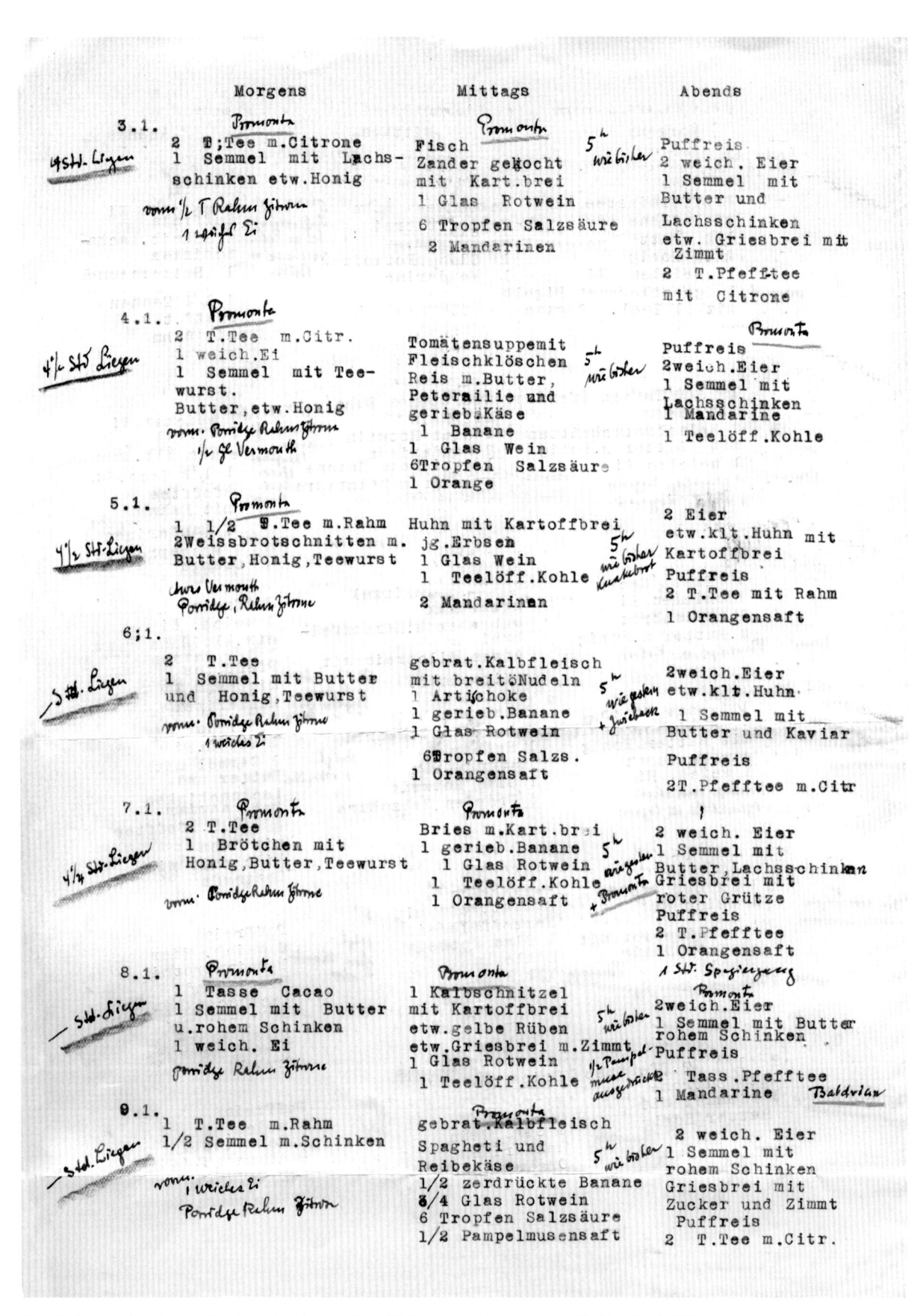

	Morgens	Mittags	Abends
3.1. *4Std. Liegen*	*Promonta* 2 T.Tee m.Citrone 1 Semmel mit Lachsschinken etw.Honig *vorm 1/2 T Rahm Zitron 1 weiches Ei*	*Promonta* Fisch Zander gekocht mit Kart.brei 1 Glas Rotwein 6 Tropfen Salzsäure 2 Mandarinen	5h *wie bisher* Puffreis 2 weich. Eier 1 Semmel mit Butter und Lachsschinken etw. Griesbrei mit Zimmt 2 T.Pfefftee mit Citrone
4.1. *4 1/2 Std. Liegen*	*Promonta* 2 T.Tee m.Citr. 1 weich.Ei 1 Semmel mit Teewurst. Butter, etw.Honig *vorm. Porridge Rahm Zitron 1/2 Gl Vermouth*	Tomatensuppe mit Fleischklöschen Reis m.Butter, Peterailie und gerieb.Käse 1 Banane 1 Glas Wein 6Tropfen Salzsäure 1 Orange	5h *wie bisher* *Promonta* Puffreis 2weich.Eier 1 Semmel mit Lachsschinken 1 Mandarine 1 Teelöff.Kohle
5.1. *4 1/2 Std. Liegen*	*Promonta* 1 1/2 T.Tee m.Rahm 2Weissbrotschnitten m. Butter, Honig, Teewurst *1/2 Vermouth Porridge, Rahm Zitrone*	Huhn mit Kartoffbrei jg.Erbsen 1 Glas Wein 1 Teelöff.Kohle 2 Mandarinen	5h *wie bisher Knackbrot* 2 Eier etw.klt.Huhn mit Kartoffbrei Puffreis 2 T.Tee mit Rahm 1 Orangensaft
6;1. *5 Std. Liegen*	2 T.Tee 1 Semmel mit Butter und Honig, Teewurst *vorm. Porridge Rahm Zitron 1 weiches Ei*	gebrat.Kalbfleisch mit breiteNudeln 1 Artischoke 1 gerieb.Banane 1 Glas Rotwein 6Tropfen Salzs. 1 Orangensaft	5h *wie gestern + Zwieback* 2weich.Eier etw.klt. Huhn 1 Semmel mit Butter und Kaviar Puffreis 2T.Pfefftee m.Citr
7.1. *4 1/2 Std. Liegen*	*Promonta* 2 T.Tee 1 Brötchen mit Honig,Butter,Teewurst *vorm. Porridge Rahm Zitrone*	*Promonta* Bries m.Kart.brei 1 gerieb.Banane 1 Glas Rotwein 1 Teelöff.Kohle 1 Orangensaft	5h *wie gestern + Promonta* 2 weich. Eier 1 Semmel mit Butter, Lachsschinken Griesbrei mit roter Grütze Puffreis 2 T.Pfefftee 1 Orangensaft
8.1. *5 Std. Liegen*	*Promonta* 1 Tasse Cacao 1 Semmel mit Butter u.rohem Schinken 1 weich. Ei *Porridge Rahm Zitrone*	*Promonta* 1 Kalbschnitzel mit Kartoffbrei etw.gelbe Rüben etw.Griesbrei m.Zimmt 1 Glas Rotwein 1 Teelöff.Kohle	*1 Std. Spazierg.* *Promonta* 5h *wie bisher* 2weich.Eier 1 Semmel mit Butter rohem Schinken Puffreis *1/2 Pampel-muse ausgedrückt* 1 Tass.Pfefftee 1 Mandarine *Baldrian*
9.1. *5 Std. Liegen*	1 T.Tee m.Rahm 1/2 Semmel m.Schinken *vorm 1 weiches Ei Porridge Rahm Zitron*	*Promonta* gebrat.Kalbfleisch Spagheti und Reibekäse 1/2 zerdrückte Banane 3/4 Glas Rotwein 6 Tropfen Salzsäure 1/2 Pampelmusensaft	5h *wie bisher* 2 weich. Eier 1 Semmel mit rohem Schinken Griesbrei mit Zucker und Zimmt Puffreis 2 T.Tee m.Citr.

Fig. 62. Page 2 of a diet plan for the period January 3–9, 1936, presumably prepared by Lily Klee for Paul Klee

and lymph vessels through the intestine ('malabsorption'), and to diarrhea.[227] Another result is weight loss. However, Klee once again made a good recovery while he was staying in Faoug beside Lake Murten in Autumn 1939.[228] While they were there, he and Lily paid several visits to a former Masters student in nearby Murten, Petra Petitpierre, who he had taught at the Düsseldorf Academy of Fine Arts.[229]

25% of systemic sclerosis cases present with **anemia** due to malabsorption of nutrients into the blood and lymph vessels, gastrointestinal bleeding or kidney failure.[230] Paul Klee suffered from anemia and gastric bleeding (see page 82, notes 292–301, and page 65, note 215).

[227] Cf. Mittag and Haustein/ML 1998, p. 547 (table 1), and cf. Gadola and Villiger/ML 2006, p. 87.
[228] Cf. letter from Paul Klee to Will Grohmann, Bern, November 28, 1939 (AWG).
[229] Cf. letter from Petra Petitpierre to Josef Albers, [Murten], April 20, 1942. Autograph: Yale University Library, Newhaven, Conn., quoted in Frey, Stefan, in: Klee 1990/2, note 131, p. 130.
[230] Cf. Krieg/ML 1996, p. 732.

Lung Disorders

Systemic sclerosis causes a massive thickening of the connective tissue in the pulmonary alveoli and bronchial tubes of the lungs ('pulmonary fibrosis').[231] The lung tissue hardens and the pulmonary alveoli contract. This leads to shortage of breath ('dyspnea'), particularly during physical exertion, and often to a chronic dry cough and pleurisy.[232] In serious cases of pulmonary fibrosis the facial skin appears blue ('cyanosis'). There is a higher risk of bronchial pneumonia, particularly after food inhalation. In almost half of patients, chronic pulmonary fibrosis develops into 'pulmonary arterial hypertension', a special form of high blood pressure which has a poor prognosis. It leads to 'cor pulmonale', or pulmonary heart disease, typically a change in the structure and function of the heart caused by an increase in pulmonary arterial blood pressure due to a lung disorder. This is one of the main causes of death in systemic sclerosis.[233] This increased blood pressure is mainly a result of abnormal collagen deposits in the small arteries (arterioles) of the lungs, which leads to a thickening of the arterial wall and a significant constriction of these blood vessels (fig. 56, page 63). Hypertension can also stem from the pulmonary fibrosis itself (due to the thickened lung tissue pressing on the lung arterioles). In about 40% of cases, X-ray pictures show diffuse shadows on the middle and lower portions of the lungs (fig. 63). Sometimes cysts develop, which can become a serious condition known as 'honeycomb lung'.[234]

In 1936 Paul Klee wrote to Lily while he was on holiday in Tarasp in the Unterengadin with Hermann and Margrit Rupf: 'Today I have been for a walk for the second time, yesterday I walked along the river Inn downstream, today I walked along it the other way. The paths are fairly flat, lovely to walk on, sometimes going through trees and sometimes open. There are plenty of benches for people like me. The altitude makes it a little harder for me, as do the cool temperatures, but at least I have the impetus, and it is important that the climate has an effect. […] The lift for bathers is right next to me, I never have to climb steps.'[235] But he then has to admit that the Ofenpass was physically too much for him: 'At the top of the pass (2,150 [meters above sea level]) it was too

[231] Cf. Krieg/ML 1996, p. 731.
[232] Cf. Röther and Peter/ML 1996, p. 385.
[233] Cf. ibid., p. 386, and cf. Gadola and Villiger/ML 2006, p. 87 f.
[234] Cf. Krieg/ML 1996, p. 731.
[235] Letter from Paul Klee to Lily Klee, Tarasp, June 9, 1936, in: Klee 1979, p. 1269.

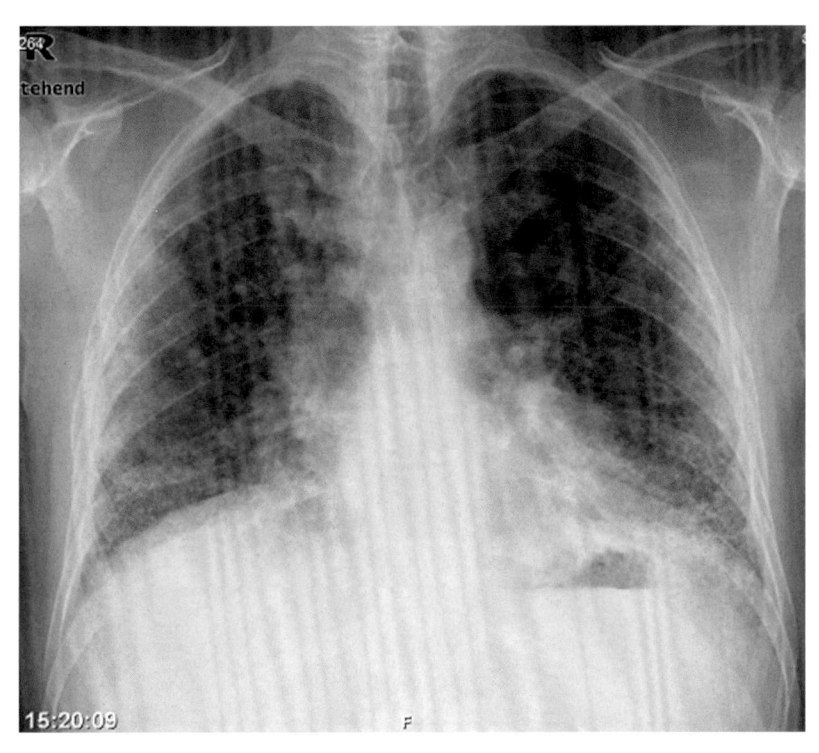

Fig. 63. Systemic sclerosis: X-ray of pulmonary fibrosis. The diffuse 'shadows' (light areas), which are most clearly seen in the middle and lower sections of both lungs, represent scarring caused by systemic sclerosis.

high, I had to stand totally still while the others walked about.'[236] 'I breathe as deeply as I can. My shortage of breath depends on the paths, whether I'm walking uphill or on the flat, and also on whether my activity is before or after the "Stifi". It also depends on the weather, yesterday during the Föhn it was not so good, but today it is better again. It also depends on whether my stomach is full or not. After "dinner" – it sounds very genteel to use the English word – is worse than before.'[237] Lily Klee observes that her husband 'has shortness of breath when climbing'[238] and that 'he walks very slowly'.[239] Klee also ironically remarks in 1939 that the slight slope on Kistlerweg outside his apartment in the Elfenau area of Bern was now 'his Matterhorn'.[240] Klee had the characteristic symptoms of pulmonary fibrosis, with shortage of breath during physical exertion, chronic cough[241], pneumonia and pleurisy. Unfortunately we do not have the results of his X-rays. After his first X-ray examination, Lily mentions the confirmation of Dr. Schorer's previous diagnosis of 'chronic double pneumonia. Pleurisy = inflammation of

[236] Letter from Paul Klee to Lily Klee, Tarasp, June 16, 1936 in: Klee 1979, p. 1272.

[237] Ibid.

[238] Letter from Lily Klee to Hermann and Margrit Rupf, Bern, September 1, 1936 (HMRS).

[239] Letter from Lily Klee to Will Grohmann, Bern, September 18, 1936 (AWG).

[240] Bürgi 1948, p. 26. The Matterhorn is the landmark of Zermatt (Valais), a huge pyramid of rock which rises to 4,478 m above sea-level, more than 1,000 m higher than the other mountains which form a ridge along the Swiss/Italian border (from: Luzern 1991–1993, vol. 4, p. 484).

[241] Letter from Lily Klee to Will Grohmann, Bern, August 24, 1936: '[…] He is also coughing a lot […]' (AWG), letter from Hermann Rupf to Wassily and Nina Kandinsky, Bern, August 9, 1937: '[…] the cough never goes away […]' (BK/CGPP), letter from Hermann Rupf to Otto and Hilde Nebel, Bern, December 19, 1937: '[…] but he is still coughing and feeling weak […].' (SLB/SLA), and letter from Hermann Rupf to Otto and Hilde Nebel, Bern, January 23, 1938: 'He [Klee] is always coughing and can only go out when the weather is fine.' (SLB/SLA).

the pleura. Cardiac dilation'[242] (fig. 37, page 47). But after his second X-ray in 1938 she only states: 'A few weeks ago he had another X-ray, at the request of the doctors, who wanted it for their studies. His case is starting to arouse the interest of the Bern medical faculty.'[243] This leads us to believe that the second X-ray was carried out in the university hospital (Inselspital) in Bern and that it produced further clues for the diagnosis – pulmonary fibrosis shows typical characteristics on X-ray pictures (fig. 63, page 71).[244] Unfortunately we have no confirmation of this. We also have no records relating to his blood pressure, so we cannot say whether Paul Klee suffered from pulmonary arterial hypertension, though based on this lack of records it is probably unlikely.

Cardiac Disorders

Patients with systemic sclerosis often have heart problems, the most common being pericarditis (inflammation of the fibrous sac surrounding the heart), but this often goes undetected.[245] The second most common heart condition is myocarditis (inflammation of the heart muscle) and thickening of the connective tissue of the heart muscle. This gradually leads to hardening ('diffuse interstitial myocarditis') and loss of elasticity in the heart muscle. The heart contractions become weaker and parts of the electrical pathways of the heart are replaced by fibrous scar tissue. As a result, the heart's function is impaired ('cardiac insufficiency', with reduced physical capacity); the cardiac conduction system is disrupted, with abnormal heart rhythms; and there are spells of rapid heartbeat ('tachycardia') and atrial fibrillation.[246] Signs of blockages also appear in the venous system: in the lungs, pleura, liver, kidneys and legs. Electrographs detect changes in over 50% of patients. As already mentioned, pulmonary fibrosis can have secondary effects: a special form of high blood pressure ('pulmonary arterial hypertension') and pulmonary heart disease ('cor pulmonale', see page 70).

In the very first year of his illness, Lily Klee noted – following Dr. Schorer's diagnosis – that 'the lungs and heart' of her husband were 'affected'[247] and seven months later, 'his heart is enlarged'.[248] Clearly Klee's shortage of breath during phys-

[242] Letter from Lily Klee to Emmy Scheyer, Bern, June 28, 1936 (fig. 37, NSMP).
[243] Letter from Lily Klee to Will Grohmann, Bern, June 29, 1938 (AWG).
[244] Cf. Mittag and Haustein/ML 1998, p. 547.
[245] Cf. Röther and Peter/ML 1996, p. 386.
[246] Cf. ibid., and cf. Krieg/ML 1996, p. 731, and cf. Gadola and Villiger/ML 2006, p. 87.
[247] Letter from Lily Klee to Rudolf Probst, Bern, November 10, 1935 (PBD).
[248] Letter from Lily Klee to Emmy Scheyer, Bern, June 28, 1936 (NSMP).

ical exertion was linked to the impairment of his lungs and heart. But unfortunately we have no X-ray pictures of his heart and no results of the electrocardiogram which was carried out in 1936 (see page 46, note 121).

Renal Disorders

It cannot be ascertained from the letters whether Paul Klee suffered from kidney disorders ('renal fibrosis') brought on by his illness. We only have one set of laboratory results from the Clinica Sant' Agnese – the results of a urine sample which showed a trace of protein in the urine, few red and white blood cells, and hyaline (homogenous) and granulated protein cylinders in the urine sediment (see pages 264 and 265, notes 13 and 23). These could indicate either renal fibrosis[249] or cardiac insufficiency with 'kidney congestion'.[250] Severe renal fibrosis leads to kidney atrophy with critical increases in blood pressure, rapidly deteriorating kidney function and a poor prognosis.[251] We have no record of this; however 10–40% of systemic sclerosis patients show clear symptoms of kidney problems.[252] And when an autopsy is carried out, up to 80% of patients are shown to have characteristic changes in the kidneys linked to sclerosis,[253] so it is very possible that Klee's kidneys were affected. Such kidney disorders result in a particularly poor prognosis for the progression of the disease and the patient's life expectancy.[254] Loss of kidney function is responsible for half of all deaths related to the diffuse form of systemic sclerosis.[255]

Death in Ticino

As Paul Klee 'had been unwell for some time'[256] (as noted by his wife), and as spending time in the mountains and in more southerly climates had always done him good, he set off on May 10, 1940, for what turned out to be his last stay at the Sanatorium Viktoria (now Clinica Santa Croce) in Locarno-Orselina (fig. 65, page 74).[257] His weak condition is evident from the postcard which he wrote to Lily the following day: 'I was well received here at the sanatorium and am gradually making myself at home. [...] Now I am busy writing this postcard [.] Yesterday that would have been too much for me.'[258]

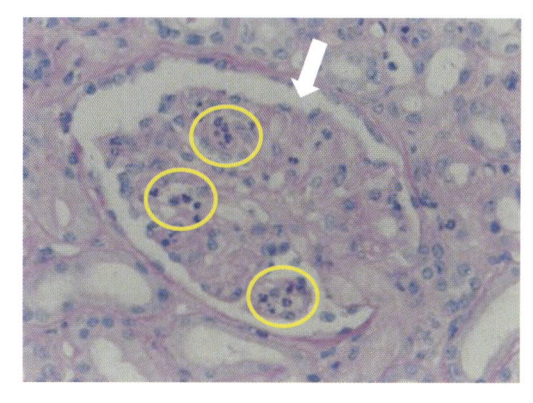

Fig. 64. Systemic sclerosis: the illustration shows a microscopic section of a kidney filter (arrow). The white blood cells, with black, round and partly-lobed nuclei (inside the yellow circles) are evidence of inflammation.

[249] Cf. Mittag and Haustein/ML 1998, p. 549.
[250] Assessment made by Prof. Alfred Krebs, specialist in skin diseases, venereology and internal medicine, Bern, personal communication to the author, Bern, November 12, 1998.
[251] Cf. Röther and Peter/ML 1996, p. 386, and cf. Gadola and Villiger/ML 2006, p. 87.
[252] Cf. Mittag and Haustein/ML 1998, p. 549.
[253] Cf. ibid.
[254] Cf. ibid.
[255] Cf. Krieg/ML 1996, p. 731.
[256] Letter from Lily Klee to Will Grohmann, Bern, July 7, 1940 (AWG), quoted in Frey 1990, p. 124.
[257] Cf. Frey 1990, p. 124.
[258] Postcard from Paul Klee to Lily Klee, Locarno-Orselina, May 11, 1940, quoted in Klee 1979, p. 1298.

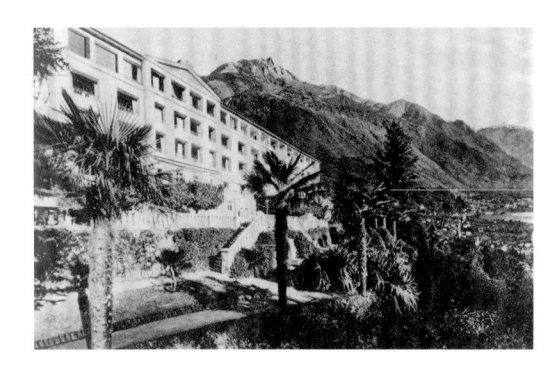

Fig. 65. Sanatorium Viktoria, Locarno-Orselina

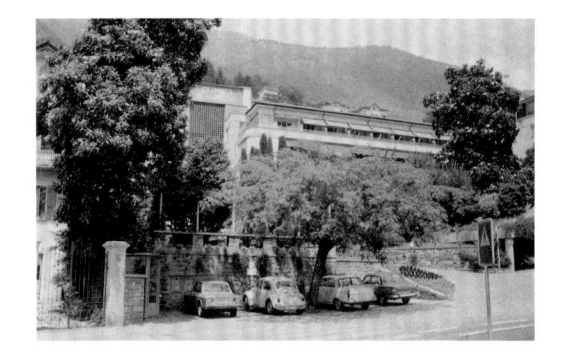

Fig. 66. Clinica Sant' Agnese, Locarno-Muralto

[259] Cf. Frey 1990, p. 124.
[260] Cf. letter from Lily Klee to Hermann and Margrit Rupf, Locarno-Orselina, May 21, 1940 (HMRS).
[261] Letter from Lily Klee to Will Grohmann, Bern, July 7, 1940 (AWG), quoted in Frey 1990, p. 124 f.
[262] Cf. Letter from Lily Klee to Hermann and Margrit Rupf, Locarno-Muralto, June 17, 1940 (HMRS).
[263] Ibid., quoted in Frey 1990, p. 124.
[264] Postcard from Lily Klee to Hermann and Margrit Rupf, Locarno-Muralto, June 23, 1940 (HMRS), quoted in Frey 1990, p. 125.
[265] 'Municipalità di Muralto. Attestato di morte. Il sottoscritto medico-chirurgico attesta che [...] Klee Paul, fu Hans, coniugato, nato nell' anno 1879, attinente del Comune di München (Germ.) domicilato in Bern, è morto il giorno 29 del mese di giugno, alle ore 7.30, in causa di malattia di cuore (myocardite) e quindi può essere autorizzata la sepoltura, passate 24 ore da quella della morte. Muralto, 29 giugno 1940[.] Il medico-chirurgo: [sig.] Dr. H. Bodmer' (photocopy: ZPKB/SFK).

(fig. 59, page 65). The sanatorium closed at the beginning of June 1940, so Klee was transferred on June 8 to the Clinica Sant' Agnese (now known as the Casa per convalescenza Sant' Agnese) in Locarno-Muralto[259] (fig. 66). This clinic was run by nuns from the order of the 'Merciful Sisters of the Holy Cross', based at the Ingenbohl Convent in the Canton of Schwyz. Here, his health deteriorated rapidly. Lily Klee joined her husband on May 18, 1940[260], and retrospectively writes to Will Grohmann: 'I followed him a week later (though I had not planned to), because I felt very worried. His condition was fair for the first two weeks, but then he suddenly became very ill. [...] He was fighting for his life. [...]'[261] The doctor treating him, Dr. Hermann Bodmer (fig. 90, page 111) called in the notable Zurich heart specialist Dr. Theodor Haemmerli (fig. 92, page 113), who happened to be staying in Locarno at the time.[262] Lily Klee notes: 'Dr. Bodmer and his assistant have proven themselves to be excellent doctors. The clinic is modern and is run by the same nuns as the Viktoria [hospital] in Bern. The standard of care is first-rate. Yesterday morning we had a consultation with the top heart specialist in Zurich, Dr. Haemmerli. He was in complete agreement with Dr. Bodmer's treatment regime, but had a few suggestions on how to improve it further. [...] It is a cardiovascular disorder, which is quite serious (that was Dr. Haemmerli's diagnosis), which corresponds with Dr. Bodmer's diagnosis.'[263] As happened so often, Klee's condition improved slightly, which gave Lily new hope: 'There seems to have been a slight improvement. Dr. Bodmer's assistant (an excellent lady doctor) was happier today [June 23]. The doctors are doing everything they can, they are really dedicated. The last few weeks have been very difficult and the situation is serious. [...] I just hope we can come back to Bern at least in the foreseeable future. But we can't think about that at the moment, we just have to wait and be patient.'[264]

Paul Klee's flame finally flickered and died on June 29, 1940. He died as he had lived: quietly and with dignity. On the death certificate Dr. Bodmer noted the cause of death as 'malattia di cuore (myocardite)'[265] (fig. 67). ('Myocarditis' = inflammation of the heart muscle.) Lily Klee writes retrospectively: 'Even the day before he died, the doctors were still

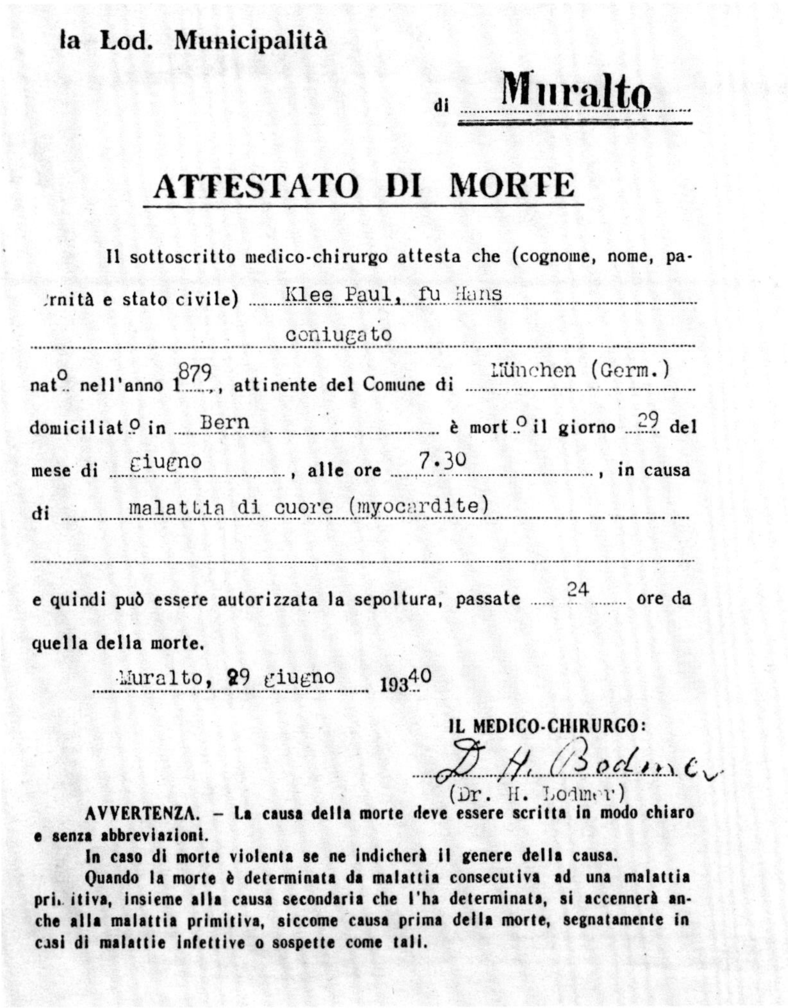

la Lod. Municipalità

di **Muralto**

ATTESTATO DI MORTE

Il sottoscritto medico-chirurgo attesta che (cognome, nome, paternità e stato civile) Klee Paul, fu Hans
coniugato
nat° nell'anno 1879, attinente del Comune di München (Germ.)
domiciliat° in Bern è mort° il giorno 29 del
mese di giugno, alle ore 7.30, in causa
di malattia di cuore (myocardite)

e quindi può essere autorizzata la sepoltura, passate 24 ore da quella della morte.

Muralto, 29 giugno 1940

IL MEDICO-CHIRURGO:

D H Bodmer
(Dr. H. Bodmer)

AVVERTENZA. — La causa della morte deve essere scritta in modo chiaro e senza abbreviazioni.

In caso di morte violenta se ne indicherà il genere della causa.

Quando la morte è determinata da malattia consecutiva ad una malattia primitiva, insieme alla causa secondaria che l'ha determinata, si accennerà anche alla malattia primitiva, siccome causa prima della morte, segnatamente in casi di malattie infettive o sospette come tali.

Fig. 67. Paul Klee's death certificate, filled out by Dr. Hermann Bodmer, Locarno-Muralto, June 29, 1940

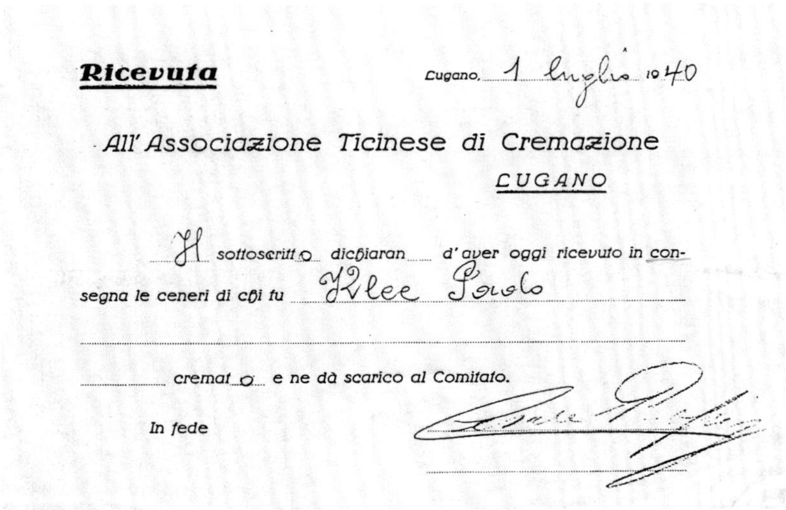

Ricevuta Lugano, 1 luglio 1940

All' Associazione Ticinese di Cremazione
LUGANO

Il sottoscritto dichiaran d'aver oggi ricevuto in consegna le ceneri di cói fu Klee Paolo

cremat o e ne dà scarico al Comitato.

In fede

Fig. 68. Paul Klee's cremation certificate, Lugano, July 1, 1940

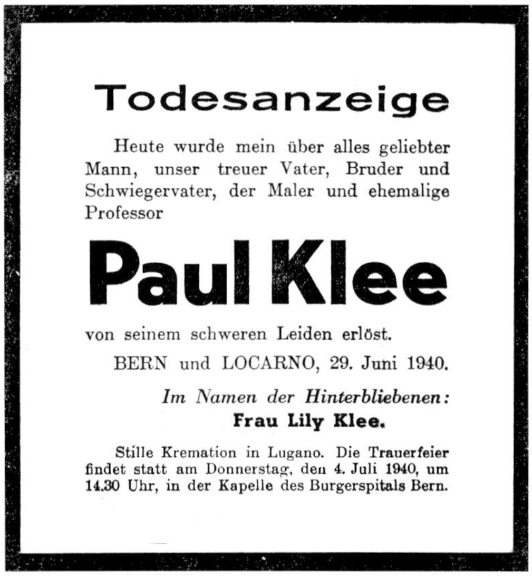

Todesanzeige

Heute wurde mein über alles geliebter Mann, unser treuer Vater, Bruder und Schwiegervater, der Maler und ehemalige Professor

Paul Klee

von seinem schweren Leiden erlöst.

BERN und LOCARNO, 29. Juni 1940.

Im Namen der Hinterbliebenen:
Frau Lily Klee.

Stille Kremation in Lugano. Die **Trauerfeier** findet statt am Donnerstag, den **4. Juli 1940, um 14.30 Uhr,** in der Kapelle des Burgerspitals Bern.

Fig. 69. Paul Klee's obituary notice, June 29, 1940

hopeful. [...] Everything had been done that was humanly possible (he had suffered greatly) but he was not thinking about death – nor was I, I still had hope.'[266] (It seems highly likely, however, that Paul Klee knew intuitively that the end was near; he just did not talk about this to his loved ones.) Two months later, Lily Klee looked back on it differently: 'Today it seems inconceivable that I could not see that the end was near. But I was still hoping, right to the end.'[267] The artist was laid out in the chapel at the Clinica Sant' Agnese from June 29 to July 1, 1940. His widow records: 'Ju Aichinger sent a huge bouquet of carnations, which was placed on his coffin. His body was wrapped in white and covered with a large veil. His wonderful, noble countenance was at peace, his expression otherworldly, with a hint of a smile on his lips as though to say: now I know, and I did the right thing. [...] His marvelous hands lay folded on his breast.'[268] On July 1, 1940 Paul Klee was cremated in Lugano[269] (fig. 68, page 75). The funeral was held on July 4, 1940 in the chapel at the Burgerspital in Bern. The addresses were given by the dean of Bern cathedral, Albert Schädelin, his old friend Hans Bloesch, chief librarian of the Bern City Library, and Georg Schmidt, curator of the public art collection in Basel.[270] The Bern String Quartet played two adagios from two quartets by Mozart, Klee's favorite composer.[271] His widow kept the urn in his undisturbed studio at Kistlerweg 6 in Bern, enshrined beneath a laurel wreath and flowers[272] (fig. 70). Upon the death of his wife on September 22, 1946, Klee's ashes were buried in the Schosshalden Cemetery in Bern[273] (fig. 71).

Now let us turn once more to Dr. Bodmer's certified cause of death. It could indeed be the case that Paul Klee died of myocarditis resulting from a thickening of the tissues of the heart muscle. We have already noted that 30–80% of patients with systemic sclerosis are shown at autopsy to have myocardial fibrosis. It was never possible to check for changes in the internal organs or to review the cause of death because Klee was cremated without autopsy in Locarno on July 1, 1940.

---

[266] Letter from Lily Klee to Will Grohmann, Bern, July 7, 1940 (AWG), quoted in Frey 1990, p. 125.

[267] Letter from Lily Klee to Will Grohmann, Bern, September 14, 1940 (AWG), quoted in Frey 1990, p. 125.

[268] Letter from Lily Klee to Will Grohmann, Bern, July 7, 1940 (AWG), quoted in Frey 1990, p. 125.

[269] Document from the 'Associazione Ticinese di Cremazione Lugano' of July 1, 1940: 'Ricevuta Lugano 1 luglio 1940[.] All'Associazione Ticinese di Cremazione Lugano. Il sottoscritto dichiaran d'aver oggi ricevuto in consegna le ceneri di chi fu Klee Paolo cremato e ne dà scarico al Comitato. In fede [?; signature illegible]' (photocopy: ZPKB/SFK).

[270] I was not able to obtain a copy of Schädelin's funeral address. Bloesch's and Schmidt's addresses were published in 1950 (Bloesch, Schmidt 1950). Excerpts of the former are reproduced in: Grote 1959, pp. 117–119; the latter is reprinted in whole in: Mendrisio 1990, [pp. 174–179].

[271] Cf. Frey 1990, p. 126.

[272] Cf. letter from Lily Klee to Will Grohmann, Bern, July 7, 1940 (AWG): 'Until it is buried, the urn will remain in the studio beneath flowers and a laurel wreath from his old friend. The studio remains undisturbed.'

[273] Verbal communication, Felix Klee to Stefan Frey, in: Frey 1990, p. 132, note 241. However, Will Grohmann stated that the urn was buried at the Schosshalden Cemetery in September 1942, cf. Grohmann 1965, p. 88 f. This could be a mistake on Grohmann's part. It is accepted that Paul Klee's urn was buried at the Schosshalden Cemetery in September 1946. Stefan Frey made enquiries at the Schosshalden Cemetery, but was told there was no record; cf. Frey 1990, p. 132, note 241. A photo taken in 1946 by Jürg Spiller supports the supposition that the urn was buried in that year (see Frey 1990, p. 126, fig. 17), see fig. 70.

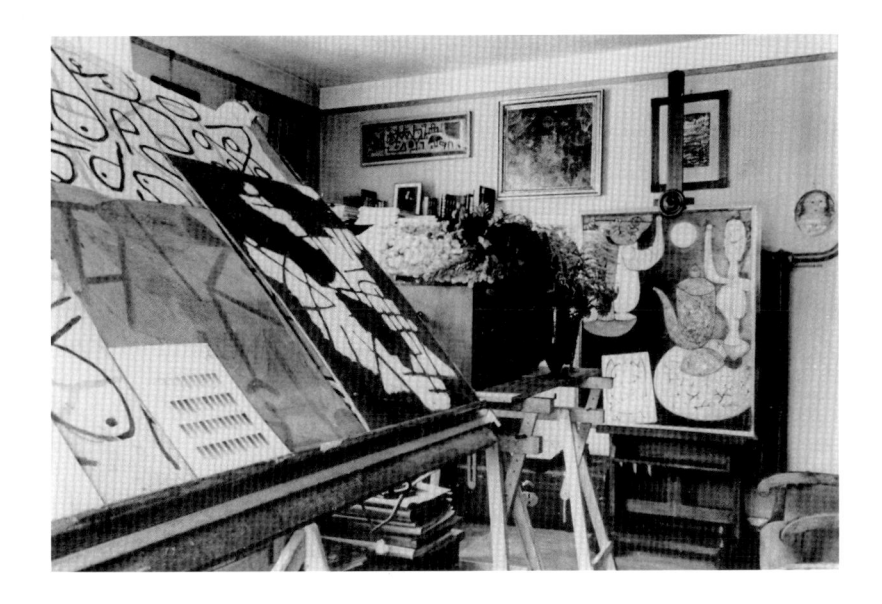

Fig. 70. Paul Klee's last studio, Kistlerweg 6, Bern. The urn has been placed under the wreath (center of picture).

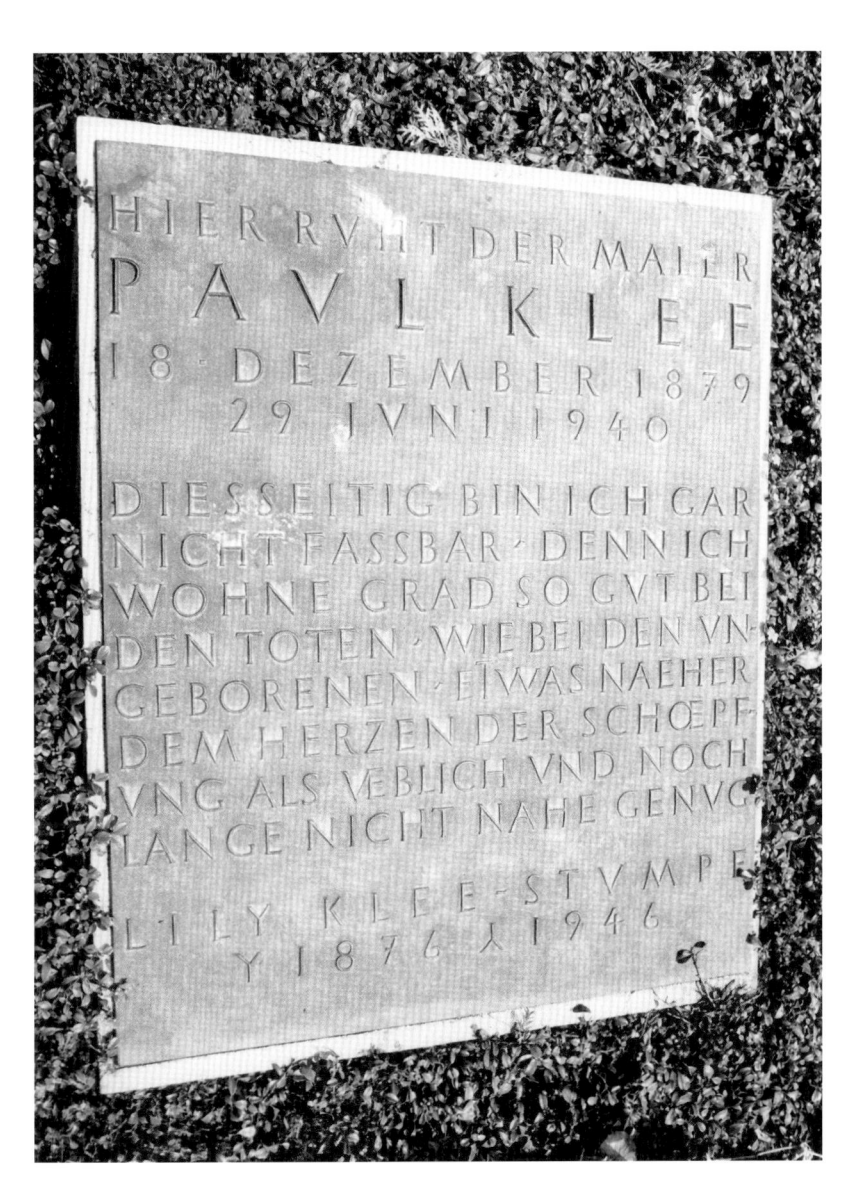

Fig. 71. Paul and Lily Klee's memorial plate, Schosshalden Cemetery, Bern

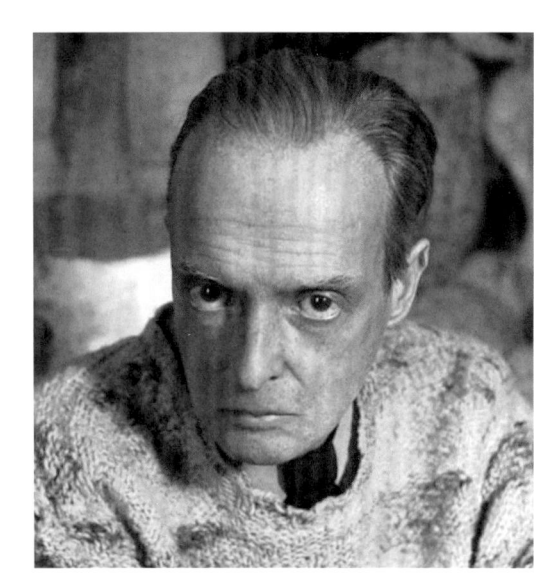

Fig. 72. Paul Klee in his living room, Kistlerweg 6, Bern, December 1939

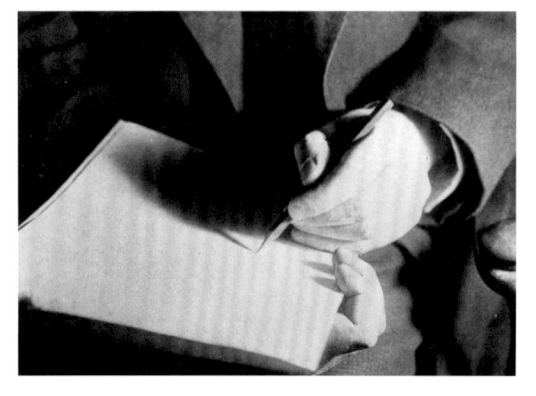

Fig. 73. Paul Klee drawing, Dessau 1931 (he drew and painted with his left hand, but wrote with his right)

[274] Cf. Masi 1980/ML, pp. 581–590, and cf. Röther and Peter/ML 1996, p. 387.
[275] Cf. LeRoy 1996/ML, pp. 4–6, cf. Castenholz/ML, pp. 138 and 139, and cf. also personal communication by Brigitta Danuser to Gabriele Castenholz, March 13, 1996, quoted in Castenholz/ML 2000, p. 137.

Discussion of the Symptoms and Course of Paul Klee's Illness

In 1980 the American Rheumatism Association established criteria for the diagnosis of systemic sclerosis.[274] These criteria are based on characteristic changes. According to the Association, the main criterion is diffuse sclerodermic changes to the skin (thickening, hardening, stiffening) 'above the fingers and toes' – so the head, neck, trunk and limbs excluding the fingers and toes. Important sub-criteria are thickened and hardened fingers ('sclerodactyly'), fingertip defects, and X-ray evidence of bilateral basal pulmonary fibrosis (thickening of the tissues of the lower lungs). As a minimum, the main criterion or two sub-criteria must be fulfilled in order to make a firm diagnosis. In Paul Klee's case we know the following: he had sclerodermic changes to his face, which, as previously mentioned, are not only evident in photos (for example fig. 72), but are also substantiated both verbally and in writing by his son. Max Huggler also confirmed these changes, and they are supported by significant statements made by Klee's dentist, Dr. Jean Charlet. In addition, Felix Klee told me that the skin on his father's neck became tight.

So Paul Klee fulfills the main criterion for a diagnosis of systemic sclerosis. This diagnosis is supported by Dr. Schorer's comment that he was suffering from a 'vasomotor neurosis' (see page 60).

But on the other hand, Paul Klee did not suffer from sclerodermic changes to the fingers, contrary to speculation which was only based on interpretations of photographs, and therefore insufficient for a diagnosis.[275] The artist had naturally strong hands and fingers (figs. 73 and 74). Based on a photo taken in July 1939 they could be construed as thickened and with bend contracture (figs. 81 and 82), but it should be stressed that Klee's fingers did not thicken or harden. Felix Klee and Max Huggler both attest that his fingers did not curl inwards, his fingers remained mobile and he did not suffer from slow-healing wounds, skin flaking or calcium buildup. On this basis, and taking into account the relatively early affliction of the internal organs and the rapid progression of the disease, we can rule out the limited form of systemic sclerosis.

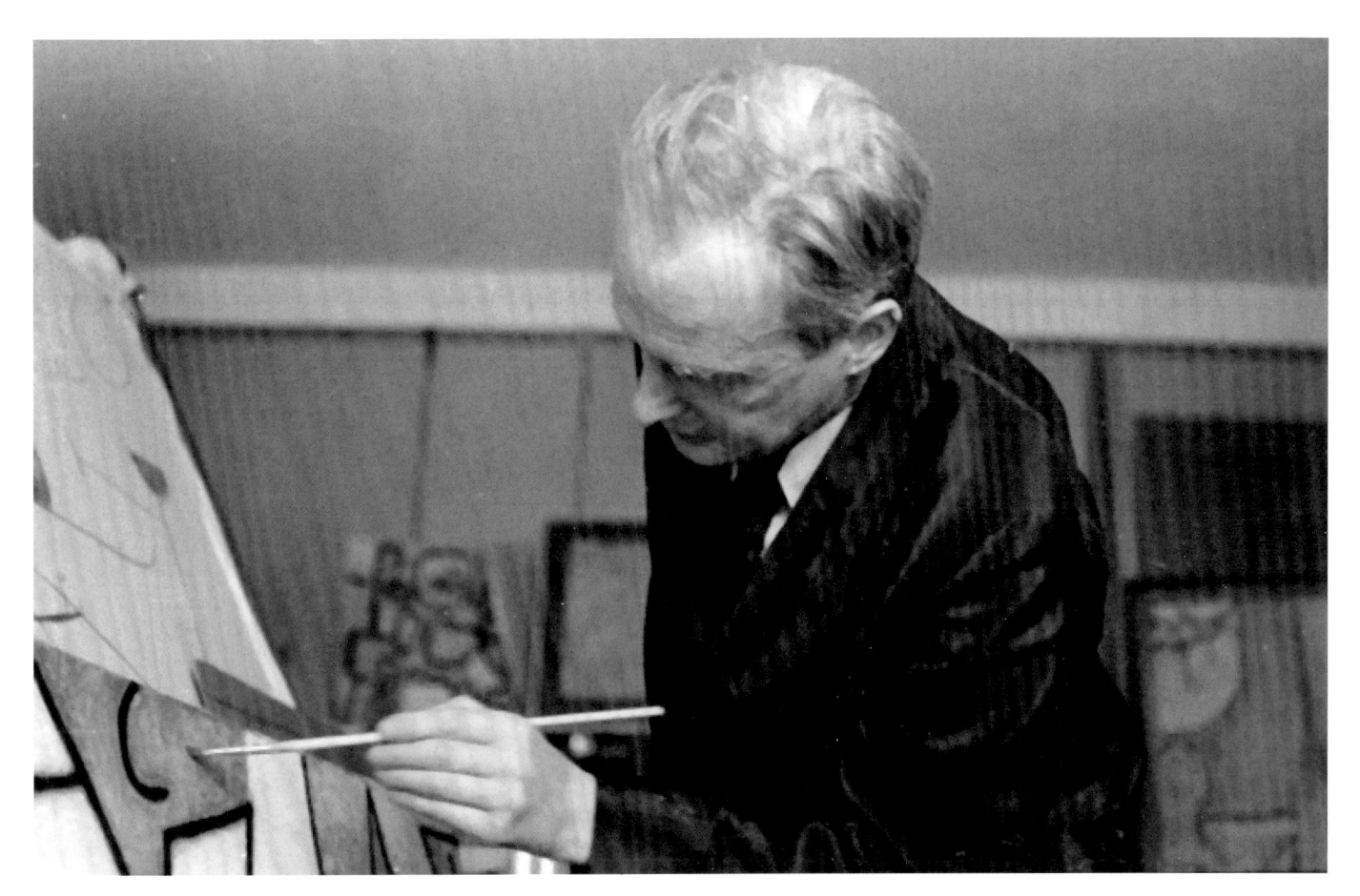

Fig. 74. Paul Klee painting in his studio, Kistlerweg 6, Bern, 1939

Is there any evidence that he had the diffuse form of systemic sclerosis? Unfortunately we do not have any conclusive evidence, but there are some strong indications. A characteristic symptom is difficulty in swallowing due to the narrowing of the esophagus, and Paul Klee suffered badly from this. Another indication of diffuse systemic sclerosis is the long-lasting preliminary phase, with mild fever, chronic fatigue and debility,[276] weight loss,[277] and chronic bronchitis with pneumonia and pleurisy. Added to this is the cough which plagued him for years, his shortage of breath during physical exertion, the evidence of heart problems, the gastrointestinal symptoms (possible lack of gastric acid, gastric ulcer with bleeding, tendency to diarrhea) and anemia. We can only surmise from Paul Klee's symptoms that he suffered from pulmonary and myocardial fibrosis. His heart and lungs were X-rayed, but unfortunately we have no record of the exact results, so fibrotic disorders of the lungs and heart remain hypothetical.

[276] Cf. Krieg/ML 1996, p. 729.
[277] Klee 1989, p. 46: 'He [Paul Klee] has lost weight, his skin has grown tight and his appearance has changed.'

The results of the urine test could suggest renal fibrosis, but they are not conclusive.

Taking Klee's sclerodermic facial changes as the main criterion, and adding to that the other symptoms mentioned above, there is strong evidence to support a diagnosis of diffuse systemic sclerosis.

The leading causes of death for patients with diffuse systemic sclerosis are lung disease, kidney disease and heart disease, in that order.[278] Unfavorable[279] prognostic factors are advanced age, reduced pulmonary function, renal malfunction and anemia. Women with diffuse systemic sclerosis usually live longer than men; patients with concurrent lung, heart and kidney problems have a particularly bad progression of the disease with reduced life expectancy.[280] The fact that Paul Klee died just five years after the onset of his illness is another indicator that he suffered from this severe form of the disease.

There is no evidence that Paul Klee suffered from any of the other possible symptoms of systemic sclerosis (cataracts, hoarseness due to hardening of the vocal cords, painful inflammation of the muscles, joints and tendons, bone changes).[281]

Nowadays it is possible to carry out immunological, genetic and other blood tests which are helpful in determining a diagnosis of systemic sclerosis. These tests also help to distinguish it from other connective tissue disorders.[282] For example, the most common autoantibodies in diffuse systemic sclerosis (as an autoimmune disease) are the 'Scl-70' antibodies, while in the limited form they are the so-called 'anti-centromere antibodies'.[283]

How Was Paul Klee's Illness Treated?

Lily Klee writes very little about how Paul Klee's illness was treated. On October 30, 1935, she told Nina Kandinsky: 'My husband is taking two medications. One for the heart. One for his cough (chronic bronchitis), which has an indirect effect on the heart.'[284] In the detailed temperature chart which

---

[278] Cf. Mittag and Haustein/ML 1998, p. 550.
[279] Cf. ibid.
[280] Cf. Mittag and Haustein/ML 1998, p. 550.
[281] Cf. Krieg/ML 1996, p. 731 f.
[282] Cf. Mittag and Haustein/ML 1998, p. 545 f.
[283] Cf. ibid., p. 546, and cf. Gadola and Villiger/ML 2006, p. 87.
[284] Letter from Lily Klee to Nina Kandinsky, Bern, October 30, 1935 (BK/CGPP).

she kept on her husband between October 18, 1935, and April 18, 1936, she notes a prescription of 'Theominal' and a 'new medication in powder form', without giving its name (fig. 35, page 43). As mentioned on page 42, she was referring to the drug 'Theominal' which is no longer on the market: a combination of theobromine and luminal. This drug was used among other things for the treatments of heart disease (see page 42 and note 103, page 267). It is quite likely that Dr. Schorer also prescribed digitalis glycoside (a preparation still commonly used today), a cardiac stimulant obtained from foxglove. This, at least, is the opinion of Gabriele Castenholz.[285] In a letter to Nina Kandinsky on October 30, 1935, Lily says she is considering 'radiation treatments' with their own radiation lamp – by this she no doubt means an ultraviolet lamp. (This form of light therapy was frequently used in winter to improve the body's defense mechanisms.) She wanted to talk to the doctor about whether it should be used on her husband,[286] but we have no evidence as to whether this treatment was subsequently carried out.

One year later – after his examination by Professor Naegeli, and presumably on his recommendation – Paul Klee was administered injections of an unnamed drug.[287] Klee had a feverish reaction. His wife notes: 'It has now been definitely confirmed that the fever was a result of the injections. [...] The fever lasted 3 days until Sunday morning, and it was a really high fever.'[288] Was the fever really a reaction to the drugs? 'Drug fever' is a common occurrence, and indeed in the past such drugs were intentionally injected in order to use the fever as a stimulus on the immune system. Could this have been the case with Paul Klee? This is a possibility, as around 1935/1940 and also even later, 'Terpichin' or 'Olobinthin' in the form of intramuscular injections were recommended treatments for scleroderma and for other chronic infectious diseases, metabolic disorders and chronic muscle and joint rheumatism; they involved a dilution of turpentine oil in olive oil.[289] They were used as 'nonspecific stimulants' in order to 'retune' the organism through localized inflammation around the area of the injection and through fever as a general reaction. The dosage was low to begin with, and then it was increased until it triggered the above-mentioned reactions.[290] It was a controversial

[285] Cf. Castenholz 2000, p. 131.
[286] Cf. letter from Lily Klee to Nina Kandinsky, Bern, October 30, 1935 (BK/CGPP).
[287] Cf. letter from Lily Klee to Gertrud Grote, Bern, February 11, 1937 (ZPKB): 'He has a problem with his glands which is very hard to treat! He had a special injection for it, but it didn't agree with him.'
[288] Letter from Lily Klee to Hermann and Margrit Rupf, Bern, November 25, 1936 (HMRS).
[289] Mayr/ML 1935, p. 74, and Bernoulli/ML 1955, p. 250: 'Oleum Terebinthinae rectificatum for intramuscular injections 0.1–0.5 in 10% dilution with olive oil. Used mainly for skin diseases, gonorrhea, sepsis, etc.; e.g. Terpichin (Oestreicher, Berlin): 15% dilution of turpentine oil in olive oil with 0.5% each of quinine and Anaesthesin. 10 ampoules/1 ml'.
[290] Cf. Bernoulli/ML 1955, p. 247.

treatment, as exogenous, 'toxic' substances were used which often led to allergic reactions. Was Paul Klee's treatment with injections discontinued because he reacted too violently? Unfortunately we have no information in this respect. At the beginning of the last century, scleroderma was also treated with injections of 'thiosinamine'. This medication, which was also available as an ointment, was supposed to have a softening effect on scar tissue (scars are composed mainly of connective tissue).[291] It caused too many side effects and, at the time of Klee's illness, it was no longer used as an injection.

We also know that Paul Klee's doctor prescribed two other remedies to prevent anemia and to act as a restorative:
– The German arsenic-iron preparation known as 'Arsen-Triferrol'[292], a liquid combination of iron and arsenic (which Lily Klee called 'Arsen-ti-ferrol'[293])
– The liver preparation 'Campolon'[294] (which Lily Klee called 'Campollon intramusculaire'[295]), a controversial animal liver extract

Paul Klee took a solution of Arsen-Triferrol from July to September 1936, a medication '[…] of which my husband drank 3 bottles, as he was anemic after his illness'[296], as Lily Klee writes.[297] As the blood contains iron, the most common form of anemia, iron deficiency anemia, can be cured through intake of iron. In former times, small doses of arsenic were commonly used both as a restorative and as a treatment for anemia.[298]

Campolon was given to the invalid from the beginning of June 1937 probably until the end of August/beginning of September 1937, in the form of intramuscular injections.[299] Dr. Schorer administered the first injections himself, then Lily Klee took them over, saying: 'The doctor has taught me how to give the injections and tomorrow [July 9, 1937] I'm doing one on my own for the first time.'[300] One month later she states more precisely: 'I give him [Paul Klee] an injection of Campolon every 2 days, which seems to be doing him good.'[301]

---

[291] Cf. Lesser/ML 1900, p. 105, and Bernoulli/ML 1955, p. 352: 'Thiosinamine (allylsulfocarbamide), is prescribed to soften scar tissue, but its effect is unreliable.'

[292] See Appendices: Composition of and Medical Indicators for the Drug Arsen-Triferrol (p. 267).

[293] Letter from Lily Klee to Will Grohmann, Bern, September 18, 1936 (AWG): '[…] Arsen-ti-ferrol/German medicament […].'

[294] See Appendices: Composition of and Medical Indicators for the Drug Campolon (p. 267).

[295] Letter from Lily Klee to Will Grohmann, Bern, July 8, 1937 (AWG).

[296] Letter from Lily Klee to Will Grohmann, Bern, September 18, 1936 (AWG).

[297] Cf. also letter from Lily Klee to Will Grohmann, Bern, August 24, 1936 (AWG).

[298] Cf. Braun Falco, Plewig and Wolff/ML 1996, p. 1307.

[299] Cf. letters from Lily Klee to Will Grohmann, Bern, July 8, 1937 and August 10, 1937 (AWG).

[300] Letter from Lily Klee to Will Grohmann, Bern, July 8, 1937 (AWG).

[301] Letter from Lily Klee to Will Grohmann, Bern, August 10, 1937 (AWG).

In 1937 Paul Klee developed a 'stomach ulcer', so Lily carefully worked out a diet plan to treat it.[302]

On June 3, 1939, the artist wrote to his wife while she was having a break at a health resort in Sonnmatt near Lucerne. At the time his health was a little better: 'I feel that I am in reasonable health. Of course we all want to feel we are recovering, so in the end, even if we exaggerate a little, everything adds up – and we are better. I started with the dentist; I felt brave enough to visit him one day. I am still playing truant from the other doctor, as things are proceeding quite nicely without him. But at the slightest setback I will be on the telephone to him once again, trying to make amends. He will just laugh about the latest phase without him and without Volz's little bottles and vials.'[303] We can gather from this that Klee had adopted a positive attitude towards his illness. We can only speculate what was contained in the 'little bottles and vials' from the Volz pharmacy in Bern. Perhaps they were tonics (= restoratives): as early as 1936, Lily Klee had commented that her husband needed these very often.[304] Incidentally, it is interesting to note that at the end of the 19th century, scleroderma was treated with 'diet, liquid food and tonics such as quinine, iron or arsenic'.[305]

According to the prescription, on August 10, 1939, Dr. Schorer prescribed the vitamin C supplement 'Redoxon' (which is still on the market today), with a dose of 3 x 1 tablet daily[306] (fig. 75). Vitamin C (ascorbic acid) is known to strengthen the immune system.

Nina Kandinsky mentions in her memoirs that her husband Wassily made a therapeutic recommendation to Paul Klee: 'Kandinsky told Klee that a "Kuhnsche mask" would help alleviate his shortness of breath. He himself had suffered with breathing problems after a bad dose of influenza in 1933, and a doctor in Berlin had prescribed this breathing mask. So he suggested that Klee should also get one of these masks. But I have no idea whether he followed Kandinsky's advice.'[307] In the past, masks were used in the treatment of throat and breathing disorders and for etherization. The mask was put over the nose and the patient inhaled through

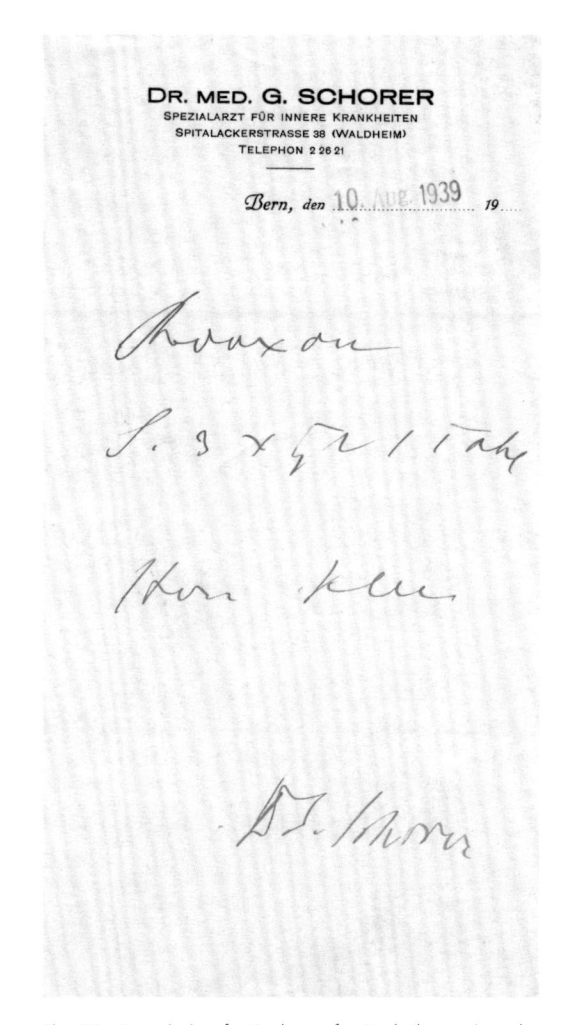

Fig. 75. Prescription for Redoxon for Paul Klee, written by Dr. Gerhard Schorer, August 10, 1939

[302] Cf. letters from Lily Klee to Will Grohmann, Bern, February 11, 1937, March 20, 1937 and May 15, 1937 (AWG), cf. letters from Lily Klee to Hermann and Margrit Rupf, Bern, February 13, 1937, February 21, 1937 and February 27, 1937 (HMRS), also cf. letter from Lily Klee to Nina Kandinsky, Bern, March 23, 1937 (BK/CGPP).
[303] Letter from Paul Klee to Lily Klee, Bern, June 3, 1939, quoted in Klee 1979, p. 1293.
[304] Cf. letter from Lily Klee to Nina Kandinsky, Bern, September 5, 1936 (BK/CGPP).
[305] Castenholz/ML 2000, p. 57.
[306] Original prescription for Paul Klee, written by Dr. Gerhard Schorer, Bern, August 10, 1939 (ZPKB/SFK, fig. 75).
[307] Kandinsky 1976, p. 201.

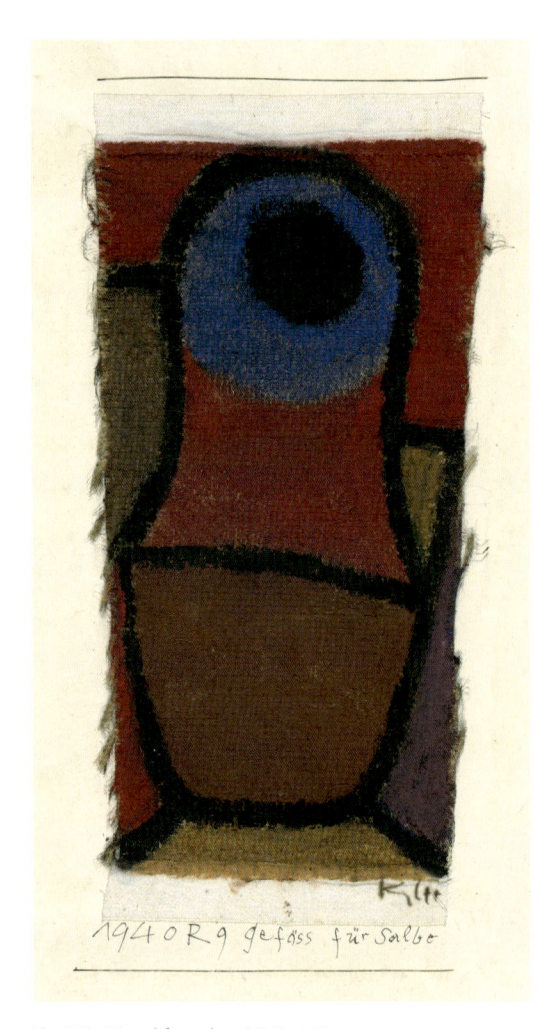

Fig. 76. Vessel for salve, 1940, 169

308 Letter from Lily Klee to Gertrud Grote, Bern, January 12, 1936 (ZPKB): 'Later he will have a change of climate, which is always the best remedy.'
309 Cf. letter from Lily Klee to Nina Kandinsky, Bern, September 5, 1936 (BK/CGPP), cf. letter from Lily Klee to Will Grohmann, Bern, October 13, 1936 (AWG), cf. letters from Lily Klee to Hermann and Margrit Rupf, Bern, October 29, 1937, and October 14, 1938 (HMRS), and cf. letter from Lily Klee to Gertrud Grohmann, Bern, November 28, 1939 (AWG).
310 Ju Aichinger-Grosch, in: Grote 1959, p. 52 f.
311 Letter from Lily Klee to Hermann and Margrit Rupf, Locarno-Orselina, May 21, 1940 (HMRS).

a layer of thin fabric. A rapidly evaporating liquid was trickled over the mask and the patient inhaled the active ingredient as a mist. These liquids were probably substances which dilated the bronchial tubes; nowadays aerosols sprays are commonly used.

Both the patient and his doctor had high hopes that mountain air and a southerly climate would help his rehabilitation and recovery.[308] So in summer 1936 Klee traveled to Tarasp in the Unterengadin, in autumn 1936 he went to Montana in the Valais, in autumn 1938 to Beatenberg above Lake Thun, in autumn 1939 to Faoug beside Lake Murten in the canton of Waadt, and in spring 1940 he went to Locarno-Orselina. He certainly felt that his sojourns between 1936 and 1939 did him good.[309]

In the year of his death, Paul Klee painted a large 'Vessel for salve' (fig. 76). Did he use a moisturizing cream on the thickened, stiff, dry parts of his skin? This could well have been the case.

A lady friend of the Klees amusingly tells us: 'He [Klee] told us with a smile that he really loved his doctor, a lovely old professor [Dr. Schorer], because he always prescribed what he really liked, dried bilberries for example.'[310] But this prescription would have been made for a reason, as chewing dried bilberries would have stimulated the secretion of saliva and thus improved the dry mouth and swallowing difficulties which are often symptomatic of the disease.

By 1940 Klee was seriously ill, and he was treated in the Sanatorium Viktoria in Locarno-Orselina with 'massages, diathermy [a procedure which uses high frequency electric current to heat the internal tissues] and injections'.[311] We have no further details on this.

There is nothing in Lily Klee's letters to suggest that her husband took painkillers. The illness meant that Paul Klee experienced pain when swallowing, but otherwise he probably did not suffer the kind of severe pain which would have affected his quality of life. He was, however, in a lot of discomfort, but he bore this with great fortitude.[312] There is also no mention of him taking medication for high blood pressure.

At the time of Paul Klee's illness, treatment for systemic sclerosis was mainly based on alleviation of symptoms, massages, baths, physical therapy and prevention of chills.[313] Today doctors have a broader range of treatment options at their disposal which help to slow down progression of the disease and protect threatened organs.[314] The following treatments can be used: for Raynaud's syndrome and incipient fingertip damage, calcium channel blockers or prostacyclin to dilate the blood vessels; for severe lung inflammation, high doses of cortisone and cyclophosphamide pulse therapy; for pulmonary arterial hypertension, endothelin receptor antagonists (e.g. Bosentan, Tracleer), phosphodiesteraseinhibitors (e.g. Sildenafil, Viagra) and prostacyclinanaloga (e.g. Ilomedin) have been successfully introduced. ACE inhibitors play an important role in preventing kidney involvement. Bacterial overgrowths of the intestines should be treated with antibiotic cycling. For rapidly progressing forms of systemic sclerosis, in particular if internal organs are affected, bone marrow transplantation is performed.[315] However, the disease is still incurable, and diffuse systemic sclerosis still can lead to death within a few years.[316]

Re. Fig. 76
In the year of his death Paul Klee painted a large 'Vessel for salve'. The disease had caused his skin to harden and dry out. It needed to be lubricated with ointment. Although his wife did not mention this in her letters or memoirs, it is likely that her husband treated his skin with salves.

[312] See pp. 154 and 155.
[313] Cf. Mayr/ML 1935, p. 74, and cf. Kumer/ML 1944, p. 315.
[314] Cf. Krieg/ML 1996, p. 733, cf. Röther and Peter/ML 1996, p. 388 f., and cf. Gadola and Villiger/ML 2006, p. 88 f.
[315] My thanks for these up-to-date treatment protocols to Prof. Peter M. Villiger, Director and Chief Physician of the University Clinic and the Polyclinics of the Department of Rheumatology and Immunology/Allergology, Inselspital, Bern, CH–3617 Fahrni, August 3, 2005; cf. also Gadola and Villiger/M 2006, pp. 88 and 89.
[316] Cf. ibid., cf. Krieg/ML 1996, p. 728, and cf. Röther and Peter/ML 1996, p. 389.

Other Medical Opinions on Paul Klee's Illness

Summarized below are details of the current state of research into Paul Klee's illness.[317]

Introductory note: It is astonishing that it has taken 40 years since Paul Klee's death to publish what is probably the first medical study of his illness. Very little has been written by doctors on the subject. With one exception, all authors have worked on the assumption that Paul Klee's illness was probably scleroderma – without considering the specific form. One author (Dr. Gabriele Castenholz) thinks it is more likely to be a combination of two connective tissue diseases rather than systemic sclerosis.

Dr. F.-J. Beer (Versailles)

Le centenaire de Paul Klee, in: Médecine et Hygiène, 38. vol., no. 1362, January 23, 1980, p. 247 f

F.-J. Beer thinks it is possible that Klee's 'vasomotor system' was disrupted due to the anxiety he suffered in Düsseldorf in 1933 resulting from the actions of the ruling National Socialists. This could then have triggered his 'scleroderma'. The vasomotor nerves are part of the vegetative nervous system which affects or inhibits the contraction of the blood vessels. Beer is here probably referring to Raynaud's syndrome (see pages 60 and 61). He also refers to the assumption which was common in French medical circles at the time that scleroderma could be caused by hormonal hyperparathyroidism. This can cause calcium to leach from the bones, leading to skin calcification and thinning.

Commentary: The author postulates first of all that mental factors could have triggered the disease. However, there is no evidence that Paul Klee had symptoms of Raynaud's syndrome. It is no longer believed that hormonal factors can cause scleroderma.

---

[317] I have taken Philip Sandblom's opinion from his monograph (Sandblom 1990). I thank Theodor Künzi, CH–3613 Steffisburg, June 25, 2005, for providing me with this publication; also Brigitta Danuser and Gabriele Castenholz for providing me with their works, and Stefan Frey for procuring the other publications mentioned. Brigitta Danuser let me have additional publications detailing the suspected role of occupational exposure to solvents and fumed silica in the development of systemic sclerosis and pseudoscleroderma.

Drs. Lisbet Milling Pedersen and Henrik Permin (Copenhagen)
Rheumatic Disease, Heavy-Metal Pigments, and the Great Masters, in: The Lancet, June 4, 1988, p. 1267 f

Lisbet Milling Pedersen and Henrik Permin look into the question of whether heavy-metal pigments could have contributed to the onset of rheumatoid arthritis in Rubens, Renoir and Dufy and scleroderma in Klee. They compared these four artists with eight other artists who did not suffer from arthritis or scleroderma, and argue that these four made much more use of light, clear oil paints which contained toxic heavy metals such as antimony, arsenic, lead, cadmium, chromium, cobalt, copper, manganese, mercury and tin. In his paintings, Paul Klee used substantially more red and violet pigments based on manganese and cobalt than, for example, Wassily Kandinsky and Karl Schmidt-Rottluff. These two artists, along with the others in the control group, mainly used harmless 'earth pigments containing iron and carbon'. Heavy metals are toxic if ingested. The authors do not discount the possibility that the heavy-metal pigments had an effect on the onset of the diseases. Felix Klee also suspected that his father's illness could have been linked to his exposure to pigments.[318]

Commentary: Paul Klee certainly used heavy-metal pigments. In the past, painters often wetted their paintbrush with their tongue to create a fine point for detailed work, so they could have ingested traces of paint in their saliva. At that time, artists were not aware that these heavy-metal pigments were toxic. As we still know very little about the causes of systemic sclerosis, a link to the ingestion of toxic heavy-metal pigments can neither be proven nor discounted.

Here I would like to mention a point made by the Klee scholar Marguerite Frey-Surbek, told to me by the artist Bendicht Friedli[319]: She confirmed from her own experience as an artist that it was usual to wet the paintbrush with the tongue and lips (as mentioned above). She had problems with her gums and some of her teeth came loose ('periodontosis'): she later found out that this was caused by her habit of lick-

[318] Cf. Klee 1960/1, p. 110: 'To begin with, my father was ill with measles. This seemingly harmless children's disease triggered a series of other problems from which he never fully recovered. His illnesses were a bit of a riddle; perhaps it was some kind of occupational illness, perhaps the paints Klee experimented with were detrimental to his health.'

[319] Personal communication to the author by Bendicht Friedli regarding a conversation with Marguerite Frey-Surbek, CH–3800 Unterseen, February 20, 2001.

ing the paintbrush. It was thought that the periodontosis was caused by involuntary ingestion of lead from Krems white. It is interesting to note that the dentist who last treated Paul Klee, Dr. Jean Charlet, also observed early-stage periodontosis (see page 59).

Prof. Philip Sandblom (Lausanne)
Kreativität und Krankheit, Springer-Verlag, Berlin-Heidelberg 1990

In this publication, the Swedish author studies how artists are affected by physical and emotional suffering. He briefly considers Paul Klee's scleroderma (pages 155–158) and writes: '[…] Because of the gradual stiffening of his limbs, it became more and more difficult for him [Paul Klee] to paint his small, playful pictures.'[320] But it is clear from his work that the artist kept his spirits up despite his illness and carried his burden bravely.

Commentary: Paul Klee's limbs did not stiffen up. He could draw and paint freely right to the end.

Prof. Brigitta Danuser (Lausanne)
Von den Gefahren des Künstlerberufs: Paul Klee und die Sklerodermie. Arbeitsmedizinische Betrachtungen, in: Newsletter, Institute for Hygiene and Occupational Physiology, Swiss Federal Institute of Technology Zurich, 3rd edition, November 2000

Artists use organic solvents to thin their oil paints and also to clean their hands, paintbrushes and other tools. Brigitta Danuser looks at whether solvents like turpentine, benzol or benzine could have triggered Paul Klee's illness. Klee came into contact with solvents because he used oil paints, but also at times during his military service. In the summer of 1916 in Schleissheim he worked on airplane repairs, painting scaffolds, staining wall panel frames, repainting or stenciling numbers on the planes.[321] At the beginning of 1917 he was transferred to the Gersthofen flying school and once again

[320] Sandblom 1990, p. 156.
[321] Cf. Klee Diaries, nos. 1013, 1014 and 1018.

had to undertake painting duties[322], commenting as follows: 'The changing moon didn't have much effect, the air became more pungent, as did the paint. I need to bring paintbrushes from home as the Prussian hangar construction command has left, and we have no materials.'[323] Brigitta Danuser writes: 'We can assume from this that Paul Klee was working without breathing protection or skin protection, and that as a result he spent years inhaling fumes from benzene solvents. So today we have some justification for the theory that Paul Klee died of an occupational disease.'[324]

How are people affected by these organic solvents?
– Many people have an allergic reaction when they come into contact with turpentine. This manifests as contact eczema on the hands.[325]
– Benzol and benzene are 'volatile' solvents, meaning they evaporate very quickly. Inhaling their fumes can be toxic and in higher concentrations can cause nausea, vomiting, impaired concentration, cramps, agitation and overstimulation.[326] Benzol is particularly damaging to the blood-producing organs and can lead to cancer.[327]

Commentary: none of the information that we have on Klee's illness suggests that he had allergic contact eczema on his hands, or that he had symptoms of toxicity or cancer.[328]

However, if organic solvent fumes are inhaled over a protracted period, it can cause a disease which is similar to scleroderma (**'pseudoscleroderma'**). We now know that pseudoscleroderma can be triggered by compounds such as vinyl chloride (chloroethylene) and trichloroethylene. Chloroethylene is used in the manufacture of the plastic polyvinyl chloride (PVC), trichloroethylene is used as an industrial solvent.[329] This disease presents with scleroderma-type thickening of the skin, Raynaud's syndrome, finger pad defects with calcium excretion, bone cysts, osteoporosis, reduction of blood platelets (thrombopenia) and liver damage.[330]

Since 1990 various medical papers have been published which support the theory that scleroderma-type symptoms are linked to occupational exposure to toxic substances, such

[322] Cf. Klee Diaries, no. 1051.
[323] Cf. ibid., no. 1061 a.
[324] Danuser/ML, p. 20. Dr. Brigitta Danuser said the same thing in a personal communication to Gabriele Castenholz, Zurich, March 13, 1996, cf. Castenholz/ML 2000, p. 142.
[325] Burckhardt/ML 1961/1, p. 447: 'In my experience, the most common cause of allergic contact eczema among painters is oil of turpentine.' This quote is from 1961. Nowadays many painters prefer acrylic paints because they are quicker and easier to use. They do not need to be thinned with turpentine. And Cronin/ML 1980, p. 801: 'In the 1950s oil of turpentine was a frequent cause of allergic occupational dermatitis, but its gradual withdrawal from general use in many countries led to a sharp decline in the incidence of sensitization.' Indeed, turpentine contact allergies are now very rare.
[326] Cf. Pschyrembel/ML 1998, p. 185.
[327] Cf. Danuser/ML 2000, p. 20.
[328] Personal communication, Felix Klee to the author, Bern, September 20, 1983.
[329] Cf. Krieg/ML 1996, p. 733 f., and cf. Castenholz/ML 2000, p. 78.
[330] Cf. Pschyrembel/ML 1998, p. 1666 f.

as protracted inhalation of organic solvent fumes[331] (as previously mentioned), or long-term exposure to quartz dust during mining.[332] Freshly fractured quartz is a very toxic substance which affects the body's cells and damages the immune system.[333] It is therefore suspected that quartz dust can trigger autoimmune diseases such as rheumatoid arthritis, systemic sclerosis, systemic Lupus erythematosus or certain chronic kidney diseases.[334] Quartz dust permeates the skin and lungs, particularly when using pneumatic drills. The vibration in the hands and arms when drilling seems to stimulate the onset of the disease.[335] It seems that miners are two to three times more likely to suffer from systemic sclerosis than the general population.[336] Many more cases of systemic sclerosis were recorded in the uranium mines of the Erzgebirge in the former German Democratic Republic (GDR) than in the coal mines of the Ruhr.[337] Quartz is much more prevalent in uranium mines than in coal mines.[338] In the former GDR, dry drilling without basic protective measures was also common.[339] In such cases the onset of silicosis was an additional factor in speeding up the progression of the diseases.[340] On the other hand, silicosis can also set off pseudoscleroderma.[341] It is significant that in the above-mentioned cases of scleroderma in the former GDR there was a preponderance of blood vessel inflammation (vasculitis), which in severe cases led to the amputation of fingers, hands, forearms and legs.[342] It is not totally clear whether the cases of scleroderma observed in miners were pseudoscleroderma or true systemic sclerosis.

Commentary: Paul Klee was exposed to solvent fumes during his military service from 1916 to 1918, but we do not have any exact details about the frequency, duration or level of exposure. His diary entries suggest that his exposure was low. When painting with oils, the artist would only have inhaled low levels of solvent fumes, as he produced relatively few oil paintings. Paul Klee would not have been affected by solvent fumes any more than many other painters who also worked in oils but who stayed healthy. So I agree with Gabriele Castenholz that Brigitta Danuser's theory is rather unlikely.[343] The artist also showed no typical signs of pseudoscleroderma. Pseudoscleroderma is apparently even less common than sys-

---

[331] Cf. Brasington and Thorpe-Swenson/ML 1991, p. 631, and cf. Bovenzi et al./ML 1995, p. 289.

[332] Cf. Haustein/ML 1990, p. 444–448, cf. Mehlhorn/ML 1994, pp. 8–11, cf. Dirschka et al./ML 1994, p. 14, cf. Wiebe/ML 1994, pp. 15–17, cf. Conrad et al./ML 1994, pp. 18–23, cf. Rihs et al./ML 1994, pp. 23–26, and cf. Degens and Baur/ML 1994, pp. 27–33.

[333] Cf. Mehlhorn/ML 1994, p. 10.

[334] Cf. Degens and Baur/ML 1994, p. 29.

[335] Cf. Dirschka et al./ML 1994, p. 13, and cf. Degens and Baur/ML 1994, p. 27.

[336] Cf. Degens and Baur/ML 1994, p. 32.

[337] Cf. Dirschka et al./ML 1994, p. 12.

[338] Cf. ibid., p. 13.

[339] Cf. ibid.

[340] Cf. Mehlhorn/ML 1994, p. 8.

[341] Cf. Krieg/ML 1996, p. 734.

[342] Cf. Mehlhorn/ML 1994, p. 11.

[343] Cf. Castenholz/ML 2000, p. 142.

temic sclerosis.[344] Klee never came into contact with quartz dust. However, the causes of systemic sclerosis are very complex, so we cannot totally discount the possibility that organic solvents acted as a trigger.

Dr. Michael Reiner (Mendrisio, Switzerland)
Dämmerblüten. Versuch einer Pathographie Paul Klees, in: Paul Klee. Ultimo decennio – Letztes Jahrzehnt 1930–1940, exhibition catalogue Museo d'arte, Mendrisio, April 7 to July 8, 1990, unpaginated [pp. 35–38]

Michael Reiner states that 'being torn away from a fertile intellectual environment and stimulating work, and losing one's circle of friends and colleagues'[345], along with professional isolation, can cause deep psychological trauma. Reiner thinks it was no coincidence that Klee succumbed to measles one year later and believes the outbreak was more likely because of his autoimmune illness. He had difficulties recovering from this virus, a typical sign of a patient with a weakened immune system. However, Reiner then asserts that measles can also be considered a causative factor in the onset of autoimmune diseases. The author rightly attaches great importance to the role of the skin as a barrier in defending against extraneous attacks from bacteria, viruses, and chemical or physical hazards. In scleroderma, a malfunction causes an overactive immune response, so that the body starts attacking its own cells. The skin reacts by thickening up, by creating a kind of 'armor' to protect it from the outside world. The faulty immune response becomes a self-harming mechanism which causes swelling of the esophagus, thickening of the lung tissues, and changes in the heart muscle and kidney tissues. The effect on the body can be devastating; it can lead to problems swallowing food, difficulty breathing and impaired function of the heart and kidneys. On June 9, 1936, Klee wrote to his wife from Tarasp: 'Intolerance to cold, difficulty breathing at altitude' (circulatory problems due to blood vessel spasms [cramps] brought on by the cold, shortage of breath from the pulmonary fibrosis, both major symptoms of scleroderma).[346] The artist's illness is apparent in the titles of his later works, which to a greater or lesser extent

[344] From 1980 to 2001 according to the Swiss National Accident Insurance Organization (Schweizerische Unfallversicherungsanstalt SUVA) there were no recorded cases of occupational pseudoscleroderma caused by chemicals (verbal communication, Dr. Hanspeter Rast, Specialist in Dermatology and Venereology, Occupational Medicine Department, SUVA, Lucerne, to the author, Lucerne, September 28, 2001).
[345] Reiner/ML 1990, no pages [p. 35].
[346] Ibid., no pages [p. 37].

clearly suggest physical suffering and anxiety. The author also confirms that there are no documents in the archives of the Clinica Sant' Agnese in Locarno-Muralto which throw any more light on the cause of death.

Commentary: As far as I know, Michael Reiner is the first doctor to consider immunological factors in Paul Klee's illness. Reiner's interpretation of the malfunctioning immune system is an interesting one. He clearly and concisely outlines the changes in the skin and organs which are linked to scleroderma. But I think he wrongly construes the intolerance to cold mentioned in the letter, for Klee also wrote: 'The altitude makes it a little harder for me, as do the cool temperatures, but at least I have the impetus, and it is important that the climate has an effect.'[347] He feels the cold much more because he is debilitated. But he does not say anything about the cold affecting his fingers with 'blood vessel spasms' (cramps caused by contraction of the arteries of the fingers, as in Raynaud's syndrome). But I agree with Reiner's assessment that Klee suffered psychological trauma because of the setbacks he experienced, and that this had a detrimental effect on his health.

Dr. Christoph Morscher, Dipl.-Psych. (Wil, Switzerland)
Paul Klee und die Hypothese der morphischen Resonanz, in: Psychotherapie, Psychosomatik, Medizinische Psychologie, Stuttgart/New York, issue 6, vol. 44, June 1994, p. 200 f

Christoph Morscher thinks that the artist had a very strong emotional attachment to his grandmother on his mother's side. She was the one who first encouraged him to draw when he was a child. When she died, the six-year old Paul 'was orphaned artistically'[348] – as Will Grohmann describes it. According to Morscher, Klee never accepted the loss of his grandmother and clung on to his: '[…] strong emotional attachment to this idealized, narcissistic and very significant person for many years to come […]. But he was quite dismissive of his parents and did not build close relationships with his wife or friends. He was himself narcissistic and he cocooned himself in his own private world of art.'[349] Morscher says: 'He

---

[347] Letter from Paul Klee to Lily Klee, Tarasp, June 9, 1936, quoted in Klee 1979, p. 1269.
[348] Grohmann 1965, p. 28: 'Grandmother Frick gave her four-year-old grandson colored pencils. […] She drew and stitched, showed him pictures of Epinal and spent so much time with him that when she died he said he felt "orphaned artistically".'
[349] Morscher/ML 1994, p. 204.

styled himself a cosmic artist, rising above earthly concerns and removing himself from involvement with his fellow men.'[350] The author ascribes Klee's social behavior to the onset of scleroderma – in the guise of a hypothetical theory known as 'morphic field' or 'morphic resonance', a theory we cannot go into here.

Commentary: Of course Paul Klee was grateful to his grandmother for helping him learn to draw. He loved her very much, and she started to awaken his great hidden talent. Many children are close to their grandparents, particularly if they spend a lot of time together, and during their life they look back and feel very thankful for having had such grandparents. This was certainly the case with Paul Klee. But it is quite out of the question that the artist or his grandmother exhibited narcissism, an exaggerated, even dysfunctional self-love. Morscher has created this theory out of thin air. There is no evidence to suggest that Klee was excessively attached to his grandmother, and he had a normal, affectionate relationship with his parents and his sister Mathilde.

As far as Paul Klee's relationship with his wife Lily is concerned, the couple's close friend Ju Aichinger-Grosch writes: 'Paul Klee was always very close to his wife and he stood by her through thick and thin all his life, perhaps because they were such opposites. She was the vibrant, funny, vivacious pianist from Munich; he was the gentle, quiet painter, always a little cut off from everyday things […].'[351] For at least ten years Lily supported the family by giving piano lessons. She lovingly cared for her husband when he was ill, trying where possible to ease his everyday life, and when he was suffering she took over most of his correspondence.[352] Their strong partnership must have been very important for the artist's psyche when he was seriously ill. Lily's loving care meant her husband was able to bear his suffering much more easily than if he had been alone or cared for by others.

Like Paul Klee, his wife Lily was also very sensitive, but unlike him she was not mentally robust. She admits this herself: 'Unfortunately I have always had very sensitive nerves.'[353] Her husband's illness put her under a lot of strain right from

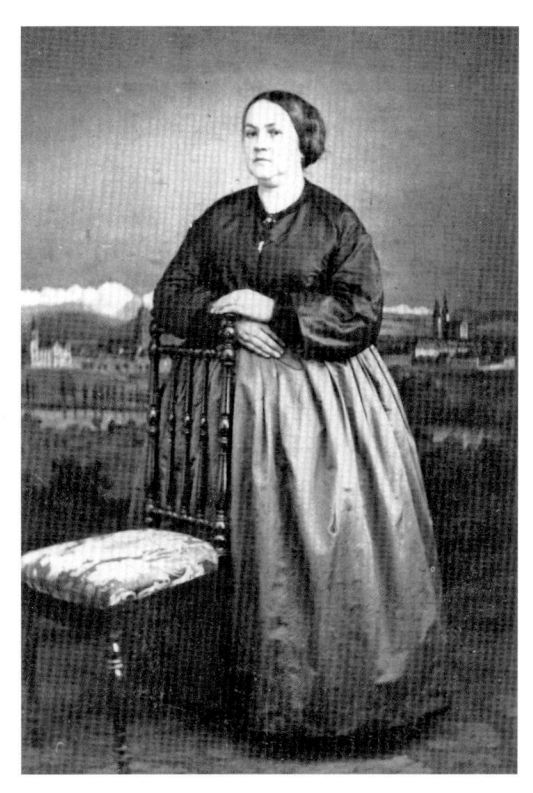

Fig. 77. Anna Catharina Rosina Frick-Riedtmann (Paul Klee's maternal grandmother), 1880

[350] Morscher/ML 1994, p. 203.
[351] Aichinger-Grosch 1959, p. 55.
[352] Personal communication, Felix Klee to the author, Bern, September 20, 1983. Cf. also letter from Paul Klee to J. B. Neumann, Bern, January 9, 1939 (photocopy: MoMAANY/NP).
[353] Letter from Lily Klee to Gertrud Grohmann, Bern, November 28, 1939 (AWG).

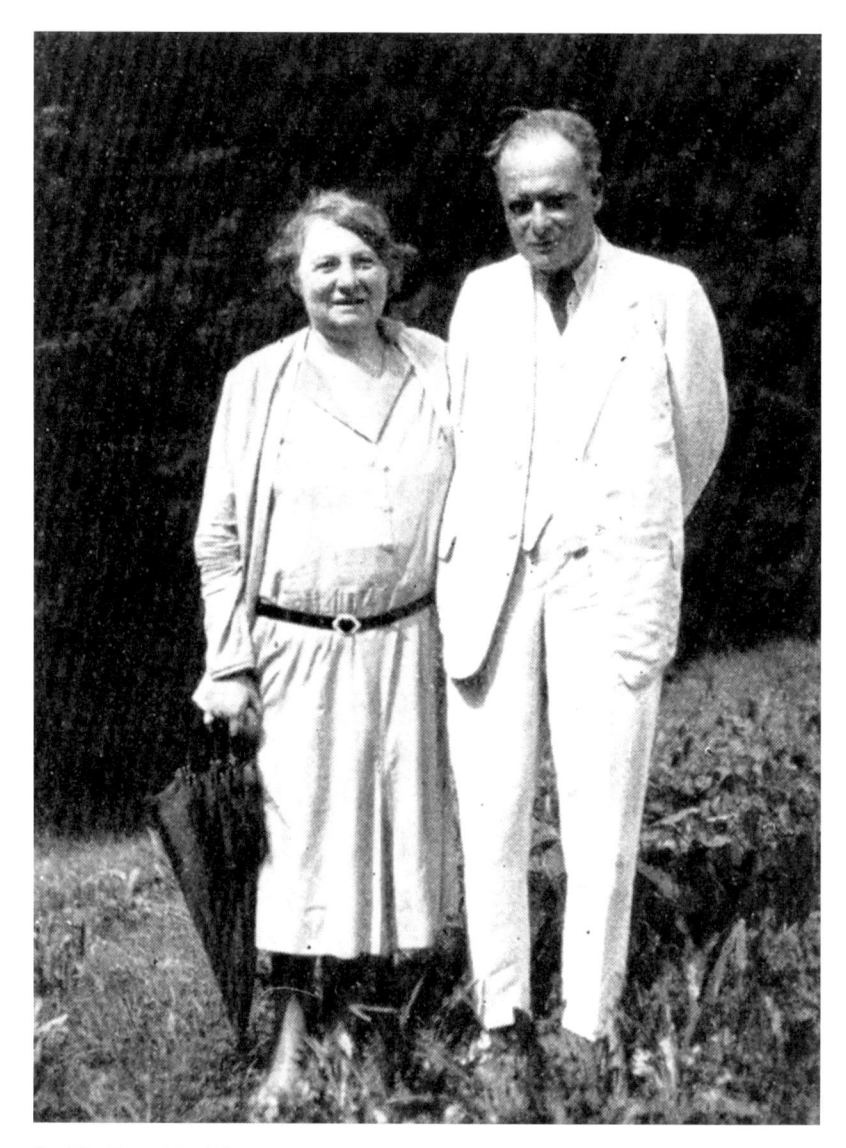

Fig. 78. Lily and Paul Klee, 1930

the start. On October 30, 1935, she writes to Nina Kandinsky: 'The last few weeks have been terrible for me. I feel eaten up with worry about my husband and my nerves are in a dreadful state.'[354] Lily generally accompanied Paul Klee when he went away to convalesce. In May/June 1939 she felt the need to take a break for the sake of her own health, so she spent two months at the Sonnmatt spa hotel near Lucerne.[355] Her husband stayed at home, but he managed very well on his own. Hermann Rupf tells Wassily and Nina Kandinsky: 'His (Klee's) health has certainly improved, but he is still very ill. [...] Mrs. Klee is in Lucerne at the moment and it is to be hoped that she is making a good recovery.

[354] Letter from Lily Klee to Nina Kandinsky, Bern, October 30, 1935 (BK/CGPP).
[355] Cf. letter from Lily Klee to Gertrud Grohmann, Bern, November 28, 1939 (AWG).

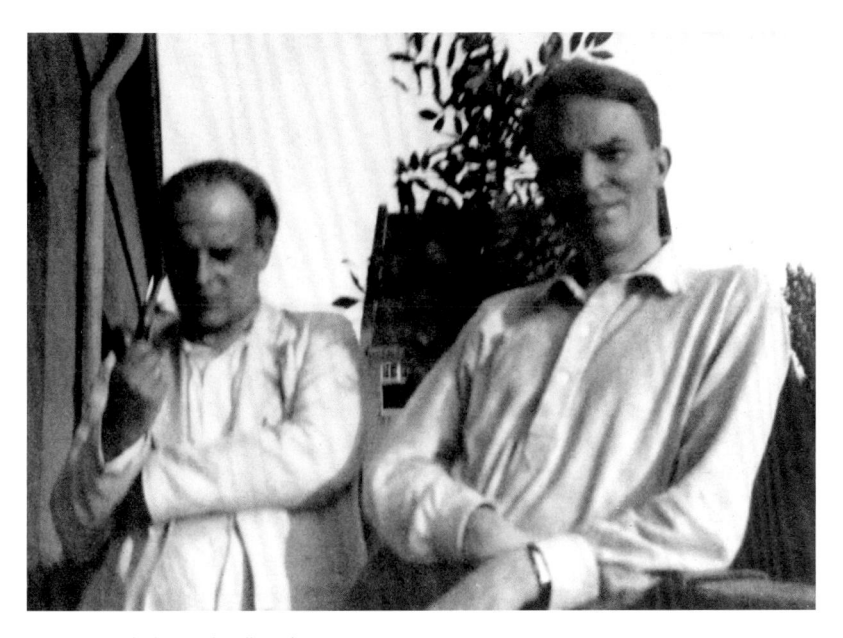

Fig. 79. Paul Klee and Will Grohmann, Bern, 1935

She has suffered greatly with her nerves as a result of her husband's long illness, and is in dire need of a rest.'[356] Even when he was ill, the artist would have been a pillar of strength for his wife: he was by nature a gentle, well-balanced man who faced life's setbacks with courage and composure. The question remains open as to whether, as Jürgen Glaesemer claims[357], the predominantly music-loving Lily had little understanding of her husband's art in his later years. But we know from Felix Klee that whenever he visited his parents in Bern, Paul Klee talked very little about his work and hardly ever mentioned his illness.[358]

It is a fact that, during his illness, Klee devoted himself to his art and consciously withdrew into his own, private world. As his ill-health progressed, he felt less and less able to go out in public. This austere, ascetic life led outside observers to believe he was isolated and lonely, and it is sad to note that Lily also had this impression. She writes to Will Grohmann: 'I do not need to tell you that you are one of the very few people who can really understand and appreciate his creative mentality. Mentally and spiritually he is such a solitary person, and his life is lonely and austere.'[359] Jürgen Glaesemer comments on Klee's loneliness: 'She [Lily] was quite clear that there was nothing she could do about it.'[360] Personally, I think

[356] Letter from Hermann Rupf to Wassily and Nina Kandinsky, Bern, May 8, 1939 (BK/CGPP).

[357] Glaesemer 1979, p. 12: 'Her [Lily Klee's] great admiration [for her husband as a man and as an artist] does not preclude the fact that his essential nature remained a mystery to her, indeed it seemed quite inaccessible.'

[358] Ibid: 'Felix Klee also remembers that whenever he visited his parents in Bern, they did not discuss his father's work or his illness. The family's conversations were largely anecdotal, and according to Felix Klee, the atmosphere was generally lighthearted and as cheerful as possible, even in the final years.'

[359] Letter from Lily Klee to Will Grohmann, Bern, October 9, 1938 (AWG).

[360] Glaesemer 1979, p. 13.

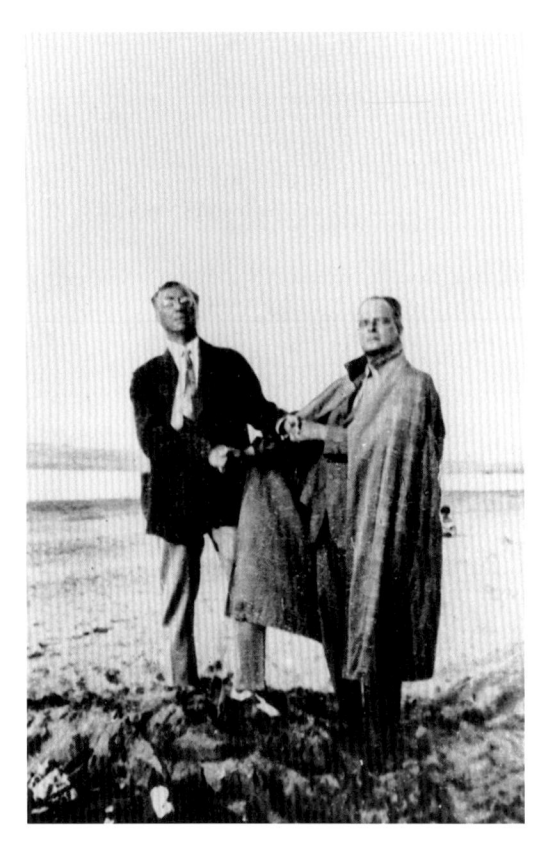

Fig. 80. Wassily Kandinsky and Paul Klee, Hendaye-Plage, 1929

we have to be more specific about the 'loneliness' which Lily Klee ascribes to her husband. Paul Klee was only outwardly lonely; beneath the surface he was totally consumed by his work and living a rich inner life. Mentally and spiritually he was far from lonely.

Although Paul Klee tended to avoid social occasions, it was important to him to stay in contact with his friends.[361] This is shown in a letter he wrote in December 1934 to his artist friend, Wassily Kandinsky, who had been his next door neighbor in Dessau from 1926 to 1933: 'And finally, I have one more wish: that we could all sit together again for one of our cozy chats, surrounded by beautiful pictures, the ladies happily chatting, all of us laughing together – it is a hardship to do without something which was so habitual for us, yet always so refreshing.'[362] He also particularly valued his friendship with the German art historian, Will Grohmann, as shown in a note he received from Lily Klee: 'You and my husband are soul mates, and other relationships revolve around your axis.'[363] During his last years in Bern, the artist's ill-health largely prevented him from visiting friends or attending social occasions.[364] As a result of this and the artistic isolation which was forced upon him as World War II drew closer, his circle of friends shrank to just a few people.

There is no doubt that in his artistic life he created a 'cocoon' for himself where he would withdraw to do his work. But once he had laid aside his pen or paintbrush he would emerge once again, ready to interact with his family, friends and the outside world.[365] It seems to me that in his analysis, Christoph Morscher has placed too much weight on the critical comments contained in the young artist's diaries, and has not taken into consideration Klee's strong character in view of the social and health-related constraints he faced during the last years of his life. I therefore cannot seriously take Morscher's rather overworked theory into account when considering the causes of Paul Klee's illness.

[361] Personal communication, Felix Klee to the author, Bern, September 20, 1983.
[362] Letter from Paul Klee to Wassily Kandinsky, Bern, December 3, 1934 (BK/CGPP), quoted in Kuthy 1984, p. 13.
[363] Letter from Lily Klee to Will Grohmann, Bern, October 9, 1938 (AWG).
[364] Personal communication, Felix Klee to the author, Bern, September 20, 1983.
[365] As above, Bern, September 20, 1983.

E. Carwile LeRoy, MD, and Richard M. Silver, MD (Charleston, South Carolina)

Paul Klee and Scleroderma, in: Bulletin on the Rheumatic Diseases, vol. 45, no. 6, 1996 (Oct.), p. 4 f

E. Carwile LeRoy and Richard M. Silver studied photographs of the artist's hands from the years 1924 and 1938 (no note of specific photos) and a photograph of his face taken in 1939. From these they ascertained that his skin was taut and shiny, claiming that it was visual evidence for the diagnosis of 'scleroderma'. They then considered Klee's art both before and after the onset of his illness, referring to E.G.L. Bywaters' publication 'Paul Klee, The effect of scleroderma on his painting'.[366] Bywaters claims the artist's illness brought about a visible change in his work, from a free, lighthearted and romantic style to a dark symbolism. After a drop in productivity at the start of his illness, subsequent years saw a staggering increase in the number of works Klee produced. LeRoy and Silver, along with Bywaters, took this to be the result of a huge burst of creative energy[367] – apparently a frequent occurrence among scleroderma sufferers – which Klee experienced once he understood more about his illness and its prognosis.

Commentary: This assessment should be put into perspective. On the one hand, it is highly questionable, and indeed irrelevant, to make a diagnosis based solely on photographs. On the other hand, I would agree with the authors that the illness certainly had a significant influence on Klee's art. But I find it inappropriate to make such a definite distinction between his work before his illness and his work during his illness. For instance, the artist always retained his penchant for humor and burlesque, which sometimes went as far as sarcasm[368], and even in the darkest days of his illness he still produced some light and colorful paintings. There is no evidence for the assertion that Klee knew the diagnosis and subsequent prognosis of his illness.[369] On the contrary, I think he gauged the seriousness of his disease early on. Although he always hoped for a partial or total cure, in the last few months of his life he would have been aware that the end was near. The idea that many patients with 'progressive scle-

---

[366] Cf. Bywaters/ML 1987, p. 49 f.
[367] Cf. ibid.
[368] Personal communication, Felix Klee to the author, Bern, September 20, 1983.
[369] As above, Bern, September 20, 1983.

roderma' feel intensely driven to work and create is an interesting theory which I have not come across before.[370]

Dr. Gabriele Castenholz (Frankfurt)
Die progressive systemische Sklerose. Analyse und Geschichte unter besonderer Berücksichtigung der Krankheit des Malers Paul Klee (1879–1940), Dissertation, Marburg 2000

Gabriele Castenholz has made a thorough historical study of 'progressive systemic sclerosis' as a disease, and is the first author to really investigate, discuss[371], and ultimately call into question Paul Klee's diagnosis of 'scleroderma'.[372] She supports her arguments with extracts from Klee's diaries from 1898 to 1918, with the contents of exhibition catalogues and with various letters, which I have also used in my evaluation. She comes to the conclusion that the diagnosis of 'scleroderma' is too narrow.[373] The author believes that the artist's illness 'was in all likelihood a mixed connective tissue disease with complications from "Lupus erythematosus disseminatus".'[374] (Gabriele Castenholz presumably means by this 'systemic Lupus erythematosus'. 'Lupus erythematosus disseminatus' is used to describe a form of 'Lupus erythematosus chronicus', which affects not only the face but also other parts of the body and – in contrast to 'systemic Lupus erythematosus' – does not afflict the internal organs). This new theory requires us to examine these diseases in more detail before drawing any final conclusions.

As the name implies, **'mixed connective tissue disease'** (MCTD) is an umbrella term for the mixed range of symptoms and indications which are found in the connective tissue diseases: systemic sclerosis, systemic Lupus erythematosus, dermatomyositis/polymyositis and rheumatoid arthritis (polyarthritis).[375] The condition was first described and named as a disease in its own right in 1972 by G.C. Sharp.[376] As already noted for systemic sclerosis, there are a series of diagnostic criteria for determining MCTD, systemic Lupus erythematosus and dermatomyositis/polymyositis.[377] MCTDs begin with Raynaud's syndrome, swelling of the fingers, joint pains and an

---

[370] Cf. note 367.
[371] Cf. Castenholz/ML 2000, pp. 81–93 and 130–148.
[372] Cf. ibid., pp. 144–148.
[373] Cf. ibid., p.147.
[374] Ibid., p. 147 f.
[375] Cf. Peter/ML 1996, p. 373, and cf. Maddison/ML 2000, p. 111 f.
[376] Cf. Sharp/ML 1972, p. 148 f.
[377] Cf. Peter/ML 1996, p. 375.

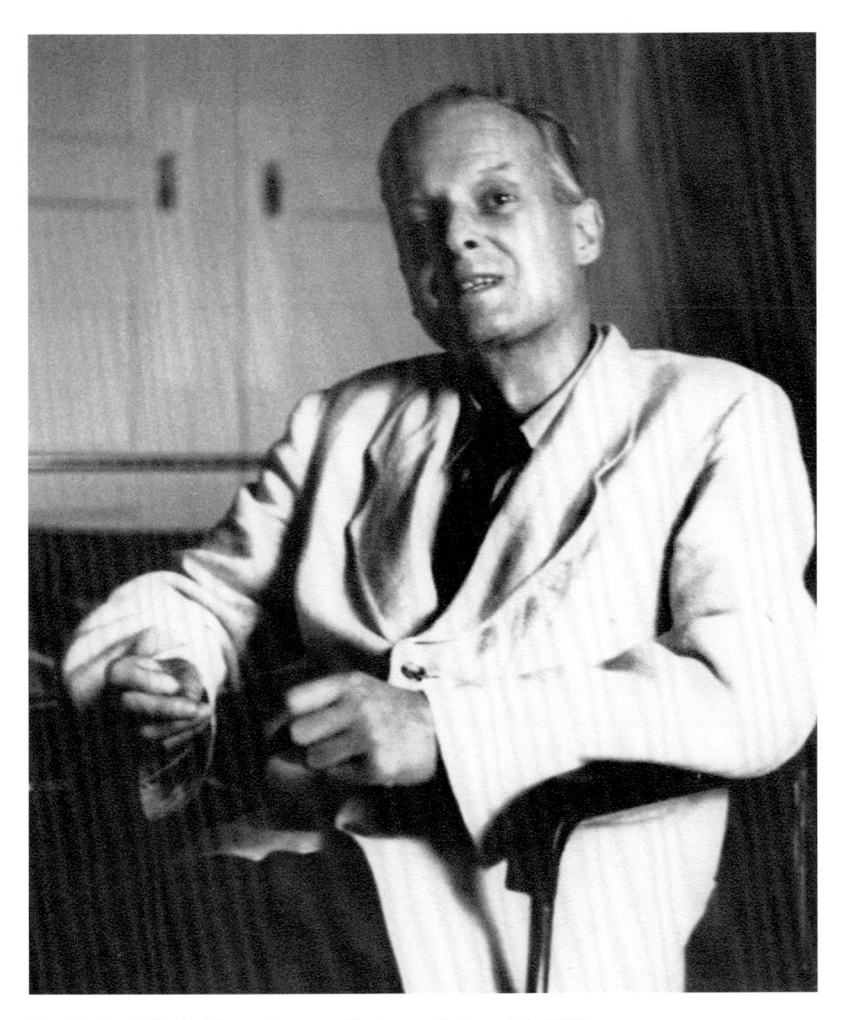

Fig. 81. Paul Klee in his music room, Kistlerweg 6, Bern, July 1939

inflammatory skin rash.[378] Further symptoms of collagen diseases and rheumatoid arthritis appear later.[379] Major symptoms of MCTDs are: Raynaud's syndrome (in 90% of cases), polyarthritis (in 85%), swallowing difficulties (in 80%), swollen fingers and/or hands (in 75%), breathing difficulties (in 75%), muscle pain (in 70%), inflammatory skin rashes, such as redness of the face (in 50%), swollen glands (in 50%), painful disorders of the oral mucosa (in 45%), sclerodactyly (in 40%), knotty growths on the skin (in 40%), pleurisy (in 30%), pericarditis (in 20%).[380] The main criteria for MCTD diagnosis are Raynaud's syndrome and swollen fingers/hands, along with two or three of the other symptoms as sub-criteria.[381] I will consider Gabriele Castenholz's contention that Paul Klee was also suffering from 'Lupus erythematosus disseminatus' and 'systemic Lupus erythematosus' a little later.

[378] Cf. Maddison/ML 2000, p. 114.
[379] Cf. ibid.
[380] Cf. ibid., p. 115.
[381] Cf. Peter/ML 1996, p. 375.

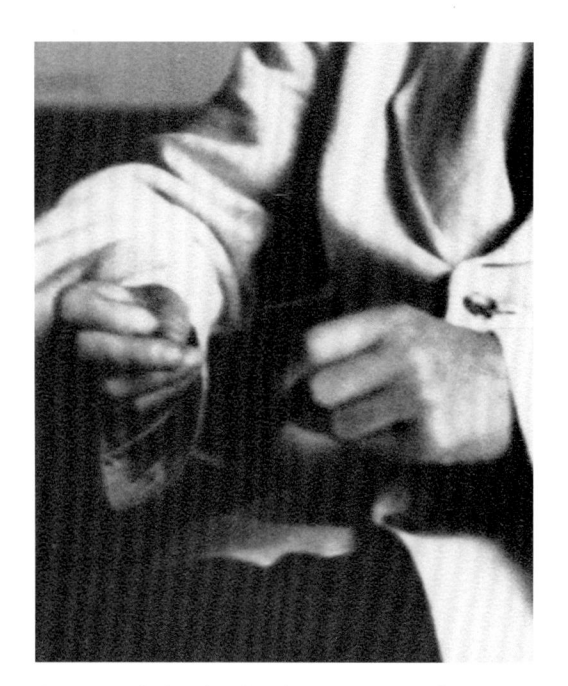

Fig. 82. Paul Klee's hands, July 1939, section of the photo shown in fig. 81

Commentary: Paul Klee displayed no symptoms of Raynaud's syndrome and had no swelling of the fingers or hands.[382] The main criteria for an MCTD are therefore not fulfilled. We can also exclude sclerodactyly, polyarthritis and redness of the face.[383] As far as the sub-criteria are concerned, we only have evidence of swallowing difficulties, shortage of breath during physical exertion and pleurisy combined with pneumonia during the initial phase. It therefore seems highly unlikely that Paul Klee was suffering from a mixed connective tissue disease.

Gabriele Castenholz also believes she can discern a thickening of the finger joints and a tapering of the fingertips in a photo taken in 1939 (figs. 81 and 82: Paul Klee in the music room of his residence in Bern, Kistlerweg 6, dated end July 1939, photo by Charlotte Weidler [Rye], reprinted in: Klee 1990/2, page 118). She is of the opinion that this could '[…] either be an indication of sclerodactyly as a symptom of scleroderma, or of arthritis as a symptom of systemic Lupus erythematosus.'[384] But she had no doubt that it caused '[…] restricted movement in P. Klee's hands.'[385] She continues: 'From 1935 onwards he only very occasionally dealt with his own correspondence, and he had to give up playing the violin on doctor's advice. Both he and his wife often mentioned the fact that he had difficulty writing. But strangely enough, it did not have an adverse affect on his art. Why this should be will probably remain a mystery to us. There is no evidence that he suffered from Raynaud's phenomenon, which can be very painful, or that he had arthritis in his joints due to systemic Lupus erythematosus. The evidence of the photographs is not conclusive enough for us to be able to include finger and hand swelling in the list of his symptoms.'[386]

Commentary: Gabriele Castenholz's assertion that Paul Klee had problems writing is based on three letters, two written by Lily Klee and one by the artist himself. In January 1937 Lily writes to Gertrud Grohmann: 'Unfortunately he [Paul Klee] cannot write to you himself. […] He still [after a bout of flu] does not have the strength.'[387] So it was not problems with his hands, but general debility that prevented him from writing the letters himself. Moreover, in the few last years of his life, he generally left letter writing to his wife, so that he could

---

[382] Personal communication, Felix Klee to the author, Bern, September 20, 1983.
[383] As above, Bern, September 20, 1983.
[384] Castenholz/ML 2000, p. 138.
[385] Ibid.
[386] Castenholz/ML 2000, p. 138 f.
[387] Letter from Lily Klee to Gertrud Grohmann, Bern, January 24, 1937 (AWG). Lily Klee had told her the same thing in a letter the previous year, Bern, January 25, 1936 (AWG). Gabriele Castenholz refers to these two letters and to the letter from Paul Klee to Felix Klee of November 29, 1938 (fig. 83).

conserve his dwindling energies and direct them exclusively towards his art.[388] He confirms this in a letter dated January 1939 to the New York art dealer J.B. Neumann: '[...] my wife has recently been looking after all my correspondence and paperwork. After all, I am an artist, and as such I work with concepts. I am not so young any more, but there are still things that I wish to achieve. This means that I always have to be ready to seize the moment. I have to be able to concentrate. My powers are dwindling, and today I feel they have deserted me.'[389] Hermann Rupf also bears this out: 'He is however working hard and well and conserving his strength.'[390]

In a last birthday letter to his 31-year-old son, the artist writes in November 1938: 'Dear Felix, as your birthday is approaching, I am taking the opportunity to put pen to paper. This is quite astonishing to me too, and I am staring at my pen as it dips itself in the ink, even though it is actually a fountain pen, and watching as it moves across the beautiful paper, even producing for the most part legible script, not the usual mysterious symbols. Now you can read that I wish you all the best for your birthday and the coming year, Your loving father'[391] (fig. 83). In my view, Klee is not here referring to his actual ability to write. He could be expressing his pleasure that he is writing this special letter in 'for the most part legible script', and by 'the usual mysterious symbols' he could mean creative expression, such as drawings. Jürgen Glaesemer shares this opinion, for he comments on Klee's last birthday letter to his son as follows: '[...] he [Paul Klee] here clearly details how he overlays writing with drawings. [...] It is true that he refers to his drawings with their "mysterious symbols" as illegible script, but he also characterizes them as the only normal form of communication. As a result, writing has become for him a strange and alien process.'[392] In a letter to his wife in April 1939, Paul Klee comments in this respect: 'I am writing these words in a less controlled way, just letting my hand run free, as if it were a drawing.'[393] On the occasion of his 60th birthday in December 1939 he received almost one hundred letters of congratulation, and he replied to them all personally, as Lily was in poor health at the time. These letters are clear evidence that his handwriting was not affected by physical limitations.[394]

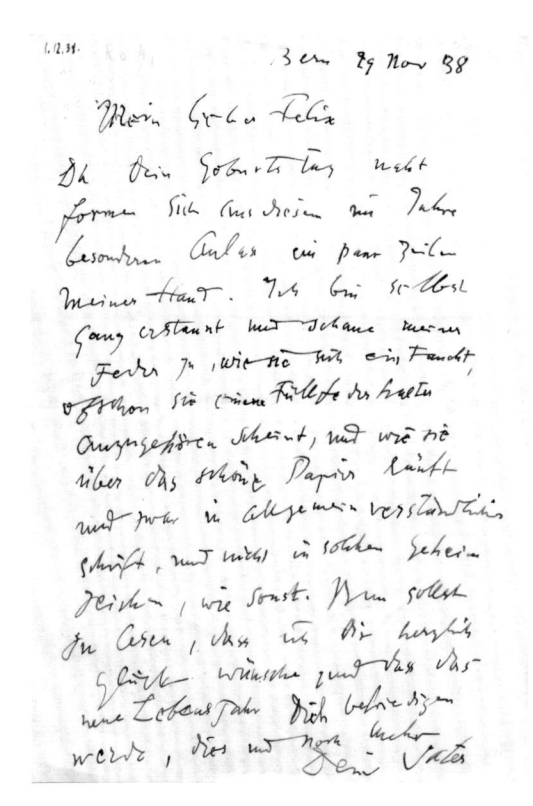

Fig. 83. Letter from Paul Klee to his son, Felix Klee, Bern, November 29, 1938

[388] Personal communication, Felix Klee to the author, Bern, September 20, 1983.

[389] Letter from Paul Klee to J.B. Neumann, Bern, January 9, 1939 (photocopy: MoMAANY/NP), quoted in Frey 1990, p. 115.

[390] Letter from Hermann Rupf to Wassily and Nina Kandinsky, Bern, March 12, 1939 (BK/CGPP).

[391] Letter from Paul Klee to Felix Klee, Bern, November 29, 1938, quoted in Klee 1979, p. 1282.

[392] Glaesemer 1979, p. 25 f.

[393] Letter from Paul Klee to Lily Klee, Bern, April 25, 1939, quoted in Klee 1979, p. 1286.

[394] Cf. Frey 1990, p. 121.

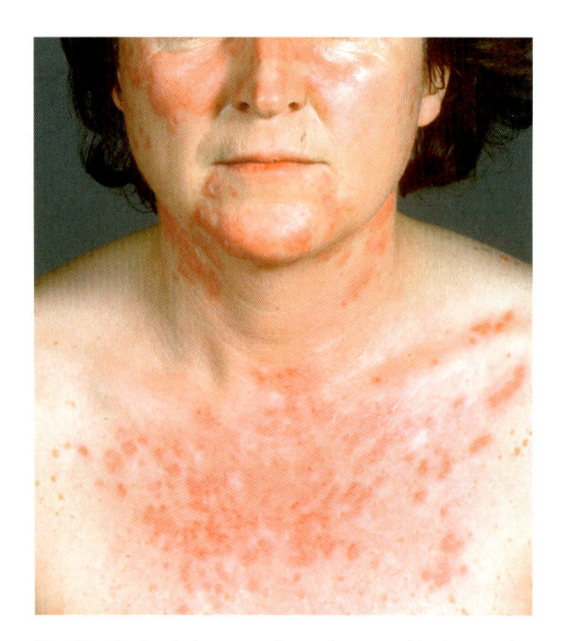

Fig. 84. Systemic Lupus erythematosus: reddening on the face, on the neck and around the neckline

Paul Klee's handwriting did not deteriorate during his illness. This is evidenced by his handwritten notes in the catalogue of works[395], the titles written under his drawings and the handwritten biography[396] written on January 7, 1940 (pages 32–35).

Lily Klee tells us that he was forced to give up playing the violin not because of problems with his hands but because the physical exertion was too great: 'He is still not allowed to play music because it is physically too much for him.'[397]

As already noted, both Felix Klee and Max Huggler confirmed that Paul Klee's fingers remained unchanged and pain-free, and that he had total use of them right up to the end. This would certainly not be the case if he had been suffering from sclerodactyly or arthritis in the finger joints.

With regard to **systemic Lupus erythematosus** (lupus, from the Latin meaning wolf, erythema, from the Greek meaning reddening), in 1982 the American College of Rheumatology (formerly American Rheumatism Association) compiled a list detailing eleven criteria for this second connective tissue disease. At least four of these criteria must be fulfilled in order to make a diagnosis of systemic Lupus erythematosus[398]: (1) redness (fig. 84); (2) often long-term characteristic changes to the skin on the face, upper chest and back (fig. 84), backs of the hands and fingers, elbows and knees; scarring (definitive) alopecia; (3) increased sensitivity to light; (4) painful disorders of the oral mucosa; (5) joint pain and arthritis; (6) pericarditis and/or pleurisy and/or peritonitis; (7) nephritis; (8) neurological symptoms; (9) blood disorders (anemia, decrease in white blood cells and platelets); (10) immune disorders and formation of certain 'autoantibodies'; (11) attacks by antibodies on cell nuclei. Other symptoms include: swollen glands, painful muscle inflammation, Raynaud's syndrome, esophageal inflammation, and general symptoms such as fatigue and elevated body temperature.[399] Gabriele Castenholz believes four of these criteria are present in Paul Klee's case: skin reddening, possible arthritis of the finger joints, pleurisy/pericarditis and anemia.[400]

[395] Location: Zentrum Paul Klee, Bern.
[396] Klee 1940 (p. 258), and pp. 32–35.
[397] Letter from Lily Klee to Emmy Scheyer, Bern, December 16, 1936 (NSMP).
[398] Cf. Tan/ML 1982, p. 1271 f.
[399] Cf. Krieg/ML 1996, p. 743.
[400] Cf. Castenholz/ML 2000, p. 137.

Commentary: There is no evidence from letters or from Felix Klee's comments to suggest that Paul Klee's skin was affected by any long-lasting redness or that his fingers were arthritic.[401] At the beginning of his illness, he certainly had a short-lived skin rash, which Lily Klee called 'measles'. As previously discussed, this was probably a drug reaction, a reoccurrence of which he also suffered towards the end of his illness. In systematic Lupus erythematosus, the skin redness is mainly confined to areas which are exposed to the sun, such as the face, in the form of a 'butterfly rash', the throat, neck, upper chest and back, forearms and hands, and it tends to be stubborn and long-lasting.[402] I do not consider Klee's pleurisy, anemia and swallowing difficulties to be sufficient to fulfill the criteria for a diagnosis of systemic Lupus erythematosus, and this illness should probably be discounted. Moreover, men very rarely – only in about 10% of cases – suffer from systemic Lupus erythematosus.[403]

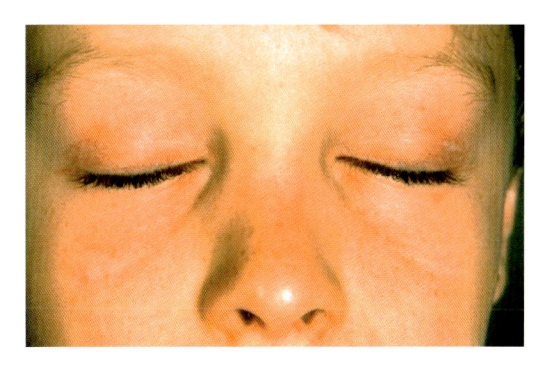

Fig. 85. Dermatomyositis: symmetrical reddening and swelling of the eyelids and the area around the eyes

With regard to the third connective tissue disease, **dermatomyositis** (derma, from the Greek meaning skin, mys, from the Greek meaning muscle, originally from a word meaning mouse, genitive form myos), the connective tissue of the skin and internal organs can thicken, just as in systemic sclerosis. But it does not lead to the mask-like face which is typical of scleroderma. The effect on the skin is clearly distinguishable from the other connective tissue diseases: it typically presents as a symmetrical lilac-colored reddening and swelling of the eyelids, the area around the eyes (fig. 85), the cheeks, backs of the fingers, elbows and knees. The face also takes on a characteristically lachrymose expression and above all there is pronounced muscle weakness and muscle pain due to inflammation of the muscles (myositis). Blood and urine tests clearly show that the muscle metabolism is malfunctioning. Immunological criteria for dermatomyositis can also be confirmed through blood testing. Other symptoms can include joint pain, internal organ disorders and anemia.[404] This autoimmune muscle disease can also present without the skin disorders typical of dermatomyositis, in which case it is termed **'polymyositis'**.[405]

[401] Personal communication, Felix Klee to the author, Bern, September 20, 1983.
[402] Cf. Krieg/ML 1996, p. 744.
[403] Cf. Welcker/ML 2001, p. 3.
[404] Cf. Krieg/ML 1996, p. 752.
[405] Cf ibid., p. 751, and cf. Gadola and Villiger/ML 2006, pp. 89–93.

Commentary: The artist showed no typical signs of dermatomyositis or polymyositis,[406] so it seems highly unlikely that he suffered from either of these connective tissue diseases.

MCTD was formerly referred to as **'overlap syndrome'** (because of the 'overlapping' symptoms of the various collagenoses).[407] Today the term 'overlap syndrome' is used when a patient presents with symptoms of two or more defined connective tissue diseases.[408] Occasionally one defined connective tissue disease can transition into another. For example, an initial presentation of systemic Lupus erythematosus can after a few years suddenly present as classic diffuse systemic sclerosis.[409] There is no evidence to suggest that there was any overlap syndrome in Paul Klee's case, or that he first presented with systemic Lupus erythematosus which later transitioned into systemic sclerosis.

Let us take a brief look at what is known in medical literature as **'CREST syndrome'**. This is a slow-progressing variant of the limited form of systemic sclerosis. CREST is an acronym for the five main features: **C**alcinosis of the skin with calcium excretion, **R**aynaud's syndrome, **E**sophageal dysmotility, i.e. a functional disorder of the esophagus, **S**clerodactyly and **T**elangiectasia (small dilated blood vessels on the surface of the skin or mucous membranes).[410]

Commentary: As previously discussed, Paul Klee did not suffer from calcium excretion through the skin, Raynaud's syndrome, sclerodactyly or obvious blood vessels on the skin surface, therefore we can also rule out CREST syndrome.

A Final Assessment of Paul Klee's Illness

Forty to sixty years after Paul Klee's death, I have tried to fully exploit every source and gather together as much information as possible which could help form an assessment of this famous artist's illness. I have also painstakingly researched the extensive literature on the painter and his work in order to extract any relevant information. I have then compared the results of my research with the latest medical knowledge relating to the diseases which seem the most likely cause of his ill-health.

---

[406] Personal communication, Felix Klee to the author, Bern, September 20, 1983.
[407] Cf. Peter/ML 1996, p. 373.
[408] Cf. Gadola and Villiger/ML 2006, p. 94.
[409] Personal communication, Prof. Peter M. Villiger, Director and Chief Physician of the University Clinic and the Polyclinics of the Department of Rheumatology and Immunology/Allergology, Inselspital, Bern, to the author, Bern, September 20, 2005.
[410] Cf. Krieg/ML 1996, p. 729.

First, a brief recap of the symptoms and findings:
- Initial phase: sudden severe onset of illness, protracted bronchitis, long-term slightly elevated body temperature, three-month confinement to bed, constant fatigue, weight loss and debility, leading to a severe deterioration in overall health
- Skin disorders: mask-like face with taut, inelastic skin, reduced facial expression, reduced eyelid mobility, pointed nose, narrowing of lips and mouth, tightening of skin on neck
- Mucous membrane disorders: early-stage periodontosis, possible mouth dryness ('Sicca syndrome')
- Esophageal disorders: pain when swallowing, necessitating a diet restricted to small portions of liquid foods
- Digestive tract disorders: gastric ulcer and bleeding, possible lack of gastric acid, diarrhea
- Lung disorders: chronic cough, pleurisy, pneumonia, shortage of breath during physical exertion
- Renal disorders: the urine test showing a trace of protein, red and white blood cells and cylinders could be interpreted as a kidney disorder, but also as a blockage caused by cardiac insufficiency
- Anemia

It is also important to note the following symptoms which were not present:
- Skin: no inflammatory skin rashes causing reddening of face, hands or backs of fingers
- Mucous membranes: no painful oral mucosa disorders
- Fingers/hands: no swelling, thickening, hardening or contracture of the fingers, no restricted mobility, no slow-healing ulcers after injury, no finger damage with tissue or calcium excretion, no circulatory disorders (Raynaud's syndrome), no arthritis
- Muscles: no painful muscle inflammation
- No increased sensitivity to light

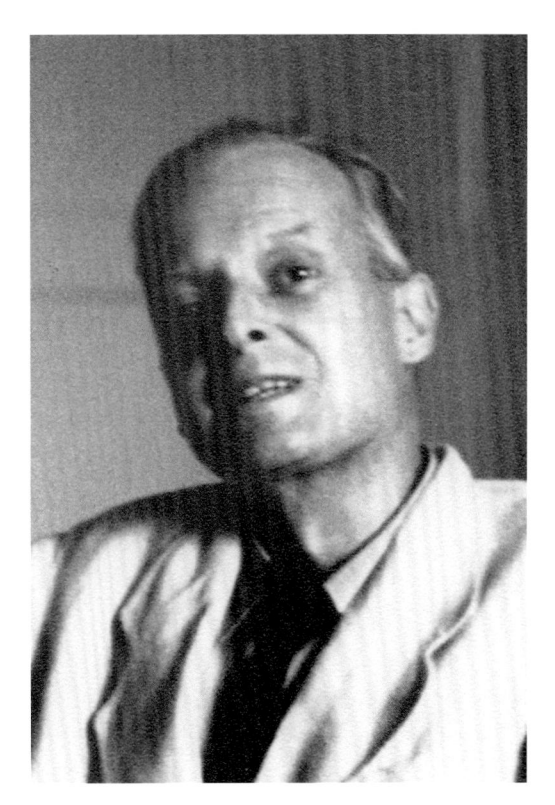

Fig. 86. Paul Klee, July 1939, section of the photo shown in fig. 81

From this we can extrapolate the following **epicrisis** (a final critical evaluation of the illness):

1. After considering all the above facts, we can conclude that Paul Klee almost certainly fell ill and died from the hypothetically diagnosed autoimmune connective tissue disease 'scleroderma'.

2. The findings allow a more precise diagnosis: it is highly likely that Paul Klee suffered from the rare and severe form of scleroderma, **diffuse systemic sclerosis**. The main indicators for this lie in the severe initial phase of the illness, the sclerodermic changes to the face (the 'mask face'), the swallowing difficulties, the cardiac and pulmonary symptoms, the anemia, the progression of the disease leading to death in only five years and the cause of death recorded as myocarditis.

3. The fact that the hands and fingers remained unaffected – no swelling, no sclerodactyly, no Raynaud's syndrome and no joint pains – refutes a diagnosis of limited systemic sclerosis, a 'mixed connective tissue disease', 'overlap syndrome' or 'CREST syndrome'.

4. The other collagenoses – systemic Lupus erythematosus and dermatomyositis/polymyositis – along with 'pseudoscleroderma' can also be discounted as they do not fulfill the necessary criteria.

5. The following statements by Lily Klee are also significant:
   – that her husband's doctor had 'finally given us a diagnosis: vasomotor neurosis',
   – and that the illness was connected to 'his [Paul Klee's] gland and skin problems', which required him to have '[…] his blood and metabolism checked for calcium and phosphorus.'

   In the 1930s 'scleroderma' was classified as a 'vasomotortrophic neurosis' and it was widely held to be a ductless gland disorder (indeed, it is still the case that the diagnosis of parathyroid disorders relies heavily on determining calcium and phosphorus levels in the serum, along with other serological tests).

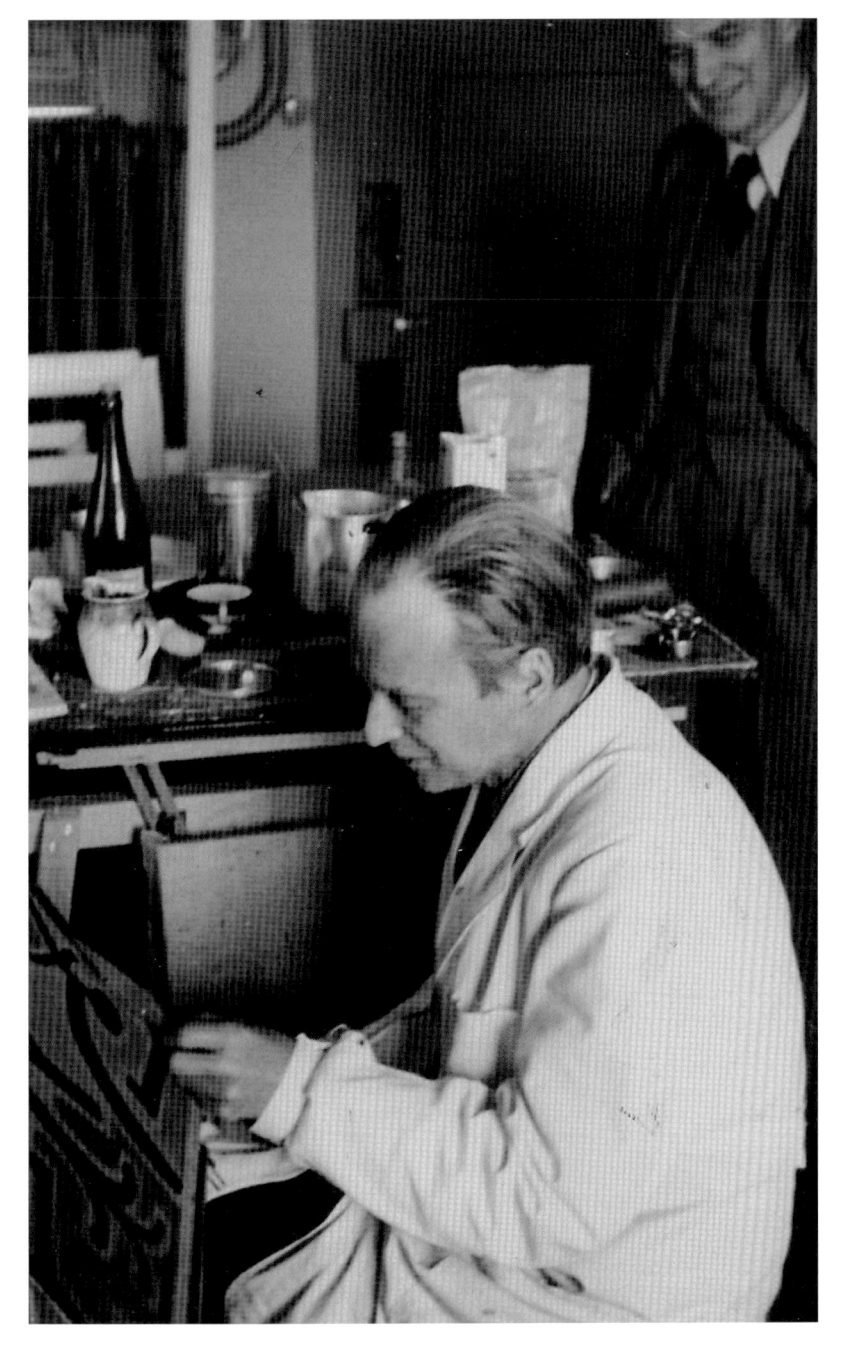

Fig. 87. Paul Klee and Will Grohmann, April 1938

6. Autoimmune diseases are very complex, so we should not totally discount the possibility of other external and internal factors playing a part in the onset of the illness, such as:
   – The inhalation of organic solvents while painting
   – The setbacks suffered in Germany and the subsequent artistic isolation that Klee experienced when he moved back to Switzerland

Paul Klee's Doctors

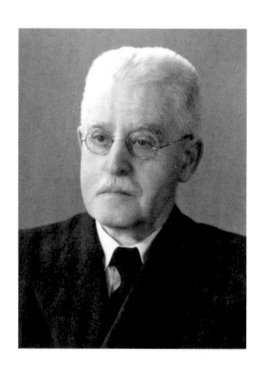

Dr. Fritz Lotmar, neurologist,
childhood friend of Paul Klee's

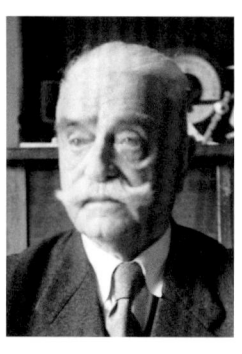

Dr. Gerhard Schorer, internist,
Paul Klee's family doctor in Bern

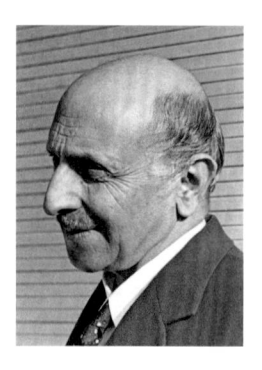

Dr. Hermann Bodmer, internist,
the last doctor to treat Paul Klee in Locarno

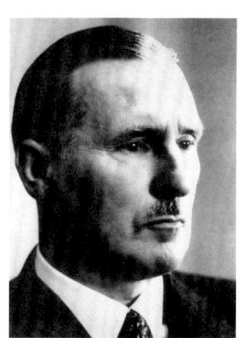

Prof. Oscar Naegeli, dermatologist,
consulting doctor to Dr. Schorer

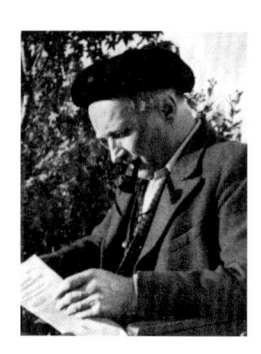

Dr. Theodor Haemmerli, heart specialist,
consulting doctor to Dr. Bodmer

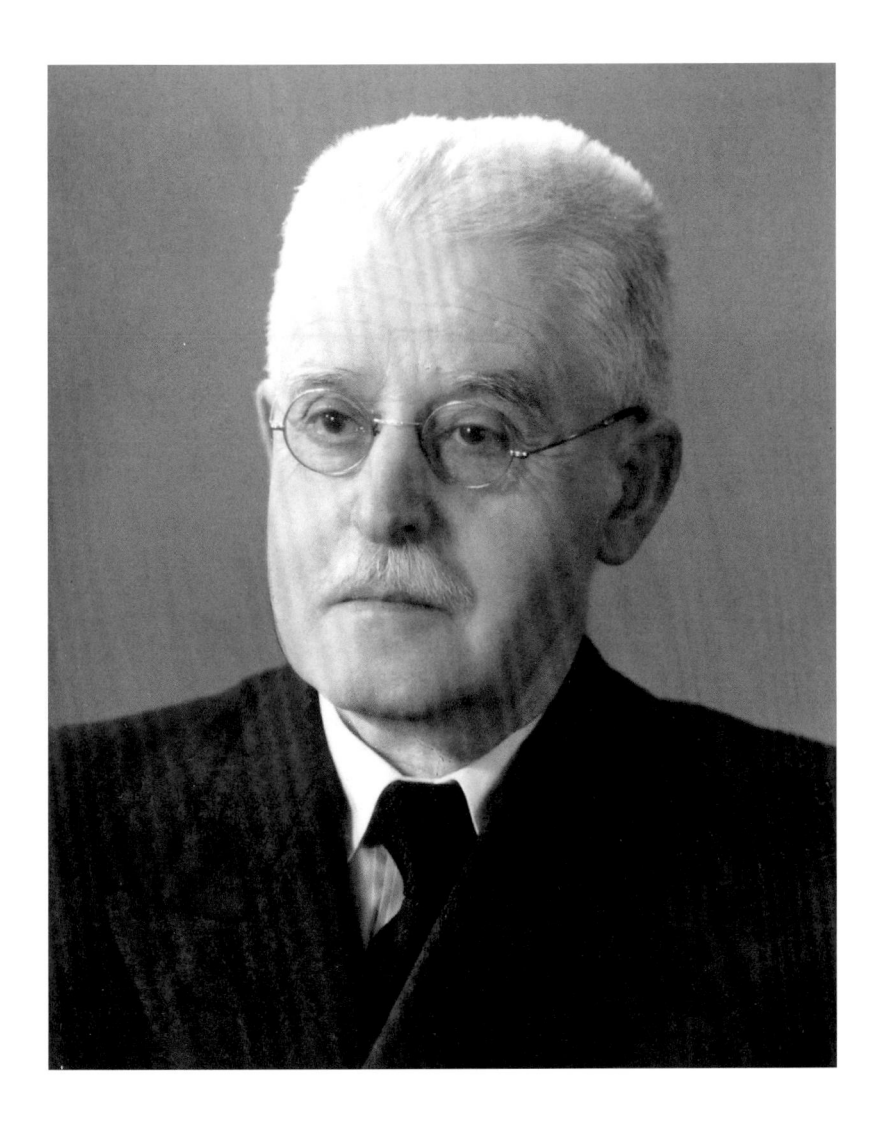

Fig. 88. Dr. Fritz Lotmar, 1878–1964

Born in Munich in 1878. 1888 moved to Bern. Attended the Progymnasium grammar school and then the Bern municipal grammar school with Paul Klee. Studied medicine in Bern, Heidelberg, Munich and Strasbourg. Further studies in Bern (under Prof. Hermann Sahli), Paris, Berlin and Munich. Specialized in psychiatry and neurology. 1913 PD in Bern. From 1918 worked at a private psychiatric and research institute in Munich. 1934 returned to Bern, practiced as a neurologist. Engaged in teaching and research. 1938 became a citizen of Bern. 1964 died in Bern. Fritz Lotmar was interested in literature, history, sociology and the visual arts; played violin in a quartet, like Klee, and had a very close friendship with Paul and Lily Klee. Dr. Lotmar did not treat Klee personally, but was constantly in contact with the Dr. Gerhard Schorer throughout his treatment of Klee's illness.

Details taken from Dr. Fritz Lotmar's obituary by Prof. Marco Mumenthaler, Bern, in the 'Mitteilungen der Naturforschenden Gesellschaft in Bern', vol. 22, Bern, September 1965, pp. 327 f. I would like to thank Prof. Urs Boschung, Director of the Institute of Medical History at the University of Bern, for providing me with a copy of the obituary, and Gerold Lotmar, Zurich, for the photo of his grandfather.

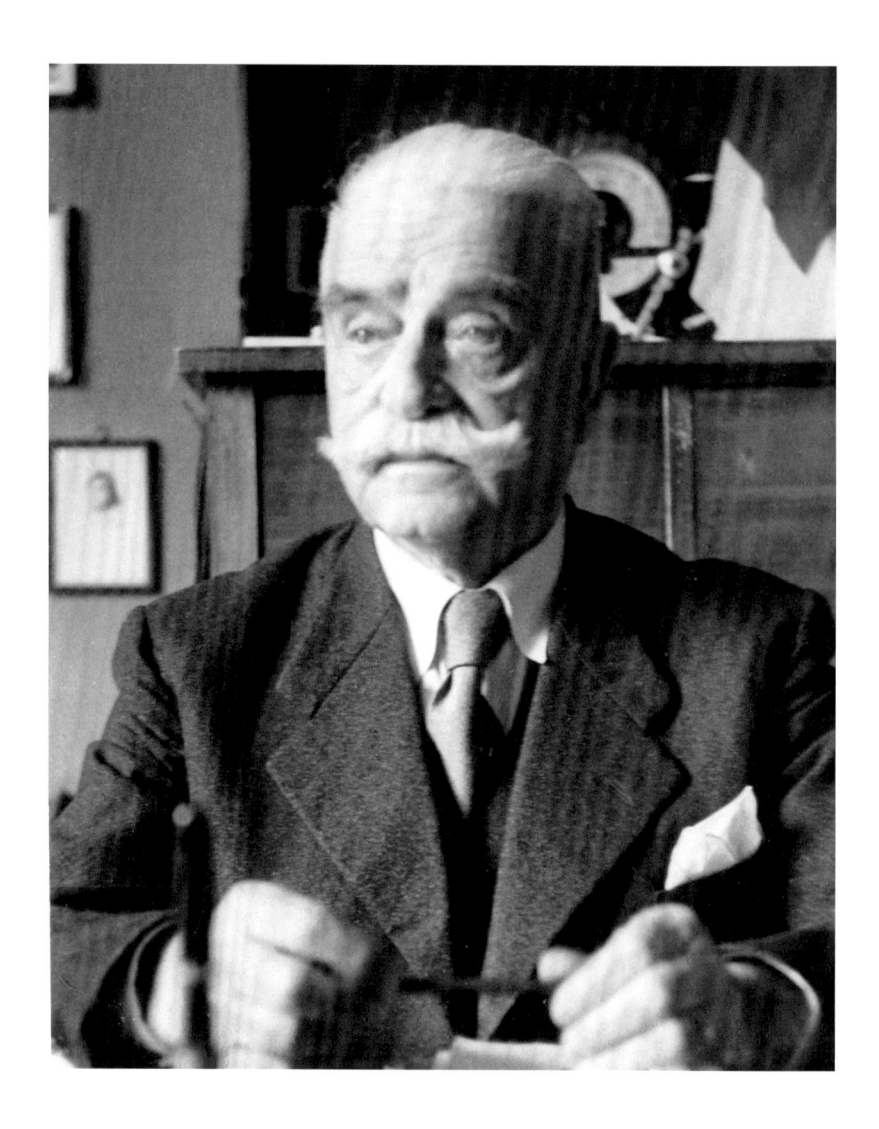

Fig. 89. Dr. Gerhard Schorer, 1878–1959

Details taken from the address given by Prof. Walter Frey, Professor Emeritus at the Medical Clinic of the University of Bern, at the funeral service for Dr. Schorer, Bern, January 9, 1959, and from Dr. Schorer's obituary by Dr. Hans W. Seelhofer, Worb (Bern), in 'Neue Berner Zeitung', Bern, January 8, 1959. I would like to thank Mrs. Marie Stössel-Schorer, Bern, for providing me with a copy of both the address and the obituary as well as the photo of her father.

Born in Heimiswil (Emmental, Bern) in 1878. Went to school in Burgdorf and Bern. Studied medicine in Bern and Berlin. Gained most of his great medical knowledge under Prof. Theodor Kocher and Prof. Hermann Sahli in Bern. From 1910 practiced for almost 50 years as an internist in Bern. From 1935 to 1940 was Paul Klee's family doctor. 1959 died in Bern. Prof. Walter Frey wrote of him: 'Gerhard Schorer was a remarkable man, powerful, genuine, idealistic. Patients found a true friend in him. He took his time when treating the sick, was dedicated, tactful and very knowledgeable. His bedside manner seemed a little influenced by the priests he had known while growing up in Heimiswil. His interests were both academic and scientific. His favorite topic was the influence of atmospheric factors on humans.'

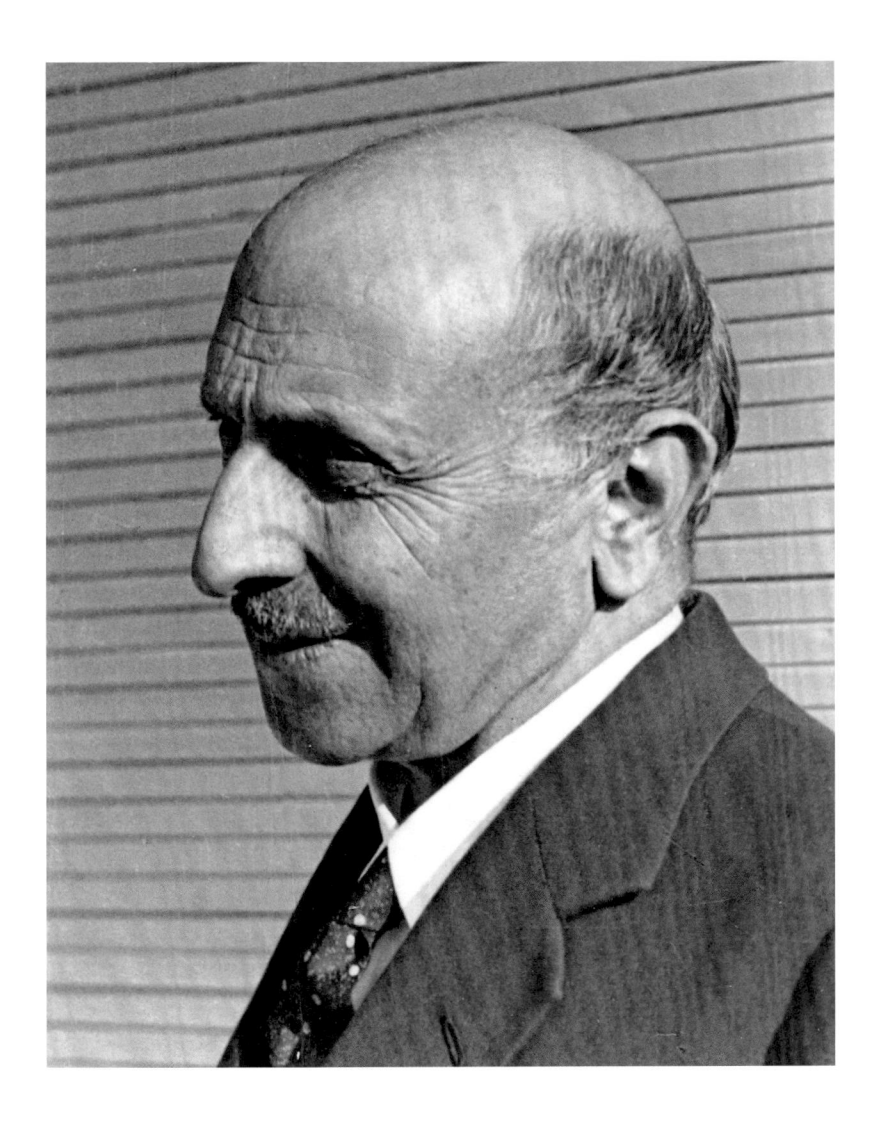

Fig. 90. Dr. Hermann Bodmer, 1876–1948

Born in Schaffhausen in 1876. Studied medicine in Zurich, Kiel and Munich. Further studies in Münsterlingen (Thurgau). Practiced as a general practitioner in Langnau (Bern). Suffered from pulmonary disease and moved to Davos for treatment. Further studies there to become an internist and specialist in pulmonary disease. Worked as a lung specialist in Davos-Clavadel and in Montana. From 1918 was chief physician at the renowned Sanatorium Viktoria in Locarno-Orselina and attending physician at the Clinica Sant' Agnese in Locarno-Muralto, where he treated Paul Klee in 1940 during his final stay there. Hermann Bodmer was active in the scientific fields of pulmonary and cardiovascular disease, infectiology, climatology and radioactivity. During the Second World War he had to give up his post as chief physician for health reasons, but continued in private practice. He died in Locarno-Monti in 1948.

Details taken from Dr. Bodmer's obituary by Dr. Otto Hug, Zurich, in the 'Schweizerische Medizinische Wochenschrift', vol. 78, 1948, no. 21, p. 523. I would like to thank Ms. Diana Bodmer, Zurich, for providing me with a copy of the obituary and the photo of her father.

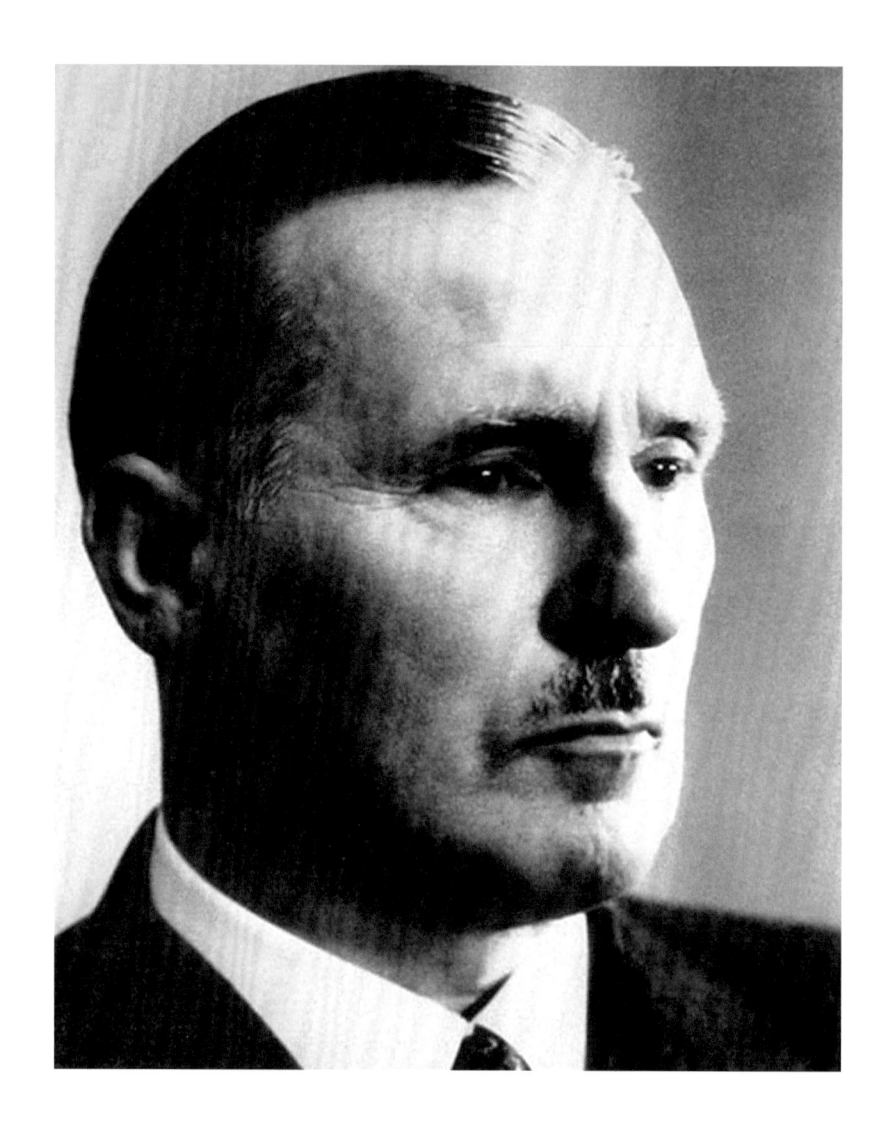

Fig. 91. Prof. Oscar Naegeli, 1885–1959

Born in Ermatingen (Thurgau) in 1885. Studied medicine in Geneva, Munich, Heidelberg and Zurich. 1909 took his state examinations in Zurich. Did his general practitioner training in Freiburg (Germany) and in Bern under the eminent dermatologist Prof. Joseph Jadassohn. 1917 associate professor, 1931 professor at the University Dermatology Clinic, Inselspital, Bern. In 1941 Prof. Naegeli had to give up his post for health reasons. He died in Freiburg (Switzerland) in 1959. Oscar Naegeli was a keen chess player and was Swiss chess champion for many years. His brother Otto Naegeli was also a professor of medicine: he gained an international reputation as a hematologist (specialist for blood disorders).

I would like to thank Prof. Urs Boschung, Director of the Institute of Medical History at the University of Bern, for providing me with biographical details about Prof. Naegeli, and Prof. Lasse R. Braathen, Director of the Dermatology Clinic and Polyclinic of the University of Bern, Inselspital, Bern, for the photo of Prof. Naegeli.

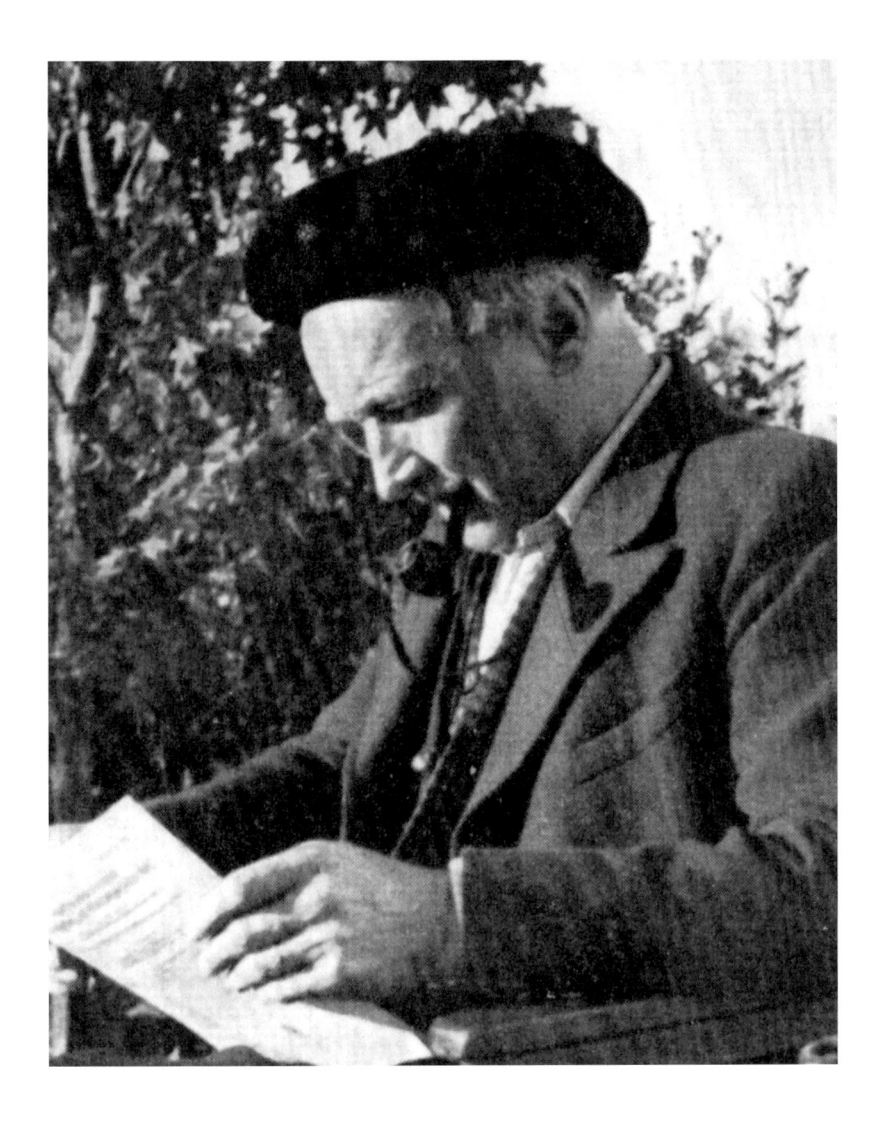

Fig. 92. Dr. Theodor Haemmerli, 1883–1944

Born in Lenzburg (Aargau) in 1883. Studied medicine in Zurich. Further studies in Munich and Zurich. Practiced as a general practitioner in Mürren (Bernese Oberland). Moved his practice to Zuoz (Grisons) before the Second World War. Later worked in the Sanatorium Valmont (Grisons). Had a particular interest in cardiovascular and circulatory diseases. Further studies in these fields in Paris, London and Vienna. 1928 opened a practice in Zurich as a specialist in cardiovascular disease. He was held in high regard for his expertise and kind, empathetic manner. He became the head of the Hirslanden Clinic in Zurich. Like Fritz Lotmar and Hermann Bodmer, he was a lover and patron of the fine arts. As with Hermann Bodmer, renowned artists would turn to him for help and advice. He died in 1944, four years after Paul Klee, also only 61 years old.

Details from Dr. Haemmerli's obituary by an unknown author with the initials 'tz' in the 'Neue Zürcher Zeitung', Zurich, July 5, 1944. I would like to thank Prof. Beat Rüttimann, Director of the Institute of Medical History and Museum of the University of Zurich, for providing me with a copy of the obituary, and Prof. Urs Boschung, Director of the Institute of Medical History at the University of Bern, for the photo of Dr. Haemmerli.

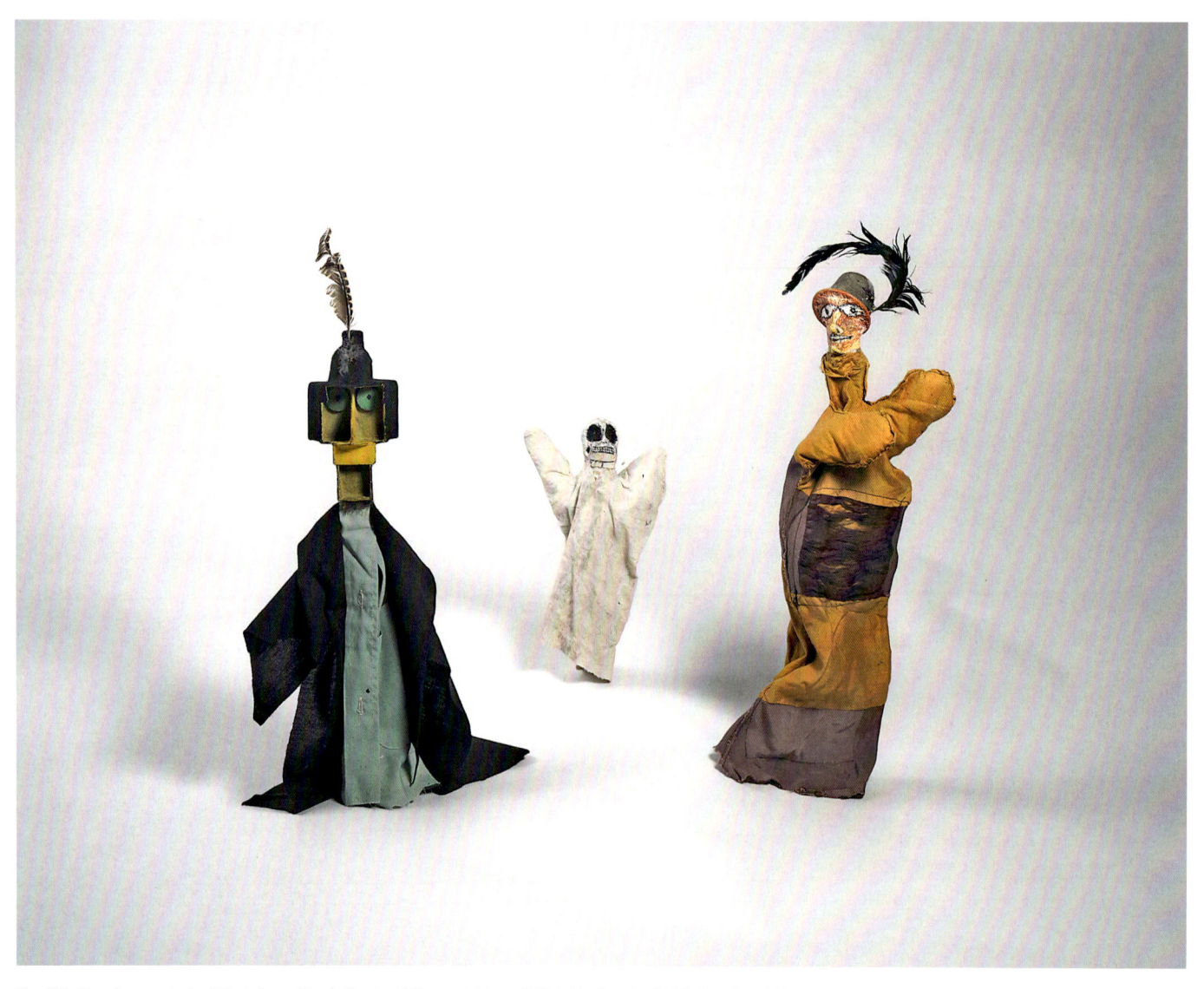

Fig. 93. Hand puppets (untitled, from l to r): Genie of the matchbox, 1925; Mr. Death, 1916; Bandit, 1923

3. Paul Klee's Personality

Before considering how his psyche and art were affected by circumstance and illness, it seems a good idea to try to put together a picture of Paul Klee's personality.

His wife **Lily Klee** writes in her 'Memoirs': 'No-one dared to behave badly in his presence, or to make low-grade conversation. He was a highly-educated man who endeavored throughout his life, alongside his immensely creative work, to further expand and develop his learning. He was a prolific reader. He worked harder than anyone I have ever met.'[411]

His son **Felix Klee** thinks back to his 'wonderful childhood': 'My father was so important as head of the family! I can never underestimate how he cared for me as a baby and how he was always at my side to offer me love and advice while I was growing up. My mother earned a living for the family by giving music lessons from morning till night in our small Munich apartment. So her husband, the unknown artist, had to run the household and look after my upbringing. He carried this out with aplomb! Our small kitchen was his domain, here he created paintings and drawings, did his etchings, developed photographs, washed the nappies and watched over the child. He was so clever at creating wonderful toys for me. I had a sailing ship, a railway station made totally of cardboard, and a puppet theater: plaster heads, puppets' clothes and scenery – he made everything himself. […] At home he always spoke the Bernese dialect including a few special 'Mattenenglisch' dialect words. He used it as a kind of secret language which people from outside Bern did not understand. His High German also bore distinct traces of his Alemannic origins. He was Bernese through and through. In later years, when he was much more comfortably off, he

[411] Klee [from 1942] (p. 258), p. 61 f.

remained the same simple, unassuming and unpretentious person he had always been. He did not spend a lot of money on himself; he just liked things that were of good, solid quality. To the outside world, he seemed a kind of reserved, slightly aloof magician, but within our little family he was always in a good mood, full of humor and jokes, a little sarcastic, with an easy-going vitality, and when he was amused he would laugh uproariously!'[412]

The art historian **Will Grohmann** describes his friend as follows: 'In his work, Klee often ties together opposites such as cold and heat, the arctic and the tropical; this juxtaposition of opposites reflects a fundamental trait of his temperament. This mixture of cold and heat lay within him, not in a discordant way but as an intrinsic part of his multifaceted personality. The mathematical existed happily alongside the fantastical, the visual alongside the musical, and the human alongside the cosmic. Indeed, these antitheses were potent forces which made up the unfathomable part of his personality. […] There was nothing Faustian about him, in fact he refused it. Growth and transformation were for him more inherent than the battle between the Absolute and the Self, and he would not have accepted the concept of the dual consciousness of the moment. He was aware of his own process of self-development, hence his calmness and assurance and the absence of dramatic or tragic complications in his life. Klee cocooned himself more and more within the life he had chosen for himself, and the emotions and agitations of his inner life came through in his artistic creation. For him, everything became an allegory, and hence his work exemplifies his life.'[413]

'He always thinks clearly, and he hates nothing more than vagueness.'[414] 'With his deep brown eyes, his hairstyle, his high forehead and olive skin, he could have been an Arab. There was something almost Oriental about him in his composure, his quiet movements, his deliberate and economical way of speaking. There was a story passed down in the family that they originated from Algiers, and this always came to mind when one was in his company, particularly when talking to him or viewing pictures together. A single word often stood for a whole sentence, and a sentence often for an al-

[412] Klee 1948, p. 14.
[413] Grohmann, 1965, p. 26.
[414] Ibid., p. 57.

legory, as is typical of the imagery-rich Orient.'[415] 'As a man and as a painter, Klee always rose above disputes and controversy. […] It is hard to say who Klee really was; he always kept his distance from life and was very reserved […].'[416] 'Klee's greatness lies in his single-mindedness and fidelity to his Self. He made great demands on himself and was always prepared to sacrifice success in order to further his personal growth. He paid no heed to success, was not carried away by fame and his only thought was how to do better. But this single-mindedness did not affect his sanguine disposition. He faced the most distressing events with equanimity and managed to turn them into something meaningful. He was also happy in his work, because it called forth his most potent forces; the more intensively he worked on an artistic level, the deeper the mysteries that were unveiled to him.'[417]

Georg Schmidt, Director of the Basel Museum of Fine Art, writes on Paul Klee: 'There is absolutely no other contemporary artist who comes close to having the richness of experience and form, the sense of realness in their work, as this most quiet, gentle, gracious and endearing artist of our time.'[418]

Ju Aichinger-Grosch, who nursed Paul Klee for several months,[419] states: 'Klee emanated a clarity, wisdom and goodness which I have never seen in another person.'[420]

Nina Kandinsky and her husband Wassily lived next door to Paul and Lily Klee at the Bauhaus school in Dessau for many years. She describes the artist as follows: 'Klee was a fascinating character. He seemed shy, because he always stayed in the background, but in reality he was not shy at all. We appreciated him for being such an attentive and patient listener, and for being such an unusually generous and helpful person. […] Paul Klee's death left a painful gap in [Wassily] Kandinsky's life that could never be filled.'[421]

Paul Klee was considerate, loyal and true. When friends advised him to consult with other doctors during his illness, he resolutely refused, continuing to place his trust in his family doctor.

[415] Grohmann, 1965, p. 64.
[416] Ibid., p. 377.
[417] Ibid., p. 382.
[418] Bloesch/Schmidt 1950, p. 10. Also quoted in Mendrisio 1990 [p. 178].
[419] Cf. Aichinger-Grosch 1959, p. 50.
[420] Ibid., p. 53.
[421] Kandinsky 1976, p. 201 f.

Hermann Rupf writes in March 1937: 'It is not possible to get anywhere with Paul Klee. The more you talk to him about another doctor, the less he wants to know about it. He even becomes angry. He says he has every confidence in Schorrer, who has experience of treating other similar cases, another doctor would not know any better, he is not prepared to lose him for the sake of having another consultation, which would not tell him anything more than he already knows, and he is not going to do anything else until he is better set up.'[422]

Wassily and Nina Kandinsky wanted their friend to have treatment from a renowned acupuncturist in Paris.[423] Paul Klee refused both this and a consultation with a homeopath in Lausanne, which was also recommended by the Kandinskys, along with Hermann and Margrit Rupf.[424] Lily Klee wrote to Nina Kandinsky in this regard: 'I spoke to my husband again at length about bringing in a homeopathic doctor. My husband doesn't want me to speak to our doctor, but he will speak to him personally as soon as he has resolved his stomach problems and diet. He does not want to start with a new doctor and new treatment at the moment, as he feels too weak and anyway he is not allowed to take medication before his stomach is fully healed. If he then feels much better and his strength has returned, he will talk to our doctor, who is the top internist in Bern, and a very illustrious doctor with great experience and totally modern methods. If our doctor agrees, then my husband would be prepared to consult the homeopathic doctor in Lausanne [Dr. Nebel]. At the moment we are not in a position financially to bring him here for a consultation.'[425]

Will Grohmann was also very worried about Paul Klee's illness. In March 1937 he tells Hermann Rupf: 'I am devastated by your news about Klee. I did not know that. The doctor [Dr. Schorer] said nothing, I have spoken to him once, Lily doesn't know, what about Klee himself? Of course I won't tell anyone but I would really like to know what it is. I never really trusted the diagnosis that Klee told me [we have no record of what Klee said to Grohmann about his illness[426]], and after my departure [end of November 1936] I was very worried and was constantly hoping that Klee would consult another

---

[422] Letter from Hermann Rupf to Wassily and Nina Kandinsky, Bern, March 22, 1937 (BK/CGPP).
[423] See Appendices: Wassily and Nina Kandinsky's Efforts to Have Paul Klee Treated by an Acupuncturist in Paris (p. 267).
[424] Cf. letter from Wassily Kandinsky to Lily Klee, Mürren, March 1, 1937, quoted in Kuthy 1984, p. 19. It referred to the homeopath Dr. Nebel.
[425] Letter from Lily Klee to Nina Kandinsky, Bern, February 28, 1937 (BK/CGPP).
[426] Verbal communication, Stefan Frey to the author, Bern, April 3, 2003.

expert. But it is Klee's opinions which count in this situation, and perhaps he is already too weak to make a decision. Is it tuberculosis.'[427] Grohmann had already written to Rupf: 'If only Prof. v. Bergmann were not so far away. He is still supposed to be the best internist.'[428]

Paul Klee's kind-heartedness and generosity are shown by how he decided to pass on his share of the inheritance to his unmarried sister Mathilde when their father died in 1940. She had stayed in the family home and looked after her father till the end, so she was given ownership of the house.[429]

Paul Klee was also held in high regard by his fellow artists and his students.

Gabriele Münter writes about Klee, who was a fellow-member of 'Der Blaue Reiter' group: '[…] he always seemed very collected, sure of himself, quietly creative, very significant, so that we immediately felt he was one of the greats who were creating a new art era at that time. […] We were drawn to his straightforward, totally genuine, diffident manner. He was not interested in widespread but insignificant concerns, and he kept out of the gossip, jealousy and resentments of his colleagues. He would quite openly refuse to get involved.'[430]

Lyonel Feininger, who was a fellow teacher of Paul Klee's at the Bauhaus school, reflects on his late colleague as follows: 'Klee was a man who possessed deep wisdom and extraordinary knowledge. He was a timeless person of indeterminate age, but he had a child-like fascination and curiosity for what his senses, his eyes and ears, his touch and taste could teach him. He was a mature person, who expected his clear intelligence to retain control at all times. Klee was always very deliberate and collected in his movements, he never lost his temper, there was no need for outbursts. […] He always seemed to be listening to an inner voice. His subtle use of irony was charming, and even when he said something mocking, he never did it unpleasantly, but with a gentle half-smile. He was very direct, but not to the point of being offensive. His personality cast a spell over people. […] We will always carry with us the clear image of Klee's enduring, simple and endearing greatness.'[431]

---

[427] Letter from Will Grohmann to Hermann Rupf, Dresden, March 16, 1937 (HMRS).

[428] Letter from Will Grohmann to Hermann Rupf, Dresden, March 10, 1937 (HMRS). Prof. Gustav von Bergmann, 1878–1955. From 1927–1945 Director of the 2nd Medical University Clinic Charité, Berlin, and from 1945–1953 Director of the 2nd Medical University Clinic, Munich.

[429] Cf. Frey 1990, p. 122.

[430] Münter 1959, p. 40.

[431] Feininger 1959, pp. 72 and 75.

Oskar Schlemmer, another Bauhaus colleague, writes about Paul Klee: 'He can convey the whole of his wisdom in just one or two lines. This is how a Buddha would draw. Serene and at peace, unmoved by passions, the least monumental of lines conveys greatness through its child-like, inquiring quality. It is everything; deep, subtle and above all, it is new. […] The acts of all great people are rooted in a simple but all-embracing knowledge. Finding this knowledge means finding oneself, and through this the world and everything in it.'[432]

Walter Gropius, the founder and head of the Bauhaus school in Weimar, which moved to Dessau in 1925, confirms that Paul Klee was valued by his colleagues for his natural authority and that he became 'a figure of moral authority at the Bauhaus.'[433]

The students revered their teacher.[434] They gave him nicknames such as 'dear god' and 'Buddha' (fig. 94).[435] Klee's charisma stemmed from his great intelligence and ability, his composure and rectitude, his calm and quiet manner, his integrity and humanity. One of his students says: 'He did not teach in the normal sense of the word. He revealed to witnesses the vastness of his thoughts and experience.'[436]

The art historian **Carola Giedion-Welcker**, who knew the Klees, describes the artist and teacher as follows: 'Paul Klee was always a loner, although he was involved in an objective way with the general artistic problems of the day; he was a quiet, inward-looking and individualistic person, but also a very dedicated and gifted teacher.'[437] And: 'His students say that outwardly his classes were quiet and peaceful. Klee emanated a sense of absorption and insularity which subconsciously affected his audience as he stood at the board, drawing simultaneously with both hands while illustrating his ideas and explaining in detail his thought and creative processes.'[438] It also seems that Rudolf Steiner and Joseph Beuys taught in a similar way.

There is no doubt that Paul Klee was a self-confident person, but when dealing with other people he always remained un-

---

[432] Schlemmer, Oskar, Diary, September 1916, quoted in Giedion-Welcker 2000, p. 161.
[433] Grohmann 1965, p. 61: 'Klee always stood above things, as Gropius says, he became "a figure of moral authority at the Bauhaus". Teachers and students all valued his quiet manner and jokingly called him "dear god".' On p. 377 Grohmann describes Klee as 'the "highest figure of moral authority" not only at the Bauhaus.'
[434] Cf. Muth 1959, Kerkovius 1959, Schawinsky 1959, Kuhr 1959, and Hertel 1959.
[435] Cf. Geelhaar 1979: 'The students at the Bauhaus supposedly gave their teacher nicknames such as "dear god" and "Buddha".' My thanks to Michael Baumgartner for the copy of Christian Geelhaar's article.
[436] Quoted by Jürg Spiller, in: Spiller 1956, p. 21 of the introduction. The name of the student is not given.
[437] Giedion-Welcker 2000, p. 8.
[438] Ibid., p. 69 f.

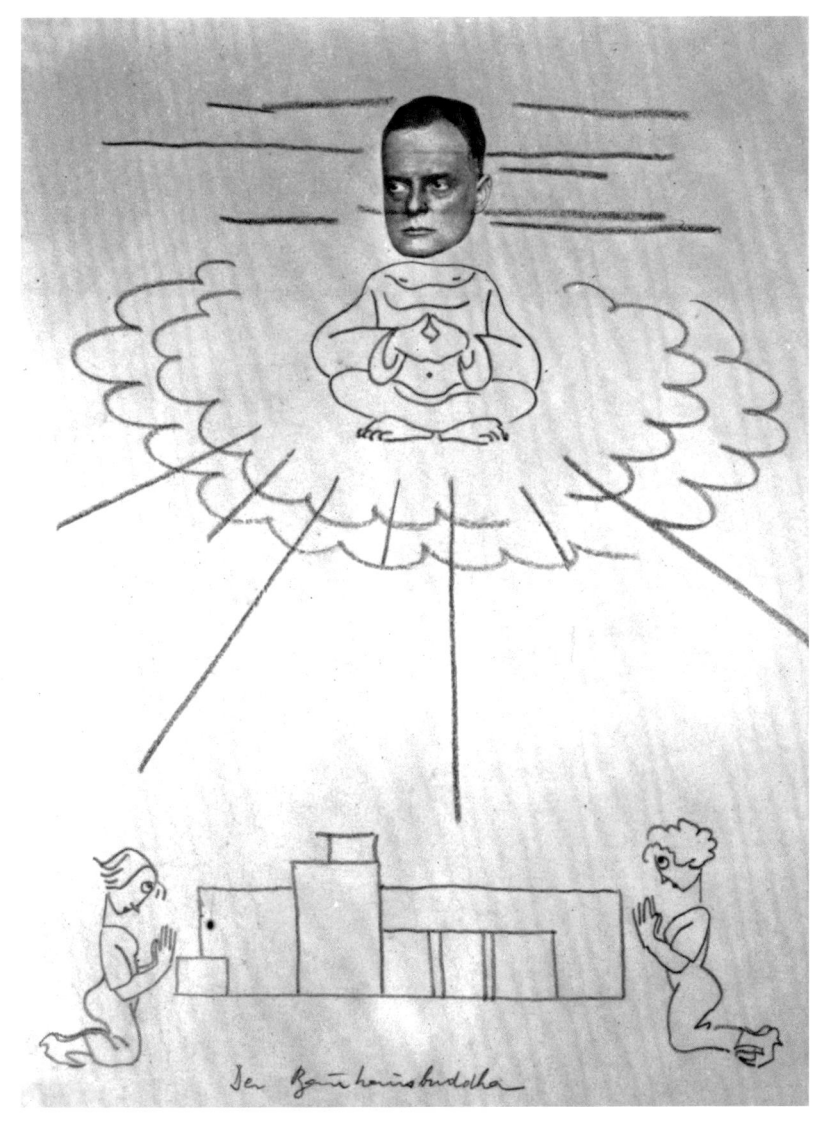

Fig. 94. Ernst Kállai, Caricature of Paul Klee. Written at the bottom is: 'Der Bauhausbuddha' (The Bauhaus Buddha), undated (Bauhaus Archive, Berlin)

assuming and tolerant. He believed his art would be considered significant in the future, so for instance he revised his diaries 'for posterity'.[439] He worked doggedly and single-mindedly to achieve his standing as an artist.

Klee also never bore grudges. This is shown in two instances: firstly, in 1935 a married couple who were slight acquaintances [Hassler-Christen, Schaffhausen] were thinking about buying the painting 'Polyphony', so they took it home with them for further consideration. They confirmed by telephone that they wanted to purchase the painting, but then wrote

[439] Hopfengart 1989, p. 216.

saying they had changed their minds. There was then a long hiatus before the painting was returned to Klee. Lily Klee was of the opinion that a verbal agreement to buy was binding and wanted to engage a lawyer. But Klee remained unperturbed and refrained from legal action.[440] In another instance, in 1940 the art collector Dr. Othmar Huber from Glarus bought the painting 'Fairy tale of the dwarf', 1925, 255, directly from the artist, but then wanted to exchange it for another picture.[441] He approached Paul Klee directly about this, as the art historian Madeleine Schuppli relates: 'He [Othmar Huber] still liked the picture. "But it has the disadvantage of not being decorative in any way. On the wall it just looks like a hole, so it spends most of its time in the cupboard, which is really a shame." Paul Klee wrote back to him, seeming in his letter to be not in the least offended, but rather showing he was prepared to cooperate with the potential buyer: "[…] and you will have the feeling that I am willing to bow to your wishes".'[442]

Fig. 95. Mourning, 1934, 8, with the dedication: 'for Lily, Xmas 1934'

A Christmas present from Paul Klee to his wife in 1934. He draws the outline of a woman, sunk in grief, with a continuous black line. Her eyes are downcast, the edges of her mouth turned down. It could be Lily herself, one year after she and her husband were expelled from Germany, her adopted home, and one year after their emigration and less-than-warm welcome in Switzerland. The base of the painting is made up of countless small, drab squares. Within the female figure itself, however, there are numerous bright red, blue and green squares among the monotone colors: perhaps he is using his art to try to cheer her up?

[440] Cf. letters from Lily Klee to Will Grohmann of June 9, 1935, September 12, 1935, October 23, 1935, and December 2, 1935.
[441] Cf. Schuppli, Madeleine, in: Glarus 1995, p. 34.
[442] Ibid., Madeleine Schuppli refers to the letters from Dr. Othmar Huber to Paul Klee, Glarus, April 9, 1940 (ZPKB/SFK), and from Paul Klee to Dr. Othmar Huber, Bern, April 14, 1940 (private collection, Switzerland).

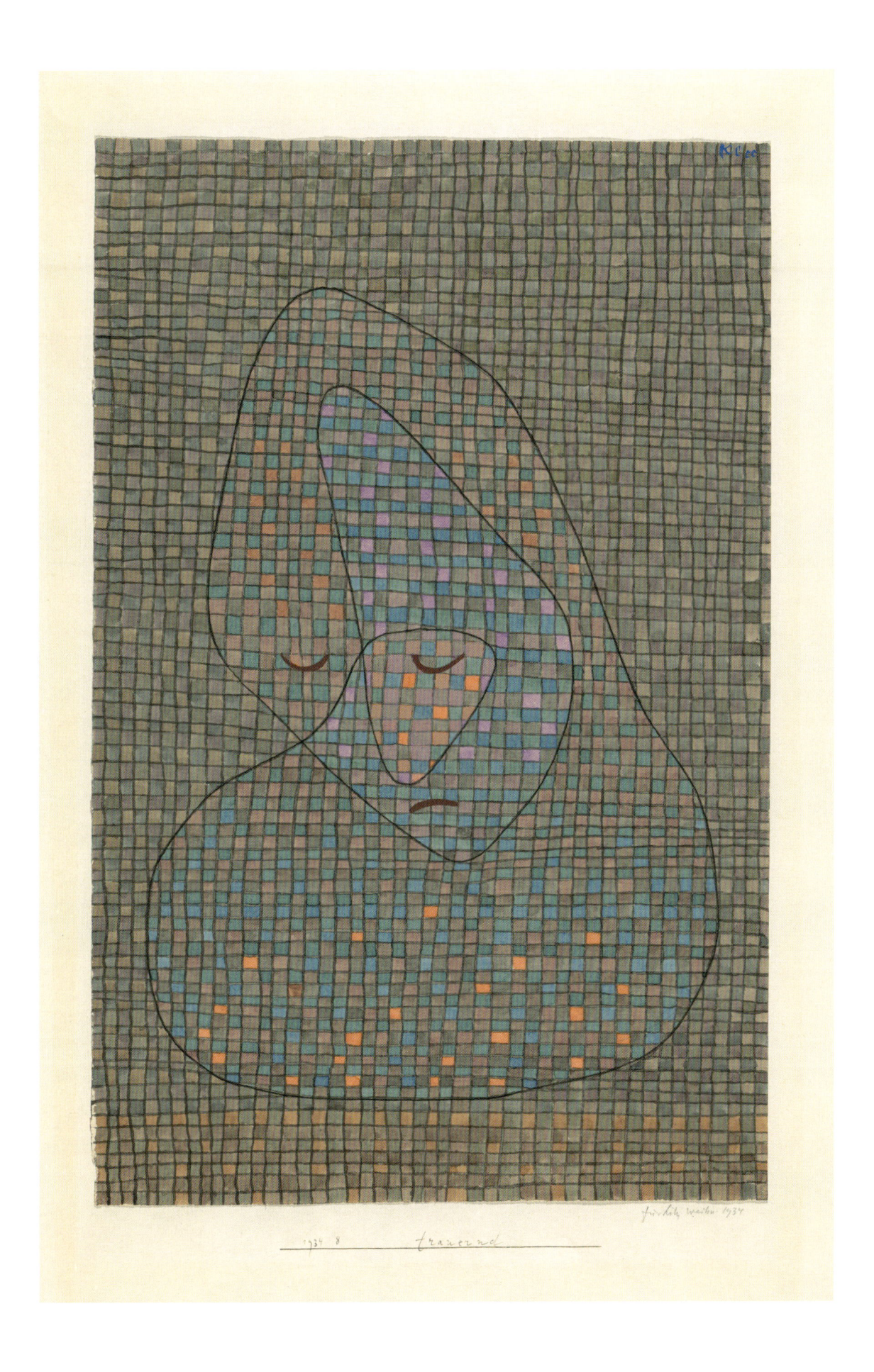

Paul Klee painted this portrait in gloomy red and black in the year that his illness started. The painting may well be a self-portrait. The artist is disappointed by his job dismissal and his defamation by the National Socialists. Perhaps he also has a sense of what his own personal fate may be. The head is shrouded in a dark hood. The large black eyes gaze at us in a serious, sad and questioning way. Klee sees himself as a 'marked man'. (Art historian Werner Schmalenbach interprets the painting in a similar way.[443]) Significantly, the only two straight lines running from top to bottom and left to right meet in the middle of the face – like in the painting 'Struck from the list' (fig. 18, page 22). Starting from these lines, we can then make out a swastika in the middle of the face. The triangular nose is mirrored by a similar isosceles triangle between the eyes. The two geometric elements make up the shape of an hour glass. Time is running out for Paul Klee.

---

[443] Cf. Schmalenbach 1986, p. 93.

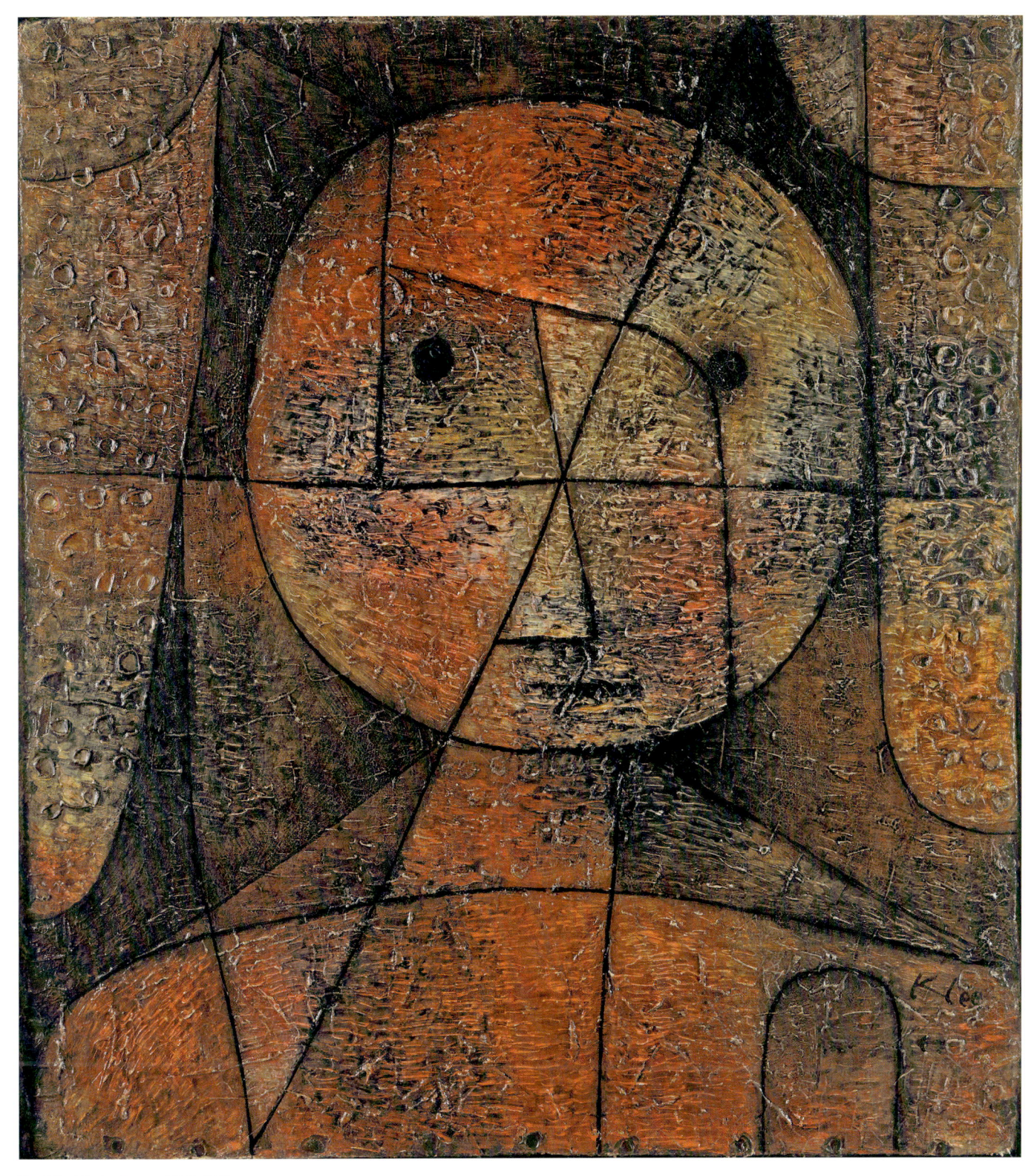

Fig. 96. Marked man, 1935, 146

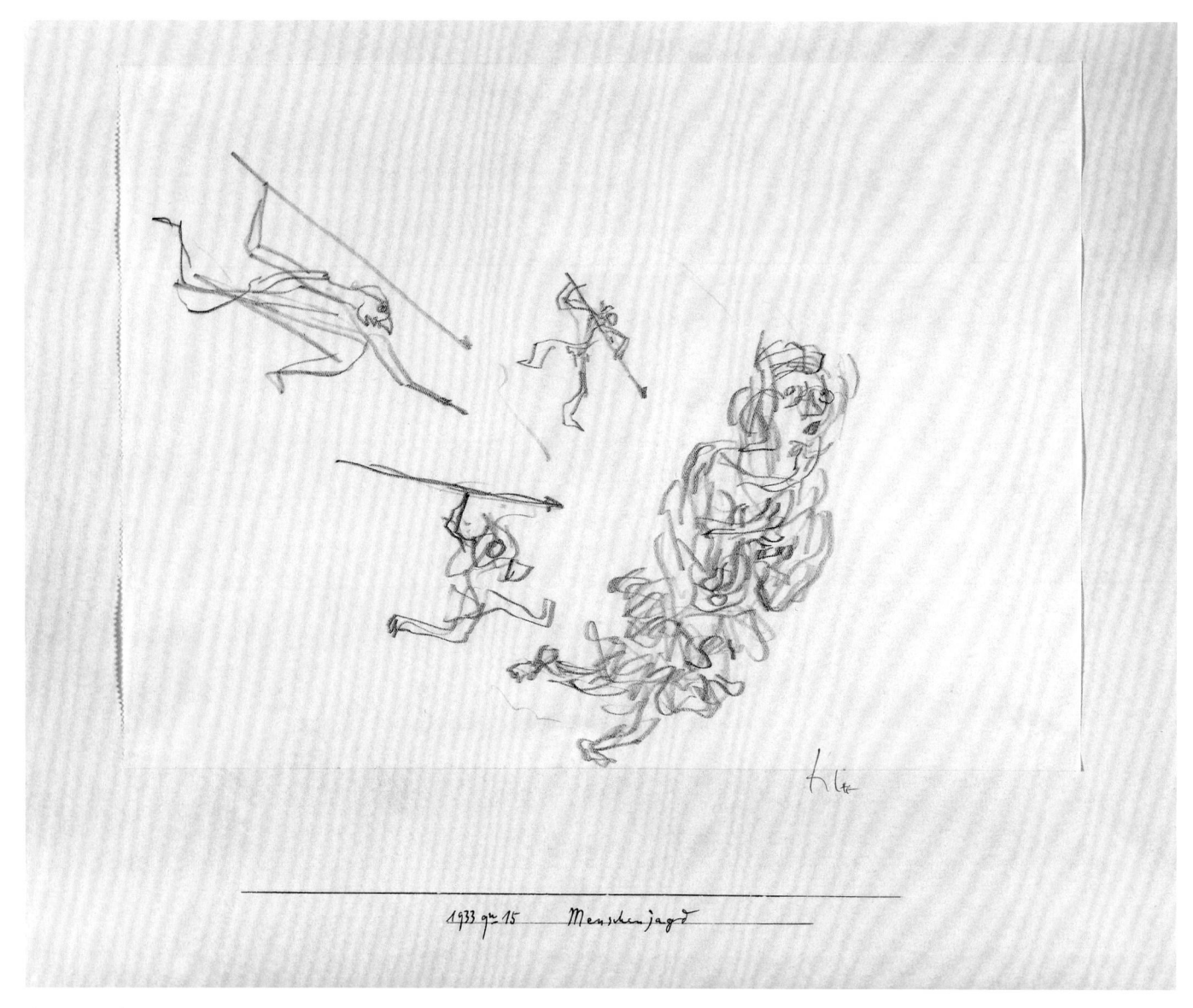

Fig. 97. Manhunt, 1933, 115

4. The Effects of Adversity and Illness on Paul Klee's Mind and Work

Robust Psyche

'I have a tendency towards ruin, but I also tend to quickly pull myself out of it,'[444] wrote the 26-year-old Paul Klee. As a highly intuitive person, did he have a premonition of the difficulties which lay ahead? The artist was clearly mentally very robust and of an optimistic disposition. Nevertheless, the events of 1933 in Germany hit him hard and undoubtedly cast a shadow over him. But, in his normal way, he kept this to himself. Even after the onset of his illness, and despite his suffering, he remained open and spontaneous, genial and even-tempered.[445] Felix Klee told me that his father did not like to speak about his illness.[446] He tried to push it to the back of his mind, as Will Grohmann also attests.[447]

In this way Paul Klee adopted an attitude which is very common among the terminally ill. The Bern psychiatrist Professor Edgar Heim describes it as follows: 'In this situation, as also when dealing with general problems in life, it can sometimes be helpful to block things out or go into denial. It is a way for the sufferer to win himself some time in order to come to terms with an unexpected situation or psychological crisis, which is always the case in the event of serious illness.'[448] The artist acted in the way that Edgar Heim described as being necessary for patients coping with serious illness: '[…] acknowledging and accepting the […] condition – the pain, disability and other symptoms of the illness or injury, […] keeping an emotional balance whereby the sufferer needs to move beyond the fear, uncertainty and confusion caused by

[444] Klee 1960/2, p. 63 (1905).
[445] Personal communication, Felix Klee to the author, Bern, September 20, 1983.
[446] As above, Bern, September 20, 1983.
[447] Cf. Grohmann 1965, p. 84.
[448] Heim/ML 1980, p. 75.

the illness, […and] calling upon the resources, reserves, help, abilities and possibilities within himself and others which could contribute to recovery, stabilization or, at the very least, a sense of inner equilibrium.'[449]

Edgar Heim writes that the seriously ill can develop an identity crisis due to their weakness and physical disability.[450] ('Identity' in this context means that which a person experiences as the 'Self'.)[451] He also notes that those with severe illnesses often are fearful: '[…] fear of losing that sense of identity, which is essential to all of us in order to feel we are both integrated and unique.'[452]

Klee had every reason to suffer a deep identity crisis, even before his illness took hold. He lost his job as a respected professor of art, he was denigrated as an artist, and he lost many friends due to his forced removal to Bern, where he also experienced a great sense of artistic isolation.

We can imagine how hard it was for him to deal with these setbacks and face up to his uncertain future. His strength of will, his optimism, his family, his few friends and his unshakeable belief in his art carried him through this difficult time. Perhaps he thought back to the note he wrote in 1900: 'The storm gives me clarity and life holds me in its thrall.'[453]

When Klee became ill in 1935, he was just 55 years old. Without the illness he could reasonably have expected to live another 20 years: a long time for such a productive artist at the height of his powers. He would have felt that he only had a relatively short time left, at most a few years. He suddenly found himself in a position where he did not know how many more works he could produce, and he was afraid he would be unable to fulfill his great artistic potential. But his mental strength enabled him to gather his energies and take a positive attitude towards the uncertainties he faced. He had withstood the crisis years of 1933–1936 through his belief in himself and his art. He now once again drew on his inner strength, and as the end approached he could be satisfied that, despite his illness, he had produced an important body of late work to round off his oeuvre.

[449] Heim/ML 1980, p. 79 f.
[450] Cf. ibid., p. 80.
[451] Cf. Duden, Fremdwörterbuch, 3rd ed., vol. 5, Bibliographisches Institut, Dudenverlag, Mannheim/Wien/Zürich 1974, p. 311.
[452] Heim/ML 1980, p. 107.
[453] Klee 1960/2, p. 21 [1900].

Jürgen Glaesemer notes: 'Scleroderma often brings about a psychopathic syndrome, which can be so pronounced, that the term "sclerodermic personality" is used in medical jargon. Anxiety, depression and nightmares are all symptoms of this "physically induced psychosis".'[454] He includes here references to W. Gottwald and J. Benos.[455] Glaesemer continues: 'In order to answer the question of whether and in what form Klee's mind was affected by specific symptoms of the disease, it would be necessary to carry out a detailed analysis of all the available facts according to neurological and psychiatric criteria. Klee suffered in no way from mental illness or even from a reduction in his mental capacities. His illness should be understood as part of his being, and thus particular characteristics of his individual psyche are realized within it.'[456] I am in full agreement with Jürgen Glaesemer on this. Serious physical illness always has psychological effects. Outwardly, Paul Klee always seemed calm and collected. He was not inclined to depression[457] and did not suffer from a 'physically induced psychosis', as described by Gottwald and Benos. (Here 'psychosis' refers to a mental disorder with loss of contact with reality. There are organic, physically induced psychoses and nonorganic functional psychoses.[458]) But Klee's works clearly show that there were times when his mental state was affected by his illness. His illness progressed in fits and starts: phases of remission would raise his hopes, only to have them dashed once more as his condition worsened, bringing attendant feelings of anxiety, despondency, doubt, despair and fear. These different states can be seen in his work, particularly in his drawings (for example figs. 98, 99, 101, 103, 104, 107, 108, 110 to 113, 117, 118, 125, 126).

Paul Klee probably knew intuitively that he had a terminal illness, but he did not resist the disease, rather he tried to accept it as his fate. However, totally honest man that he was, he did not try to conceal his anxiety and fear. Fear is a basic instinct which puts us on alert and warns us of impending danger. We feel afraid when we get a serious illness: are we going to suffer a lot of pain? Could it even be life-threatening? Edgar Heim writes in this respect: 'As the physical condition deteriorates, there is a corresponding effect on the mind, and conversely the patient's mental attitude can affect

[454] Glaesemer 1976, p. 318, note 17.
[455] Cf. Gottwald and Benos/ML 1974.
[456] Glaesemer 1976, p. 318, note 17.
[457] Personal communication, Felix Klee to the author, Bern, September 20, 1983.
[458] Pschyrembel/ML 1998, p. 1315.

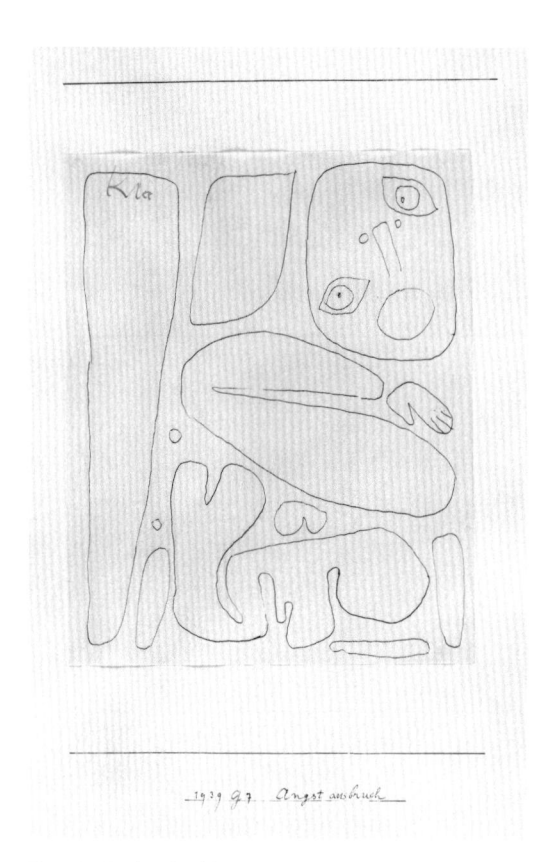

Fig. 98. Outbreak of fear, 1939, 27

the progression of the disease. A little-known study comparing one hundred terminally-ill patients with one hundred seriously, but not terminally, ill patients[459] showed the following: The terminally-ill patients were much more affected emotionally than the seriously ill. 70% suffered from anxiety states (compared to 50% of the non-terminal patients).'[460]

Klee's thoughts and feelings were taken up by his own situation, but at the same time he always felt concern about the political developments in Germany. He had experienced first hand the arrogance of the new rulers, their racist tendencies and their debasement of opponents. He avoided talking about it, as he wished to spare himself yet another burden, but as a sensitive person he could not simply sweep it under the carpet. He and his wife could not be indifferent to the political changes in Germany, as their son and several close friends lived and worked there.

I am convinced that Klee foresaw at an early stage the brutality which would emanate from the National Socialists, the suffering which would be caused, the impending war and the catastrophe which would engulf Europe. Jürgen Glaesemer points to this: 'In the days after Hitler seized power, Klee foresaw the events to come.'[461] He was not only 'avant-garde' in his art, but also in the literal sense of the word someone who was 'in advance', someone who could foresee world events. So it is very possible that the drawings and paintings he produced on the theme of 'fear' actually portend the fear, misery and desperation of those who suffered oppression and persecution in Nazi Germany. The intensity of Klee's work brings to mind works by other artists on the same theme, such as the drawings of Käthe Kollwitz, the etchings of Gregor Rabinovitch and the paintings of Edvard Munch.

Jürgen Glaesemer refers to the fact that as early as 1934, after his dismissal by the Nazis but before the onset of his illness, Klee produced a panel painting entitled 'Fear', 1934, 202.[462] He compares it with the two pen drawings 'Outbreak of fear', 1939, 27 (fig. 98)[463] and 'Outbreak of fear II', 1939, 110[464] and with the watercolor 'Outbreak of fear III', 1939, 124 (fig. 99), writing about the latter that: '[...] the move-

[459] Cf. Hinton/ML 1963, quoted by Edgar Heim in: Heim/ML 1980, p. 105.
[460] Ibid.
[461] Glaesemer 1984, p. 342.
[462] Cf. Glaesemer 1976, p. 335.
[463] Klee also gave it a subtitle: 'Screams of fear'.
[464] This pen drawing is identical to the previous one (fig. 98), but more than twice the size.

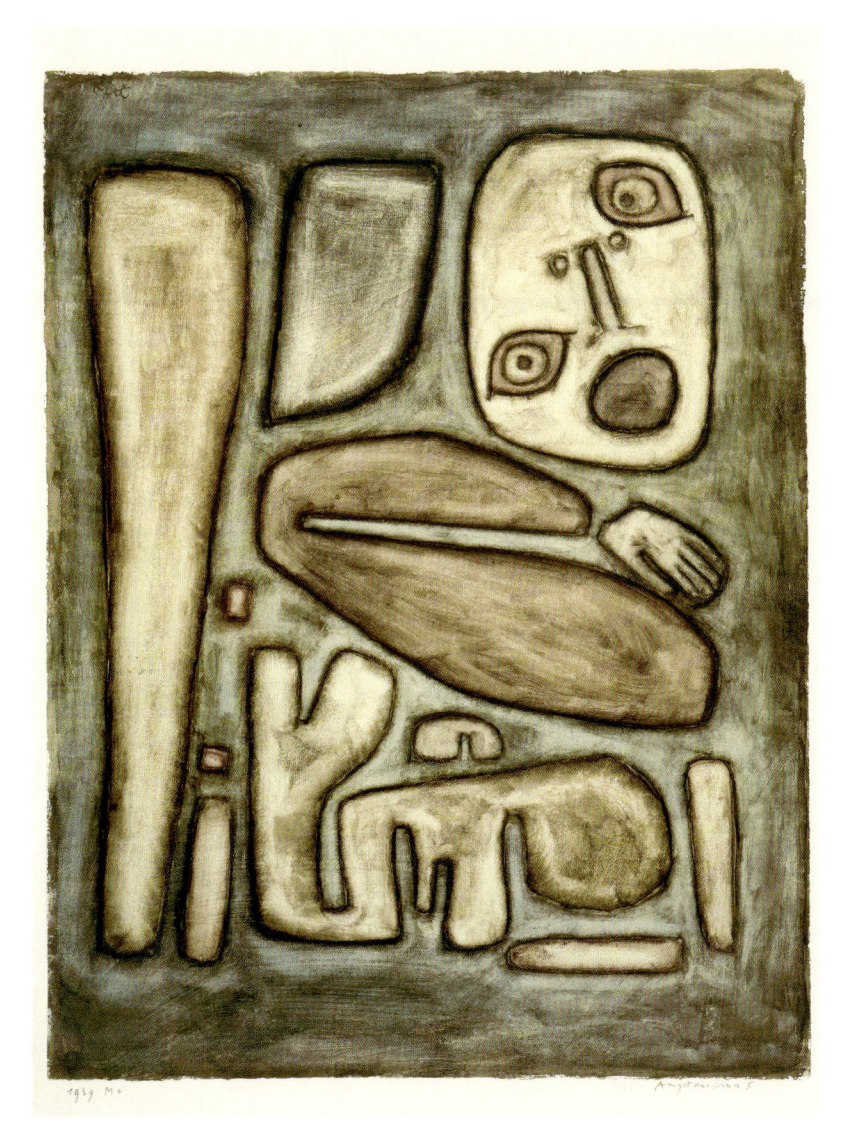

Fig. 99. Outbreak of fear III, 1939, 124

ment from abstract generalities to personal expression cannot be ignored. In his later watercolors, human despair takes on a concrete form, forcing us to make the connection between this motif and Klee's own situation. His personal suffering is reflected in certain figures, but it would nevertheless be a mistake to ascribe a very specific biographical situation to a composition such as "Outbreak of fear".'[465]

So Klee was able to conceptualize his personal experiences and transform his emotions into art. Mentally and intellectually he was able to create a kind of distance from his illness, shaping his inner trauma into drawings and paintings, trans-

[465] Glaesemer 1976, p. 335 f.

Re. Figs. 98 and 99

Paul Klee is seriously ill. It is only natural that he should experience some fear. As in many other drawings and individual paintings from the years 1937–1939, the human bodies depicted are breaking apart. Jürgen Glaesemer comments: 'At the beginning of 1939 he [Klee] did a series of drawings which mirror human suffering in an extreme way. Figures appear whose bodies break up agonizingly into different parts. Hands, arms, legs and unspecified body parts come apart and are scattered across the paper in whole pieces, like individual islands. Only the head has details drawn within its outline, causing it to stand out from the rest of the parts. But here too the large eyes, the nose and the open mouth start to slip and fall into disarray. The faces mostly appear to be suffering, despairing, distorted with pain or simply resigned.'[466]

The head, with the big eyes full of fear and the wide open mouth, is reminiscent of what is probably Edvard Munch's most famous picture: 'The Scream' from 1893.[467] This painting is also a reflection of personal experience. However, as Paul Klee was mentally much stronger than Edvard Munch, he was better able to live with his fear.

ferring his worries to paper and canvas. This meant that all through his illness he could still create works which were totally detached from what he was undergoing psychologically.

It seems that Klee had no fear of dying, as is shown by a comment he made in 1930: 'Death is nothing bad; I long ago reconciled myself to it.'[468] Edgar Heim writes that patients who believe in God are less fearful in their final days than those who are non-believers: 'There is no doubt that deeply religious people normally have less fear of dying, as they are afforded hope by their belief in the afterlife.'[469] Paul Klee was a religious man (fig. 100) and he believed in an afterlife. In 1915 he wrote in his diary: 'One leaves the realm of here and now and builds forward into the beyond which is still allowed to be an absolute "Yes".'[470]

---

[466] Glaesemer 1976, p. 334 f.

[467] Eggum, Arne (PhD, Director of the Munch Museum, Oslo), in: Eggum 1998, p. 225: 'This, Munch's best-known composition, has become a symbol of the existential angst of civilized man'. And: Chiappini, Rudy (PhD, art historian, Director of Lugano City Museums), ibid., p. 84: '[…] An inescapable earthly fate which burdens mankind and is the central theme of the section "Fear of Living" containing "The Scream" (1893), Munch's best-known work, which has become a symbol of modern man, of his alienation and existential anguish.'

[468] Quoted in Petitpierre 1957, p. 65 (see also note 573), and cf. Grohmann 1965, p. 358. Grohmann dates this quotation to 1930.

[469] Heim/ML 1980, pp. 105 and 106.

[470] Klee Diary, no. 951.

Let us briefly return to Jürgen Glaesemer's question, '[...] whether and in what form Klee's mind was affected by specific symptoms of the disease, and how this was expressed in his work [...]' (see page 129, note 456). We can now answer the question as follows: Klee's mind displays no specific scleroderma-related characteristics, and psychosis can be ruled out. However, his illness is clearly reflected in his later work (see Chapter 5). And if, as suggested by E.G.L. Bywaters, scleroderma sufferers often develop a huge burst of creative energy (see page 97, note 367), this would seem to apply to Klee: his 'hyperactivity' led to a massive increase in productivity.

Every human being is unique. This means that everyone reacts differently to trauma, misfortune and bad news. Most people are shocked if they are caught off-guard by a diagnosis of a terminal illness.

In my experience, many patients know intuitively that they have a terminal illness because of the doctor's behavior and the medical procedures they undergo. So it is astonishing that they then often do not want to be faced with a concrete diagnosis or prognosis, indeed they often try to avoid it. Times have changed, and doctors now believe that they cannot conceal a diagnosis of terminal illness. Their patients expect honesty from them so that they can prepare themselves for whatever time remains. This is the right thing to do, but the doctor must be careful to treat his patient with empathy, taking a step-by-step approach and supporting his patient's hope of recovery, even if that hope is nothing more than a glimmer. I have treated several elderly skin-cancer sufferers whose prognosis was statistically hopeless, but who nonetheless survived. I once had another patient who was dying of cancer. Her sister nursed her day and night, always there to care for her and cheer her up, and amazingly she recovered. Miracles do happen. Doctors should be a little guarded in their prognoses, as their patients' outcomes can be unpredictable.

Paul Klee had a robust constitution; he was mentally very stable and had a superior intellect. It was important to him to achieve a sense of stability, even when he was personally

Eine Art von Stille leuchtet zum Grund.
Von ungefähr
scheint da ein Etwas,
nicht von hier,
nicht von mir,
sondern Gottes.
Gottes! Wenn auch nur Widerhall,
nur Gottes Spiegel,
so doch Gottes Nähe
Tropfen von tief,
Licht an sich.
Wer je schlief und der Atem stand:
der ......
Das Ende heim zum Anfang fand.

A kind of stillness illumines the ground.
From something vague
a something shines,
not from here,
not from me,
but of God.
Of God! Even if only an echo,
only God's mirror,
God is still near
Drops from deep,
Light in itself.
Who ever has slept and breathing paused:
he ......
Has found the end to be the beginning.

Fig. 100. Poem by Paul Klee from his diary of 1914, no. 948

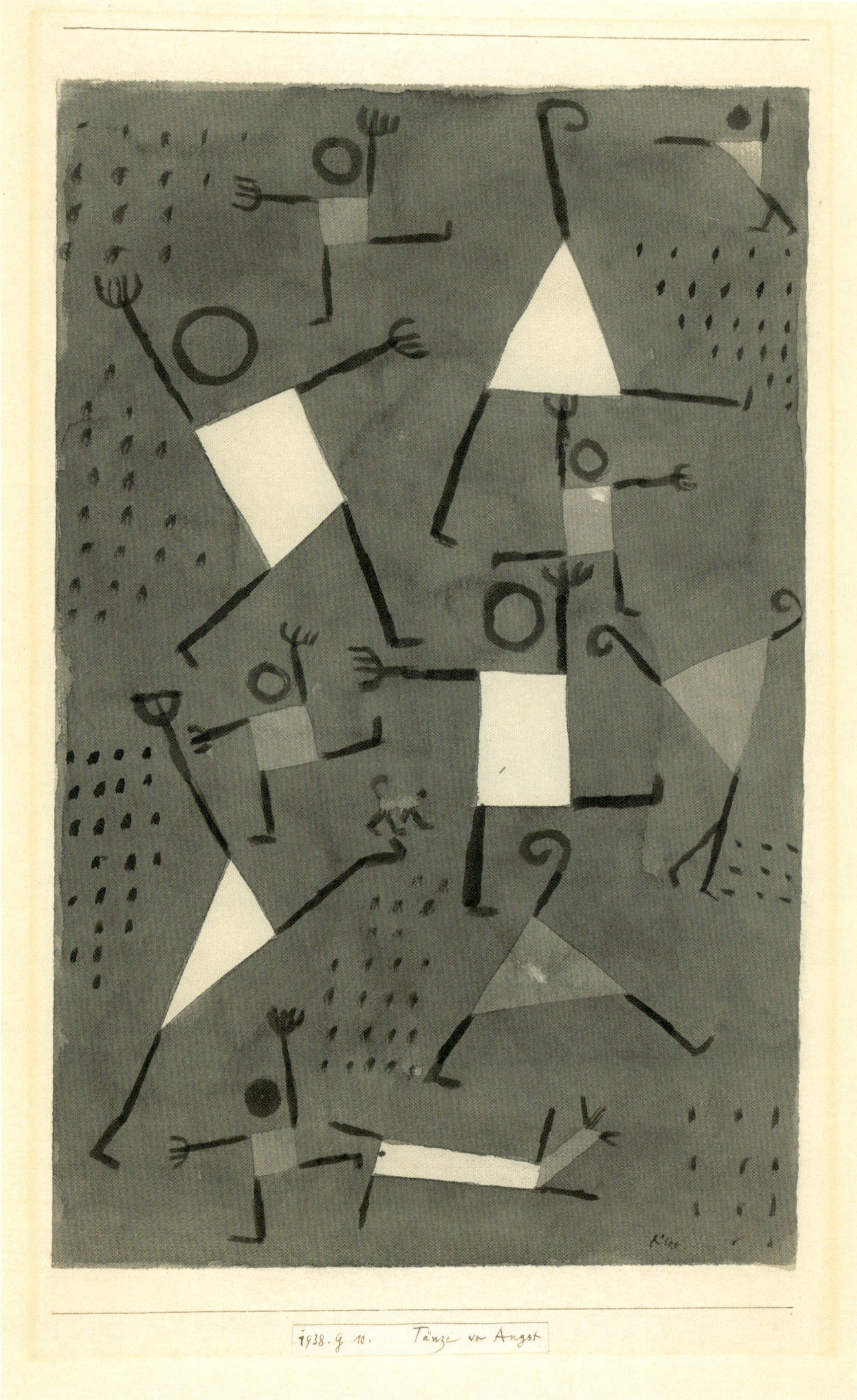
Klee
1938. g 10. Tänze vor Angst

> In this painting, people are trying to banish or master their fear through physical activity: they start to dance.

Fig. 101. Dances caused by fear, 1938, 90

suffering adverse circumstances. He strove for balance in all things, taking on the guise of a bold and confident tightrope walker. I believe he would have handled his diagnosis and the prognosis of a terminal illness in the same way that he handled his defamation and dismissal by the Nazis.

Paul Klee produced cryptic diary-like drawings which give us a clue to his mental state during the course of his illness. They show us anxiety and depression, but also a sense of hope, revival and optimism. The following drawings illustrate this.

Re. Fig. 102
The illness is affecting the artist badly. He is starting to doubt that he will ever get better. In this picture too, body parts have detached themselves, the person seems to be falling apart. In the bottom right a figure has fallen to the ground. But then this figure stands up, stretches, grabs a trumpet and blares out his name from the instrument: 'Klee'. He gathers his courage and faces up to his fate with a defiant 'so what!'. In fact his artistic output is now about to increase at a staggering rate.

Re. Fig. 103
Even though the spirit is willing, the sick body is still weak. Bringing oneself to stand up again is proving to be hard. One's belief in a cure, one's hope of recovery is gradually fading away.

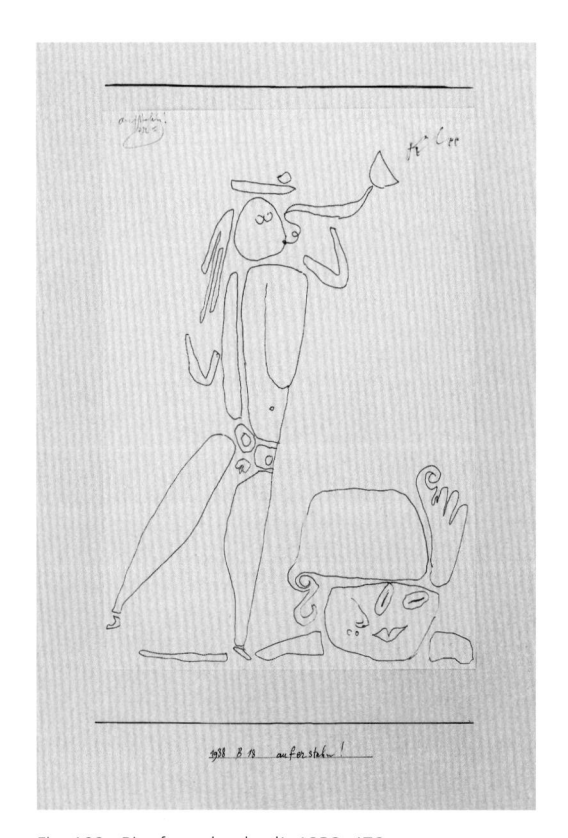

Fig. 102. Rise from the dead!, 1938, 478

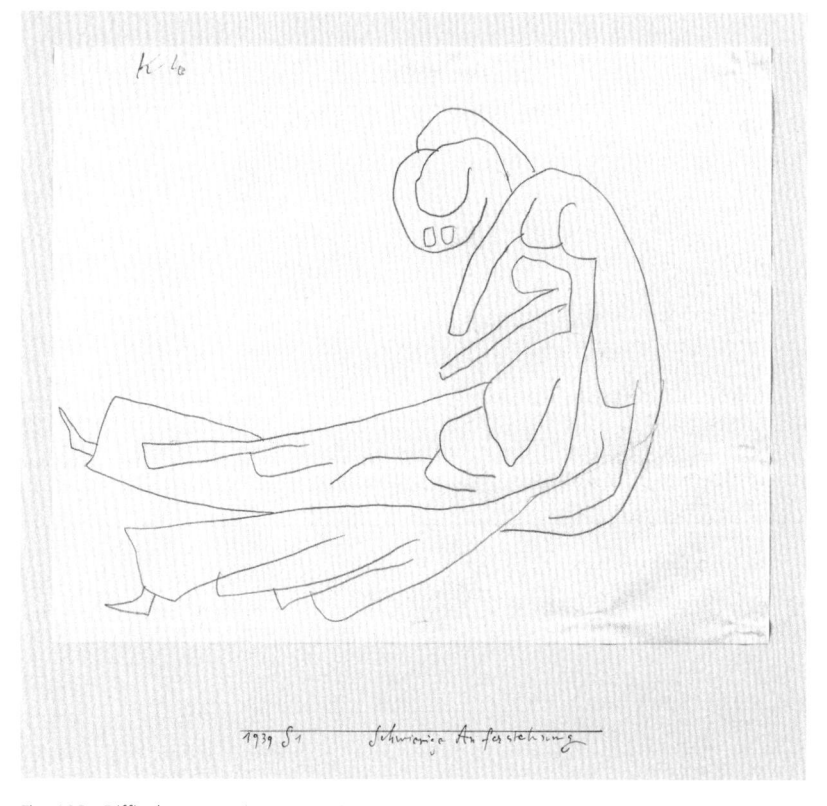

Fig. 103. Difficult resurrection, 1939, 221

Re. Fig. 104
In 'Oh! above me!' the artist is no doubt referring to himself in the title. A crude shape has formed above the sick man. It seems to be moving towards him. Klee supports his head on his right hand. His cruel fate is weighing heavily on him.

Re. Fig. 105
In the same series as 'Oh! above me!', and only three drawings later, an almost cheerful face appears. The previously oppressive shape over his head has shrunk into itself. It seems to be moving away: 'Something better is nigh'. Paul Klee's illness progressed in fits and starts. During periods of improvement, hope once again came to the fore.

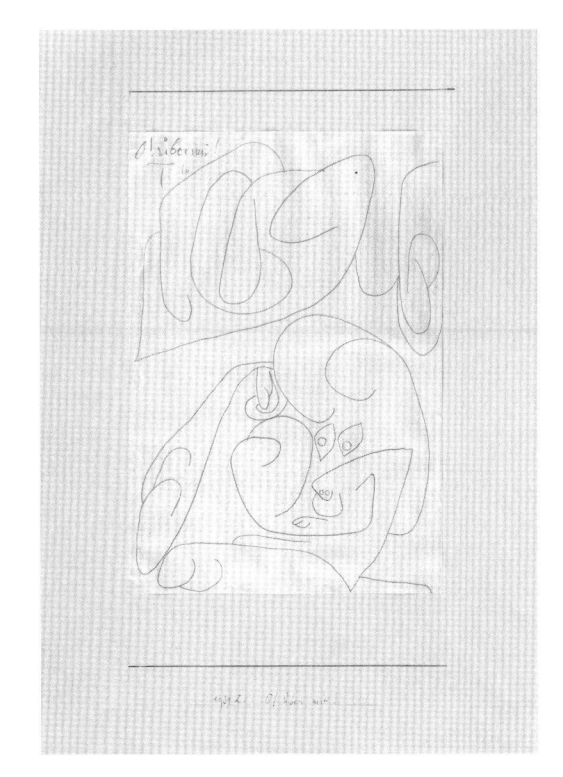

Fig. 104. Oh! above me!, 1939, 201

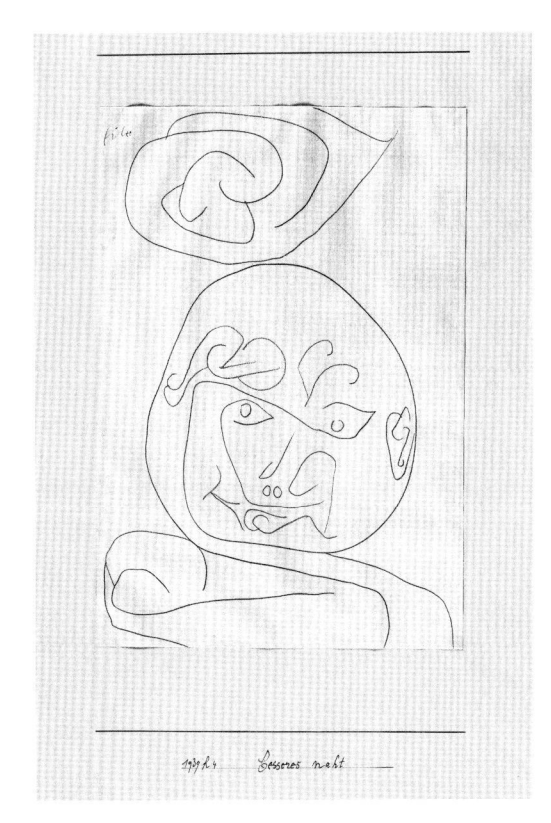

Fig. 105. Something better is nigh, 1939, 204

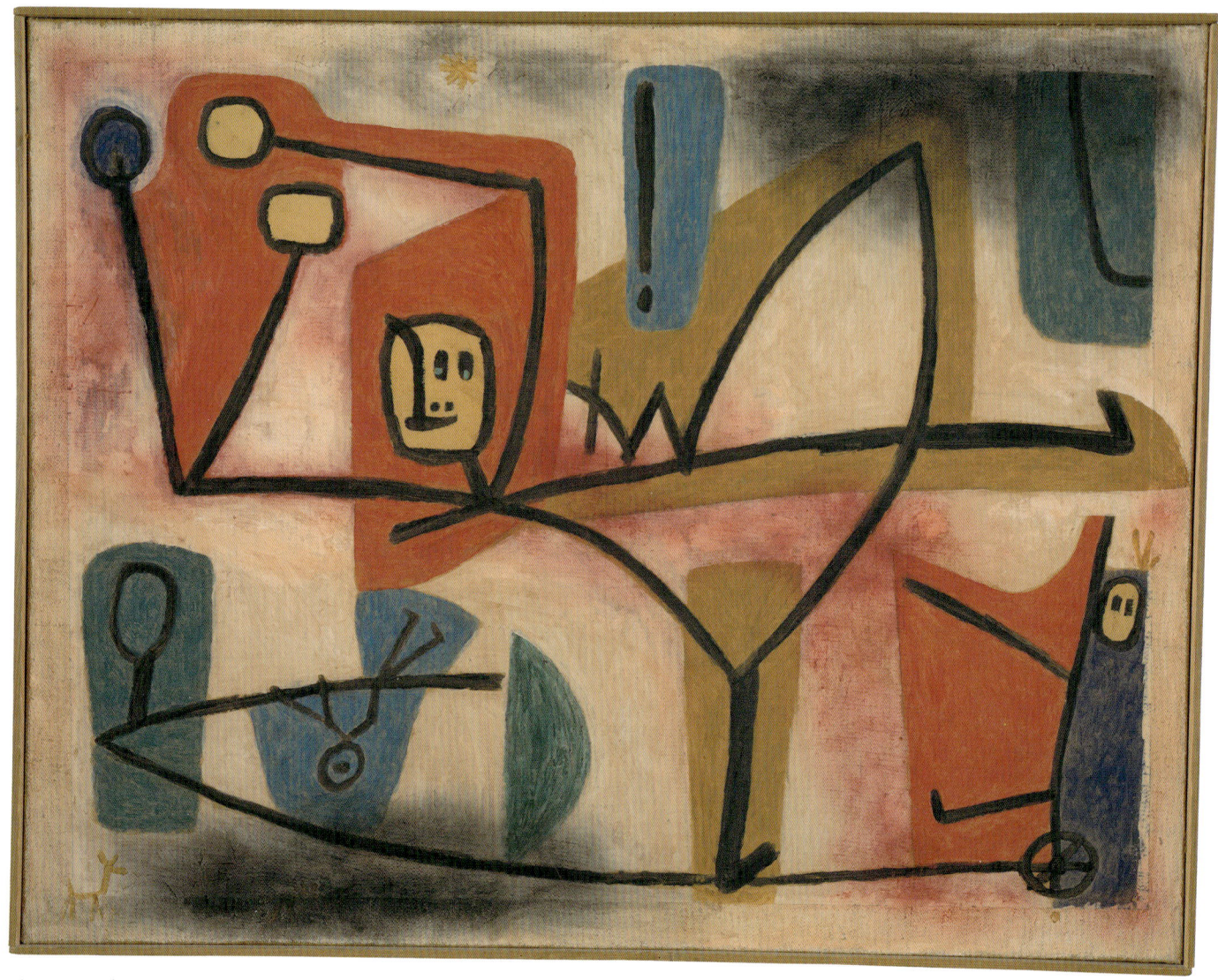

Fig. 106. High spirits, 1939, 1251

Re. Fig. 106
Jürgen Glaesemer writes: 'In the painting "High spirits" the epic qualities of the drawing define the character of the whole composition. The different colors give volume to the framework of lines and the various accents throughout give the painting a balanced tension. However they are still subordinate to the linear elements. [...] The large figure in "High spirits", juggling precariously on a thin line, brings to mind the motif of playing with fate. There are also echoes of the well-known oil painting "The tightrope walker", 1923, 121 [fig. 109]. However, in contrast to the mechanical-looking puppet of the earlier painting, the tightrope walker in "High spirits" is able to express his individual feelings. His delight at the successful balancing act is emphasized by an exclamation mark. A lucky star above his head has determined his present fate. But the black lines and pared-down form remind us that this exuberance, portrayed with such grim humor, has to prevail against dark forces and is based on the artist's personal experience. This comes across far more strongly than in the light-hearted dance of the early tightrope walker. The "exuberant man" is successfully walking the wire above the precipice of life.'[471] Wolfgang Kersten understood the painting to be 'an allegory of his [Klee's] artistic existence and an expression of his contemporary historical awareness'.[472] The following details should also be noted: the tightrope walker is cockily sticking his tongue out, in the bottom left hand corner a spellbound dog is watching the acrobatics, while in the bottom right hand corner death is lurking.

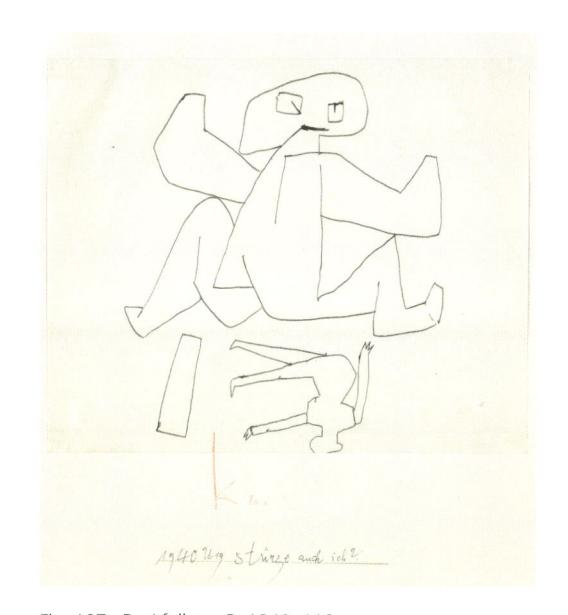

Fig. 107. Do I fall, too?, 1940, 119

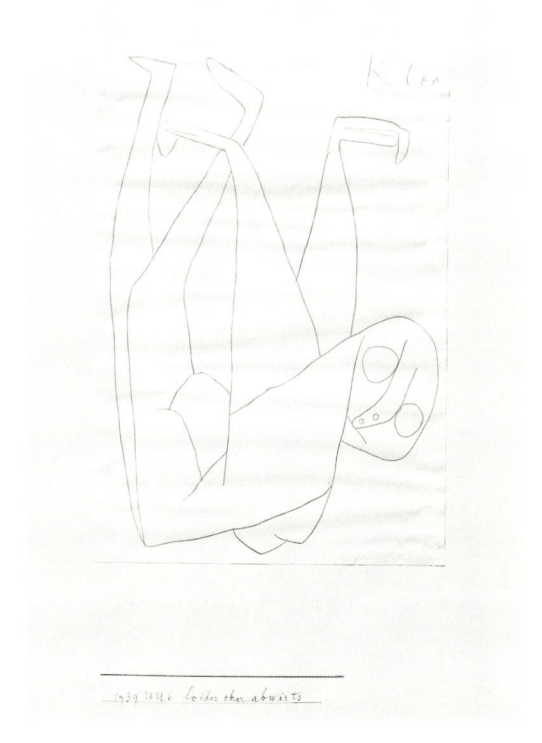

Fig. 108. Alas, rather downwards, 1939, 846

Re. Fig. 107 and 108
In the drawings 'Do I fall, too?' and 'Alas, rather downwards' Klee directly expresses his doubts about a positive outcome in the balancing act between life and death. Yet the position of the hands while falling suggests a last, faint hope: the hope of still being able to arrest the fall.

[471] Glaesemer 1976, p. 343.
[472] Kersten 1990, pp. 8 and 49.

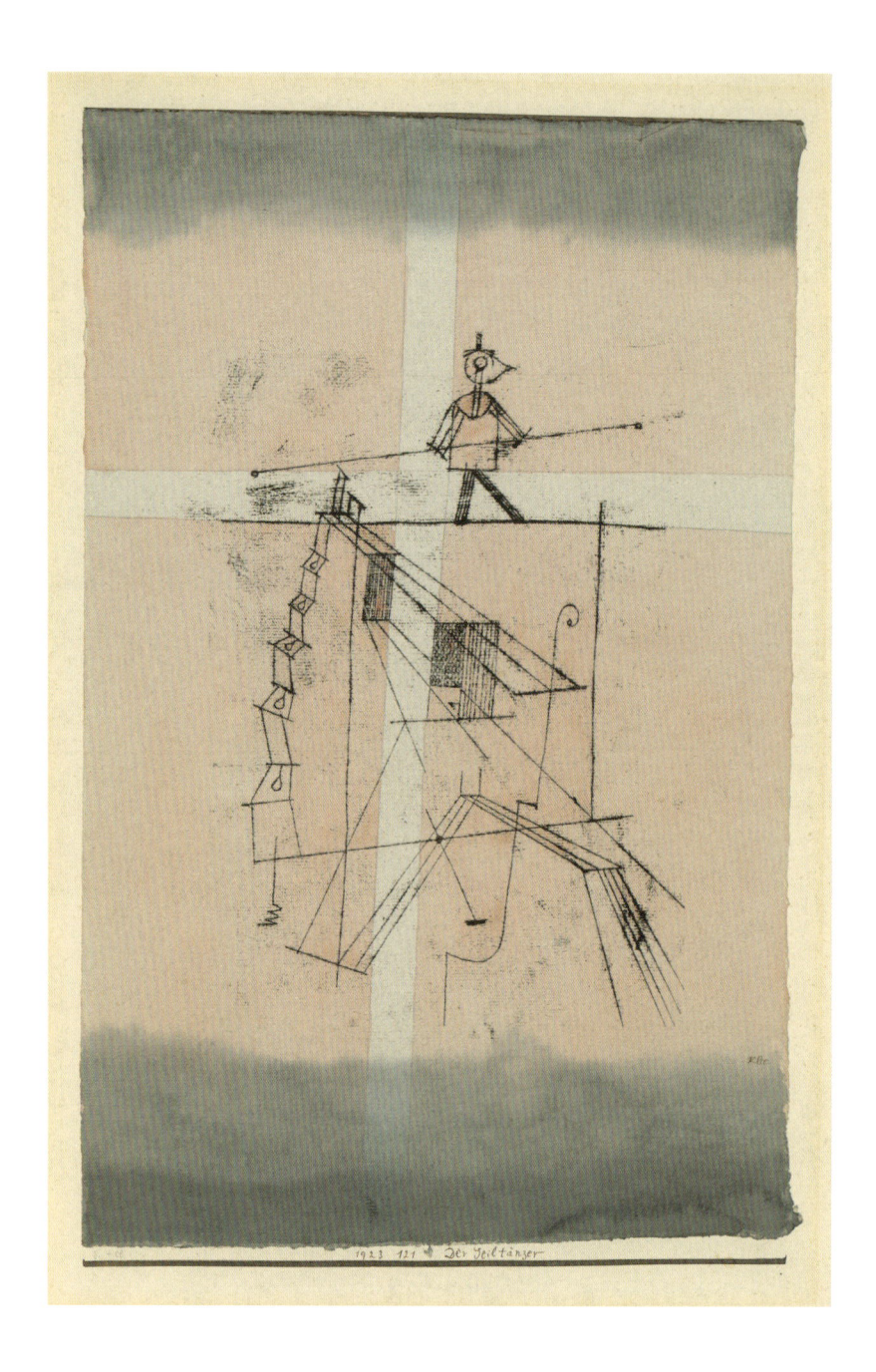

Fig. 109. The tightrope walker, 1923, 121

In the painting 'The tightrope walker' from 1923, a performer has climbed up a rope ladder onto the high wire. Carefully and deliberately he puts one foot in front of the other. A long pole in his hands makes balancing easier. The man is standing in the spotlight. A simple frame hanging from the wire offers a less-than-secure safety net in the case of a fall. Below, there is the suggestion of a face bearing an expression of intense concentration (the face of the performer magnified like a modern projection onto a screen?). Great concentration will allow the tightrope walker to reach his goal. Spellbound, we watch the circus performers swaying on the high wire. In just the same way, we gaze at Paul Klee's often precariously-balanced and tension-filled pictures. His academic papers, almost 4,000 pages of manuscript compiled in preparation for his teaching at the Bauhaus in Weimar and Dessau from 1921 to 1930 (kept at the Zentrum Paul Klee in Bern under the heading 'Pädagogischer Nachlass' [pedagogical legacy])[473], show that he attaches great importance to balance in artistic forms.[474]

◁ Christine Hopfengart comments on this work as follows: '"The tightrope walker" offers a particularly complex interpretation of the subject of "balance", combining elements of artistic theory, psychology and poetry. This striving for balance through a constant adjustment of "weights", through a balancing of picture elements and color, is a common feature of many of Paul Klee's pictures.'[475] Hans Christoph von Tavel also sees it this way: 'With Klee it is very rare to get some form of symmetrical balance; it is always about forces and movements, whose counter-effects lead to an often unstable, precarious type of balance.'[476]

Re. Fig. 110
On a thin signpost pole – it could also be a reed – Klee has attached a see-through piece of cloth like a flag. The pole is leaning to one side; its attachment to a large rock has worked loose. The signpost is unstable – like the condition of the seriously ill. The next gust of wind could knock the pole over, a flurry could cause the reed to snap – life could soon come to an end. A somber red sun shines through the transparent flag, the arrow is pointing backwards, the sky is overcast.

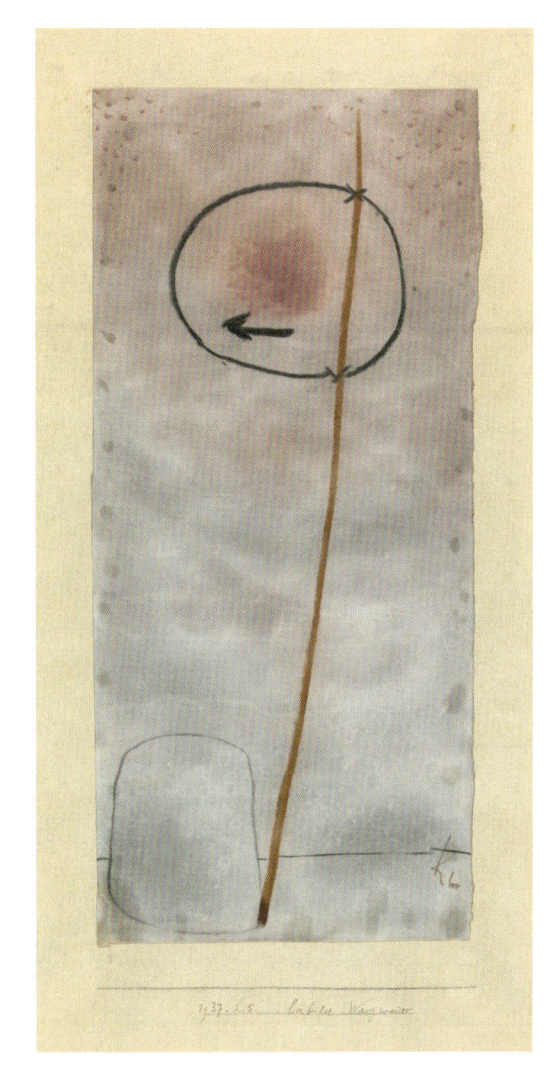

Fig. 110. Unstable signpost, 1937, 45

[473] Cf. Savelli, Rosella, in: Pfäffikon 2000, p. 9.

[474] Klee 1956, e.g. pp. 172, 176–181, 196–216, 235, 309, 386–394.

[475] Hopfengart, Christine, accompanying text to exhibition 'Paul Klee im Kunstmuseum Bern' from February 15, 2002 to May 15, 2003.

[476] Von Tavel, Hans Christoph, in: Paul Klee. Vom Leben und Sterben in seinen Stillleben, lecture, Rome, February 22, 2001, and Bologna, February 27, 2001. With thanks for providing the manuscript (12 pp.), from which I took the quotation included in the section on Klee's painting 'Unstable equilibrium', 1922, 159.

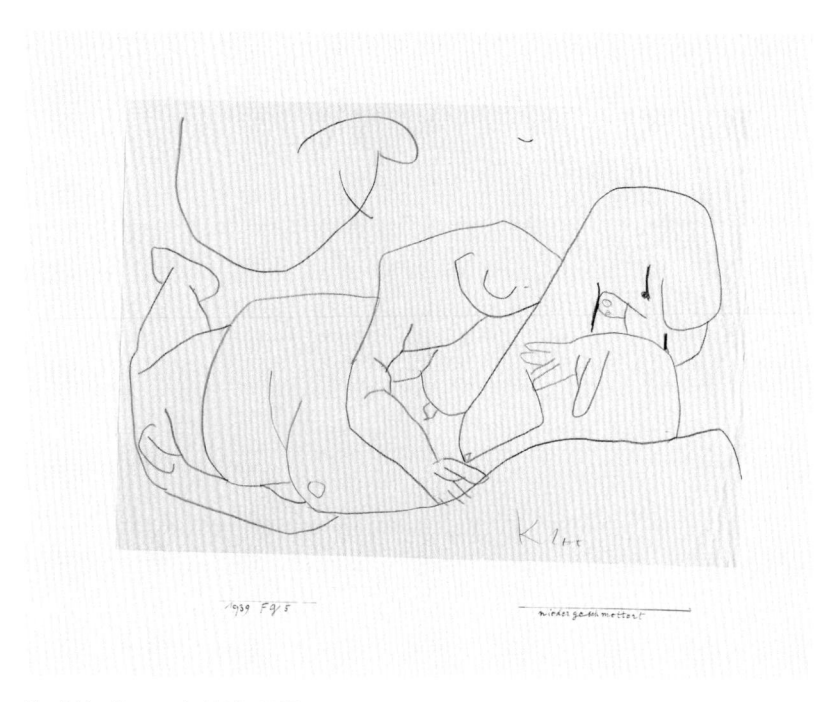

Fig. 111. Shattered, 1939, 1065

The illness has once again shattered the weakened body. The artist's new type of art is not understood in Switzerland. His exhibitions are largely ignored. Only a few friends, art collectors, art historians and other artists are standing by him. Paul Klee feels physically and mentally 'Shattered'.

Re. Fig. 112
The arm of the figure on the ground stretches vertically upwards like the periscope on a submarine. The 'shattered man' is hoping to be saved. The angled hand, waving weakly, signals 'SOS, the last signal'. It is calling for help at a time of great distress.

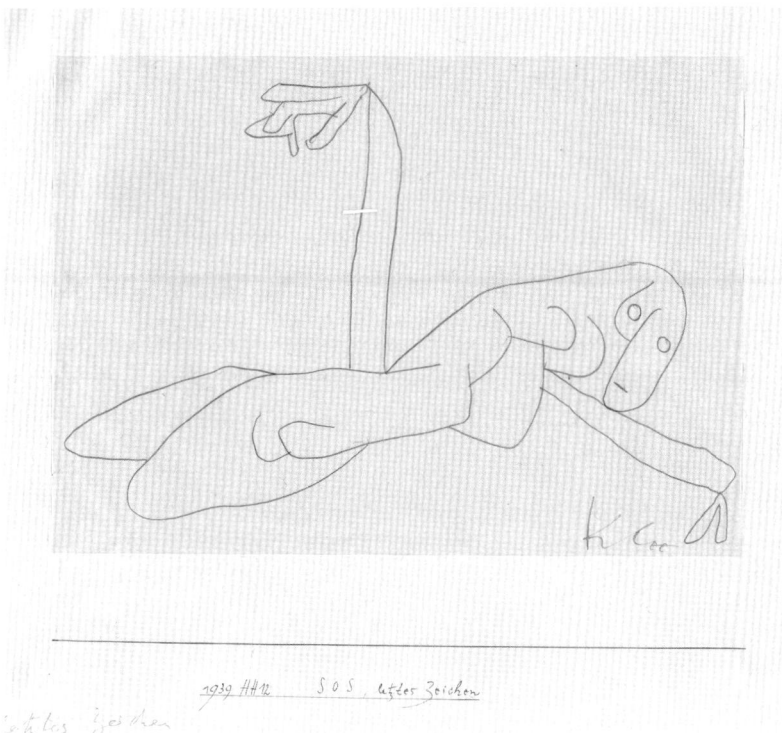

Fig. 112. SOS, the last signal, 1939, 652

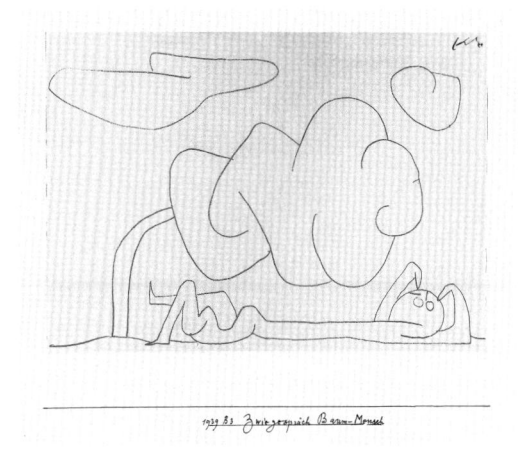

Fig. 113. Dialogue between tree and man, 1939, 403

Re. Fig. 113

In 1923 in an article entitled 'Wege des Naturstudiums' (Ways of Studying Nature) Paul Klee states: 'For the artist, dialogue with nature is a conditio sine qua non [an essential prerequisite]. The artist is man, nature himself, and a part of nature within nature itself.'[477] On the face of it, the tone of the drawing is light-hearted, but it has a more serious undertone. A tree leans dangerously close to a figure lying on the ground. The dialogue with nature, which is so important to the artist, has suddenly become dramatic. The sky is clouded and the huge treetop looks threatening. It sways like a heavy load above the figure below. How easily this load could cause the tree to break and crush the man. He clutches his hands to his head, his eyes full of fear. He wonders how he can escape from this precarious position. He lifts his right leg reflexively, wanting to use it to hold back the tree – a forlorn hope!

[477] Klee 1923, p. 24, reprinted in: Klee 1976, p. 124.

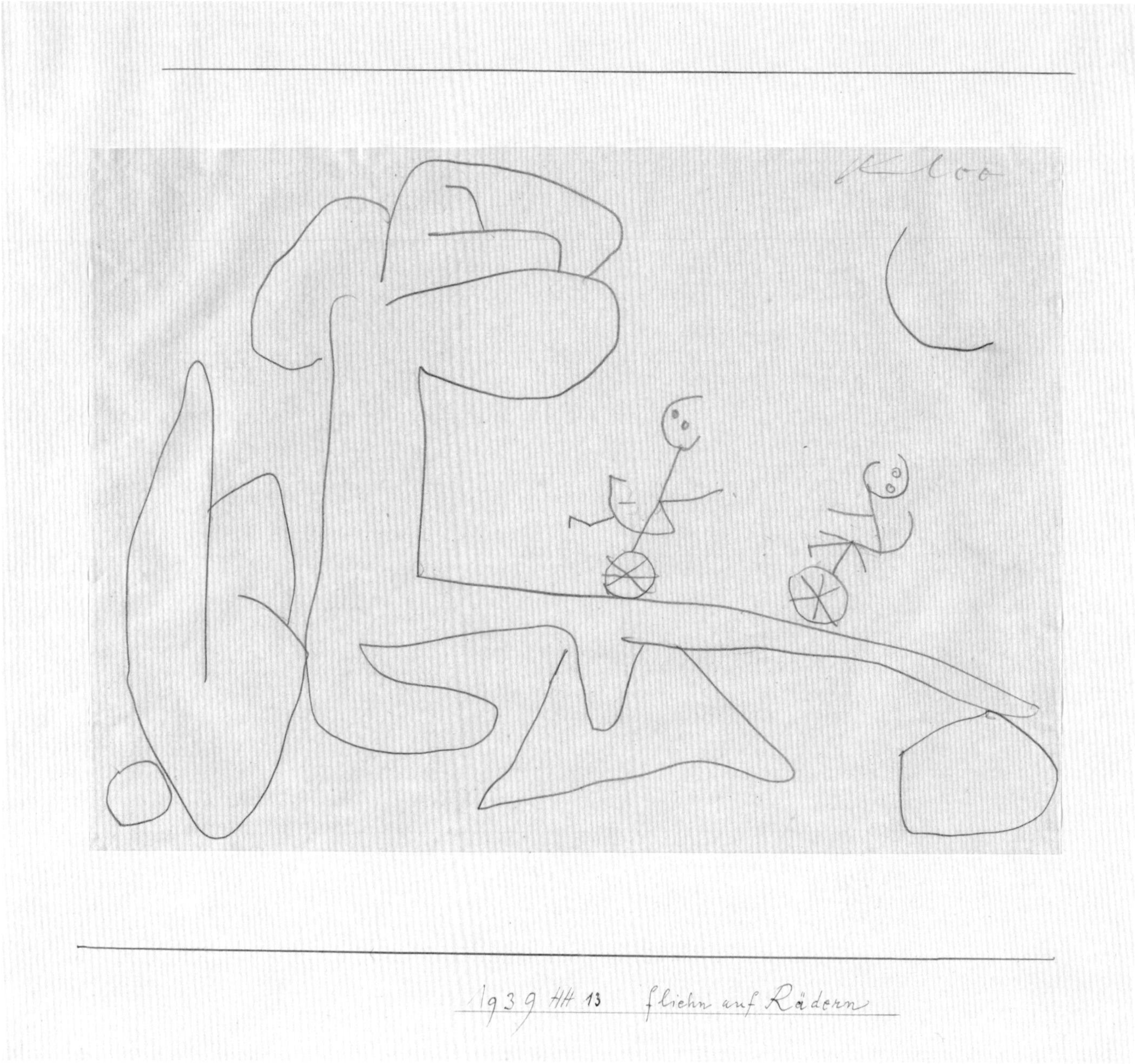

Fig. 114. Fleeing on wheels, 1939, 653

This drawing immediately follows the one with the title 'SOS, the last signal' (fig. 112, page 143). Klee is beset by illness. The outlook is bleak. Might it still be possible to escape? Preferably on wheels, together with his wife? But fate still looms large, threatening and monstrous, trying to seize the fleeing couple in its clutches. Destiny will catch up with them again.

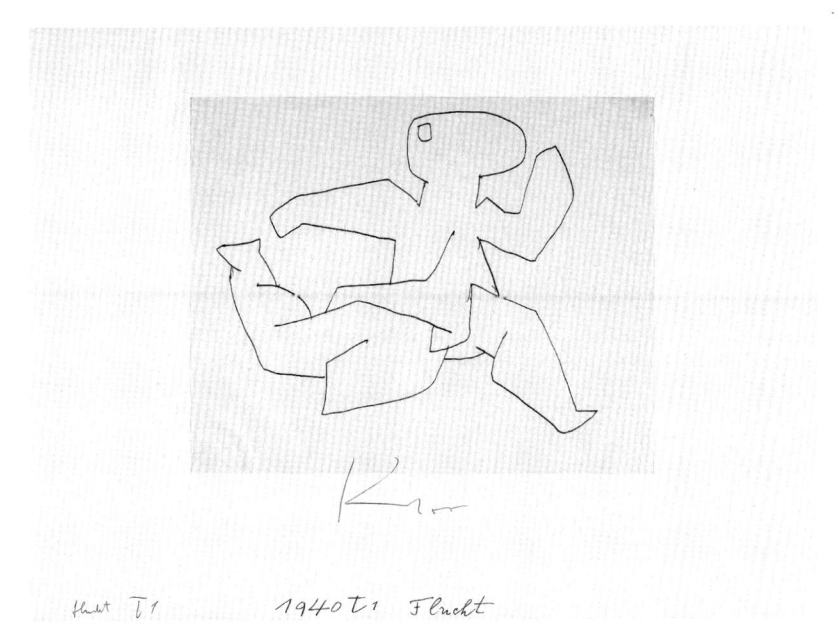

Fig. 115. Flight, 1940, 121

Here a figure is running away as fast as he can. He looks back in fear.

Re. Fig 116
Also in the drawing 'He can't escape' a man is trying in vain to flee as fast as he can. He has wrapped himself in a large coat. He has pulled the hood down over his face in order to avoid being recognized.

Re. Fig. 117
'Mon dieu!' (Oh my God!) shouts Klee. He knows his own fate. The words are literally spelled out on his face.

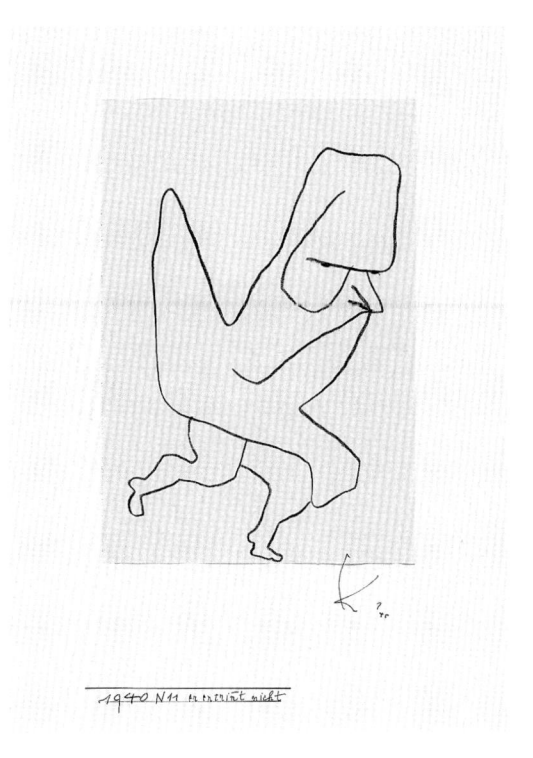

Fig. 116. He can't escape, 1940, 231

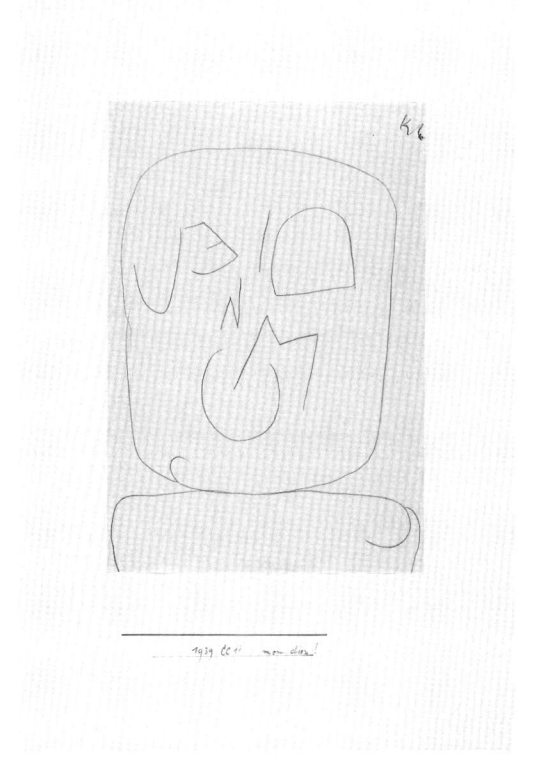

Fig. 117. Mon dieu!, 1939, 551

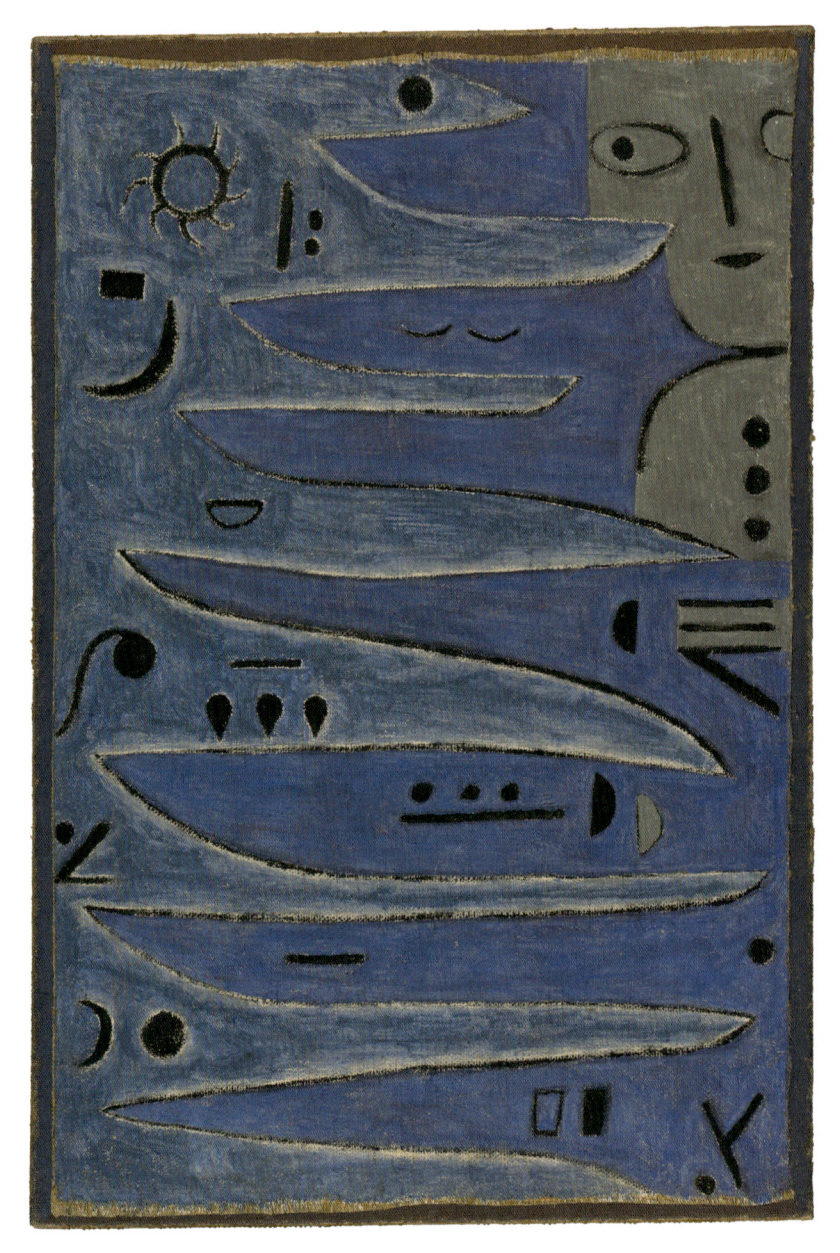

Fig. 118. The grey man and the coast, 1938, 125

We are looking down on a broken, fjord-like coast line. There seems to be a ship between two spits of land. In the top right-hand corner a figure is warily eyeing the coastal landscape. From his perspective the landscape changes dramatically: the sun and moon symbols on the left-hand side become sharks' eyes, the spits of land become the wide-open mouths of predatory fish. The figure 'goes grey' faced with these serious threats.

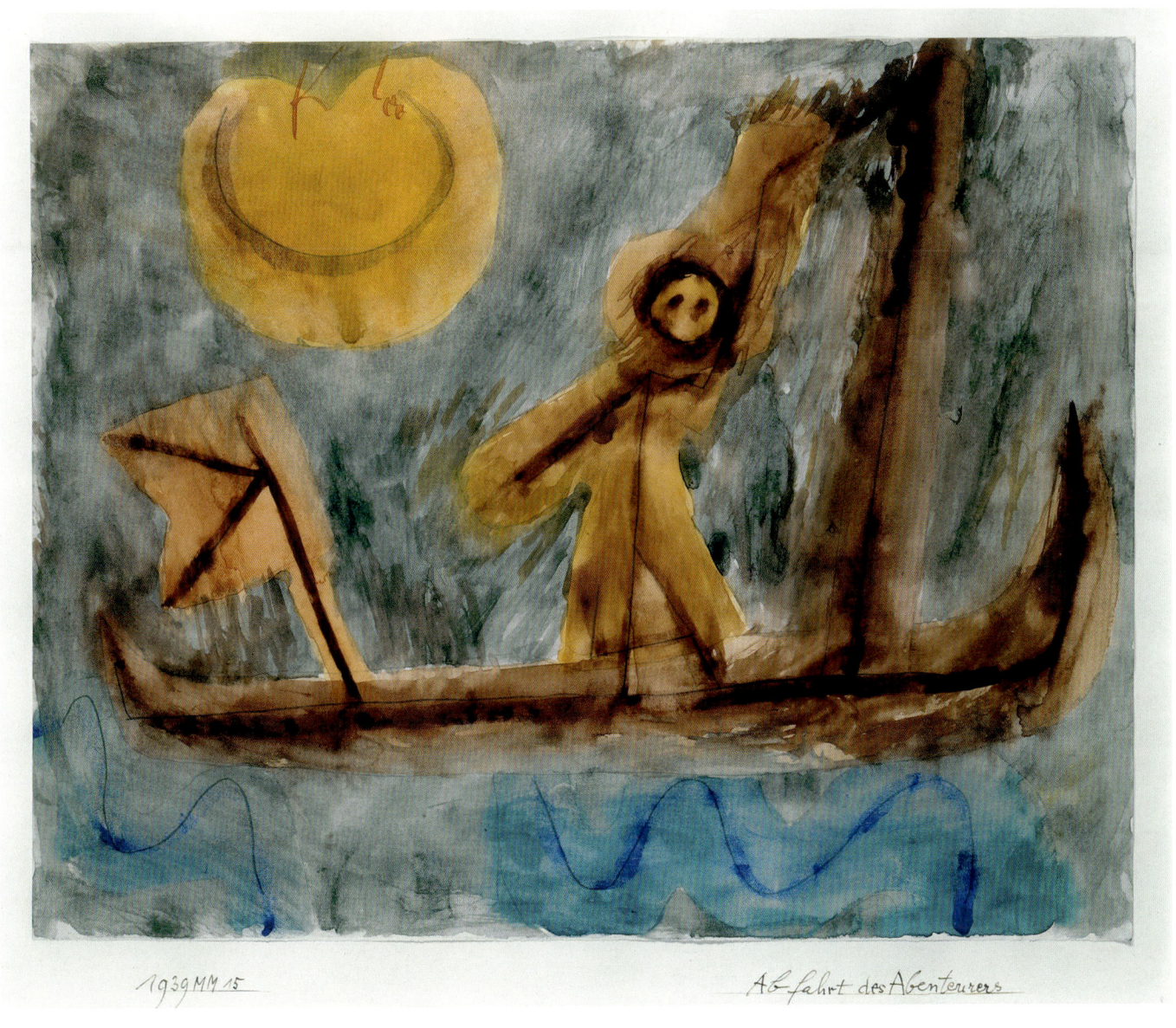

Fig. 119. Departure of the adventurer, 1939, 735

Paul Klee feels the end approaching. In the picture he is bravely setting off across the high seas in a small dugout-like sailing boat. He has raised a flag at the back of the boat. It carries the letter 'K' (Klee). The journey will be full of adventure. The sailor is waving goodbye, standing up-right in the narrow, fragile-looking boat. The outlook is not good. The sky is grey, a storm is on the way, the waves are high.

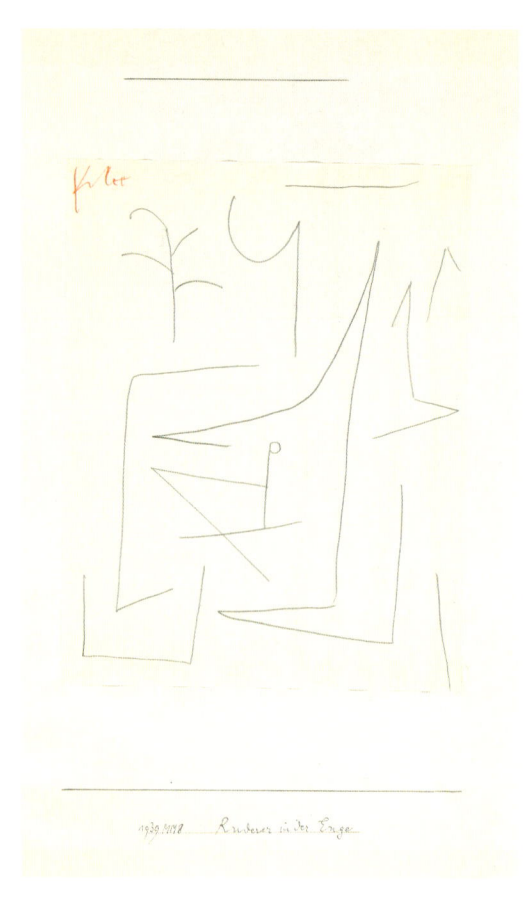

Fig. 120. Rower in the narrowness, 1939, 728

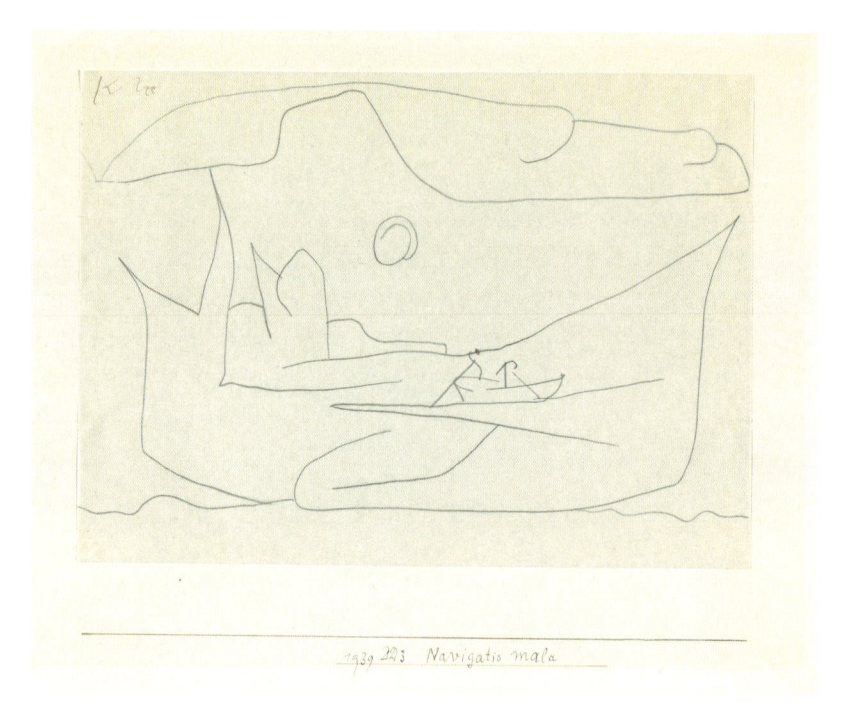

Fig. 121. Navigatio mala, 1939, 563

Re. Fig. 120
In the three drawings in this series, we are witness to the imaginary drama of a rower. He has entered a narrow passage taking him into a labyrinth. He looks desperately for a way out. He is surrounded by high obstacles. He feels trapped.

Re. Fig. 121
The rower is stranded. He gets out of the boat and tries to re-float it. The Latin title of the drawing 'Navigatio mala' (bad boat-trip) says it all: cliffs tower around the stranded sailor.

Re. Fig. 122
Suddenly the rower ends up in a narrow river gorge. He immediately recognizes the danger he is in. With all his strength he pushes an oar against the edge of the precipice to try to stop himself from falling. The rushing water thunders down the narrow gorge. It is Y-shaped. The rower will be dragged down into it.

Fig. 122. River gorge near Y, 1939, 734 ▷

1939 MM14 Strom-Schlucht bei Y

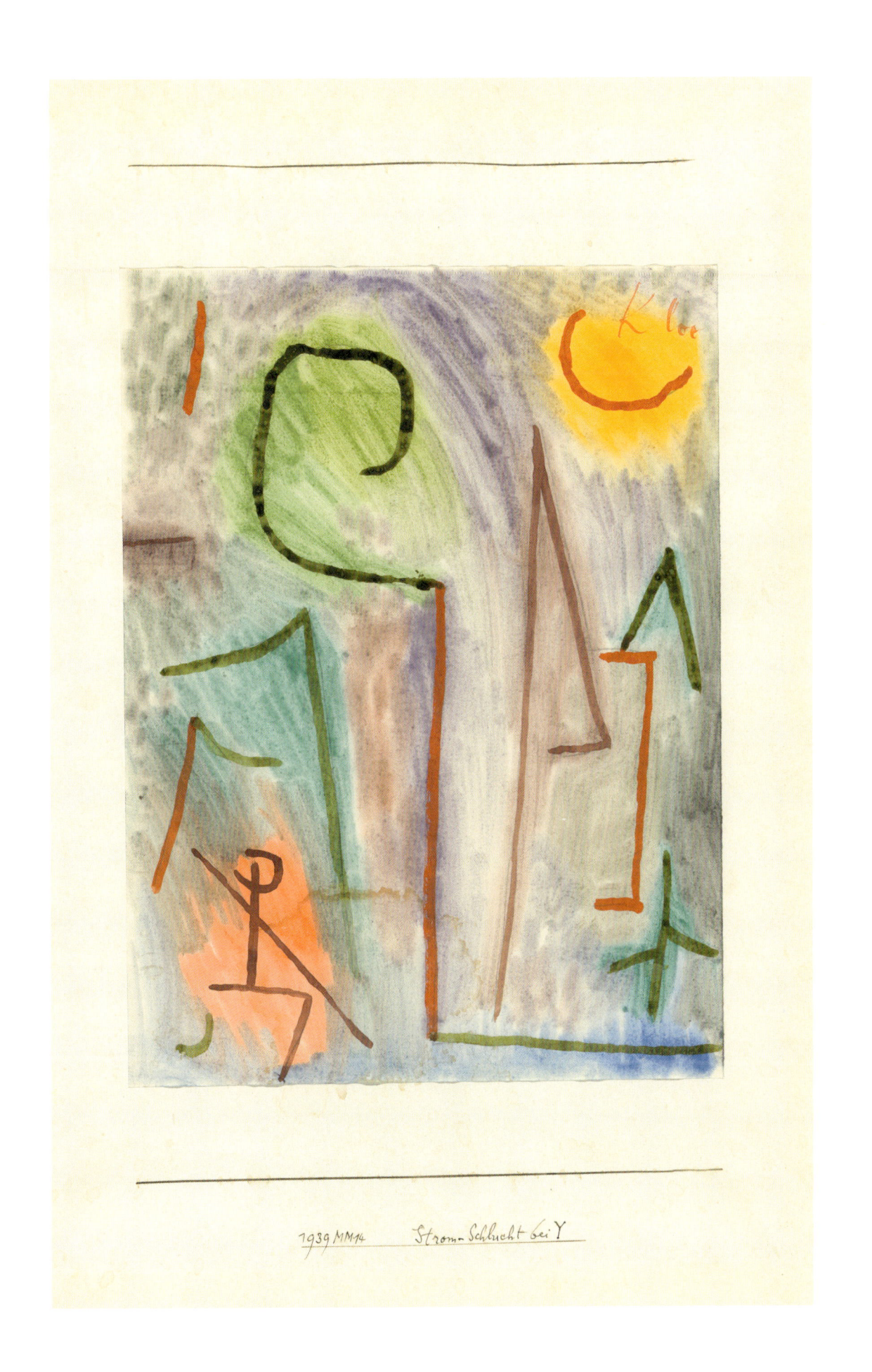

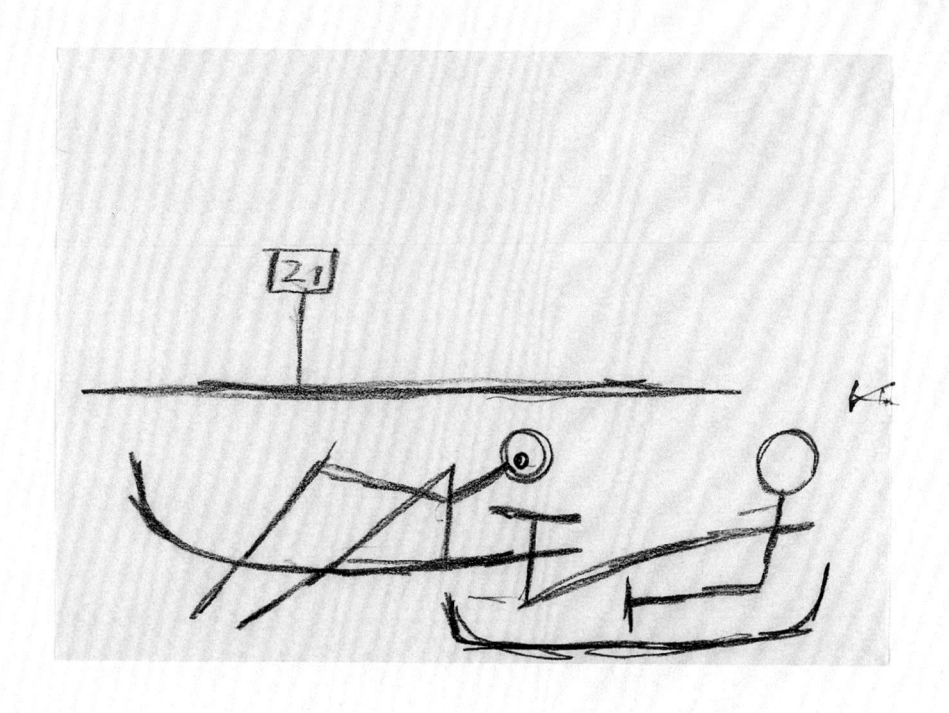

Fig. 123. Rowing competition, 1940, 172

The rower finds himself in a competition (a race for survival). Another rower comes up from behind just before the finish and rows alongside him, trying to beat him to the line. It is death, and Klee must accept that this competitor will overtake him – at the finishing line the number two will be in front of his number one. He now knows that he will lose the race with death.

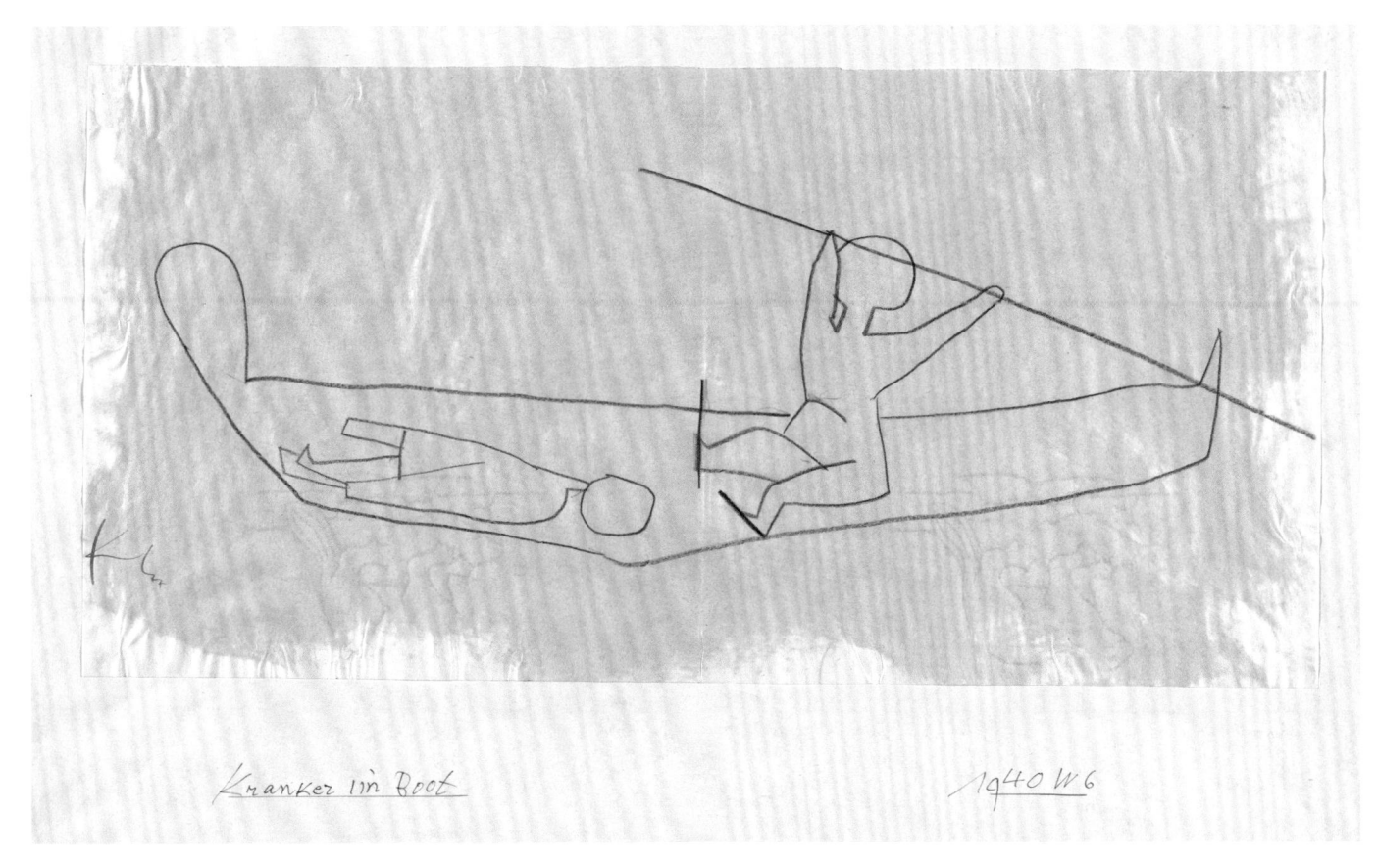

Fig. 124. Sick man in a boat, 1940, 66

This drawing reminds us of Charon, the ferryman who carries the souls of the dead across the river Acheron. But the title tells us that a sick man is lying in the boat. The seriously ill man senses that death is near. The ferryman could therefore soon become Charon. Interestingly, Paul Klee gave the title 'Charon', 1940, 58 to another drawing which he completed shortly beforehand.

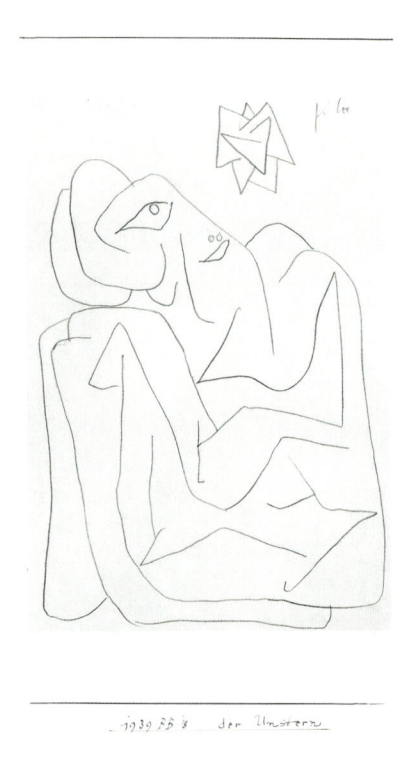

Fig. 125. The unlucky star, 1939, 538

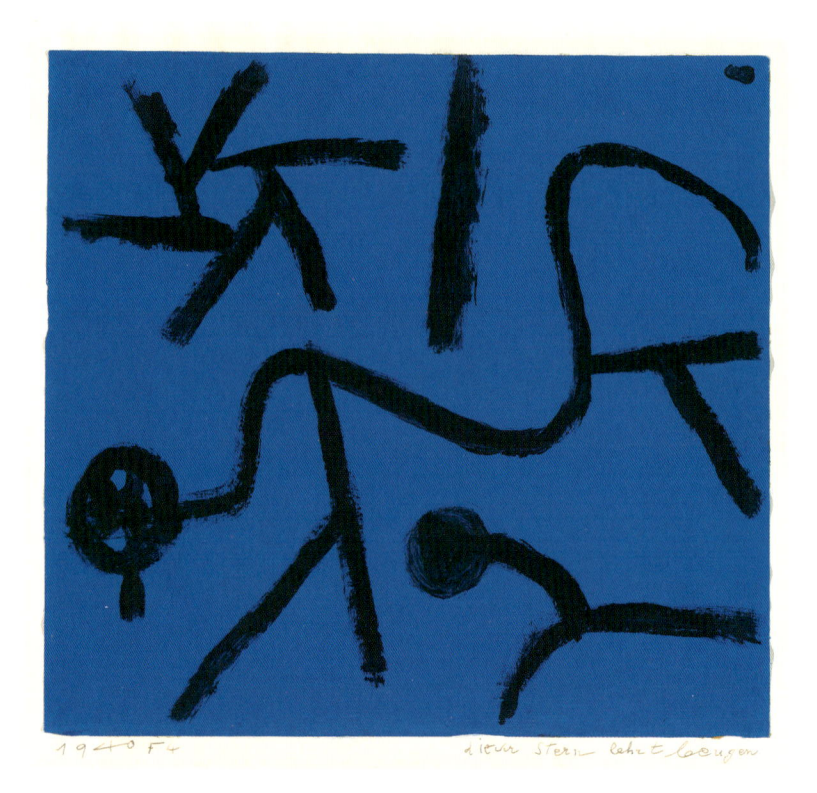

Fig. 126. This star teaches bending, 1940, 344

Re. Fig.125
A many-pointed star, spreading pain and suffering, floats ominously close to a hunched figure. The arrival of this 'unlucky star' spells the beginning of an inauspicious development. The victim wants to avoid it. He leans back imploringly in the face of looming disaster.

Re. Fig. 126
'The unlucky star' now appears as a cogwheel, which will drive his remaining life inexorably forward, tooth by tooth. Klee has bent to his fate; he has accepted it with a heavy heart. The vertical bar bearing down upon the sick man's back may symbolize the pressure brought about by his suffering, a pressure that crushes him body and soul. But a companion is striding along beside him (his loving wife?).

What Could Have Caused Such a Serious Illness?

Life is often unpredictable. There is not always an obvious reason why a person should suddenly be struck down by ill-health. Until he was 55 years old, Paul Klee enjoyed excellent health.[478] He had a robust constitution (see page 39, note 72), very rarely even suffering from influenza. On the few occasions that he came down with flu, it was only a mild dose, even when he caught it in 1937 and 1939, a time when he was already very ill.[479] In his diaries from 1898 to 1918 he mentions having the flu in 1914[480], 1916[481] and 1918. Millions of people were killed by the 'Spanish Flu' pandemic in 1918, a time when Klee was still serving in the military. On November 14, 1918, he wrote in his diary: 'I have clearly had influenza; the day before yesterday I had a fever and cough. But after a delirious night I was back to good health. It obviously wanted to break out but was not able to do so.'[482]

It is therefore strange that in summer 1935 Paul Klee should be so severely afflicted by a primary viral infection of the upper airways which at first seemed relatively minor, but which he struggled to shake off. One explanation for this could be the enforced and tragic break from his old life. I am convinced that his dismissal and banishment by the National Socialists and his emigration to Bern, the city that he described as 'really my home'[483], contributed to the onset of his illness. From being a highly respected artist and teacher in Germany, once he moved to Switzerland Klee found he was largely ignored and cold-shouldered (see pages 28–30). His life was suddenly very different. Other authors such as F.-J. Beer[484], Michael Reiner[485] and Gabriele Castenholz[486] also consider it possible or probable that the onset of his disease was linked to his defamation and dismissal by the Nazis. It is a known fact that mental pain can lead to physical pain. On April 3, 1933, Paul Klee wrote to his wife Lily: 'I have to admit that all this uncertainty about my post and income is very unsettling. But worrying does not help; in fact on the contrary it only makes one ill, putting strain on the nerves and the mind until one suffers a real misfortune in the form of the collapse of one's health.'[487]

[478] Cf. letter from Lily Klee to Rudolf Probst, Bern, November 10, 1935 (PBD), and cf. letter from Lily Klee to Daniel-Henry Kahnweiler, Bern, November 30, 1935 (location unknown).

[479–482] See Appendices: Details of Paul Klee's Flu Illnesses (p. 268).

[483] Cf. Klee 1940, p. 14.

[484] Cf. Beer/ML 1980, p. 247.

[485] Cf. Reiner/ML 1990 [p. 35].

[486] Cf. Castenholz/ML 2000, pp. 143 and 145.

[487] Letter from Paul Klee to Lily Klee, Dessau, April 3, 1933 (ZPKB/SFK), quoted in Medrisio 1990 [p. 63].

Edgar Heim believes psychological stress plays a significant role in triggering physical disease: 'A study carried out on people with physical and mental illnesses showed that the majority of the illnesses began a few weeks after the sufferers had faced a crisis of some sort in their lives.'[488] The crisis which affected Paul Klee's professional and everyday life continued for more than a year before his illness took hold.

The artist was also very distressed by the loss of several people who were close to him. In May 1933 Karla Grosch, a young gymnastics teacher at the Bauhaus in Dessau,[489] drowned while bathing during her engagement trip to Tel Aviv.[490] Lily Klee writes: 'She was [...] very dear to us. She was such a delightful, happy creature, a real ray of sunshine [...]',[491] and adds: 'He [Paul Klee] was also very melancholy after Karla's death. But now when he is working I can see a trace of brightness returning to his features.'[492] In August 1938 Hanni Bürgi-Bigler died. She was Klee's patroness in Bern, and Lily describes her as follows: 'Her friendship remained constant over the course of many years and through all of life's vicissitudes. Such a thing is very rare, because one has so few true friends. Hers is truly an irredeemable loss. [...] And so we stood together grieving over her coffin. It was a heavy blow from which we have still not recovered.'[493]

On January 12, 1940, Hans Klee, Paul Klee's father, died suddenly at the age of 91, shortly after Paul and Lily had celebrated Christmas with him, '[...] I will never forget what a pleasant, harmonious time we spent with his elderly father,'[494] comments Lily Klee.

Great Fortitude

Paul Klee displayed great fortitude during his illness.[495] After he had come through the first serious phase, his wife **Lily Klee** writes of him: 'But it is remarkable how he has borne it. He is always calm and composed, exercising his mind with reading; and he is so long-suffering! Never a word of complaint.'[496] Looking back after Klee's death, she says: 'He never once complained about his suffering. But it severely affected his quality of life.'[497]

---

[488] Heim/ML 1980, p. 36.

[489] Karla Grosch, sister of Ju (Paula) Aichinger-Grosch. She was a student of Gret Palucca and, from 1928 to 1932, teacher of ladies gymnastics at the Bauhaus in Dessau. Karla Grosch also acted at the Bauhaus theater. She [Karla Grosch] had a close friendship with the Klees' (Aichinger-Grosch 1959, p. 49).

[490] For the circumstances of her death, see Frey 2003, p. 286 (May 8, 1933).

[491] Letter from Lily Klee to Gertrud Grohmann, Düsseldorf, May 26, 1933 (AWG).

[492] Letter from Lily Klee to Will Grohmann, Düsseldorf, May 26, 1933 (AWG).

[493] Letter from Lily Klee to Will Grohmann, St. Beatenberg, August 26, 1938 (AWG), quoted in Bern/Hamburg 2000, p. 251.

[494] Letter from Lily Klee to Gertrud Grohmann, Bern, January 20, 1940 (AWG).

[495] Personal communication, Felix Klee to the author, September 20, 1983.

[496] Letter from Lily Klee to Emmy Scheyer, Bern, June 28, 1936 (NSMP).

[497] Letter from Lily Klee to Johannes Itten, Bern, October 18, 1940 (photocopy: ZPKB/SFK).

Jürgen Glaesemer interprets Klee's relationship to suffering as follows: 'Klee buried his private suffering deep within himself, and in his letters he generally hid behind a mask of inconsequentiality. […] He allowed himself only one form of expression for his feelings of sadness, despair and anxiety: his art.'[498]

Carola Giedion-Welcker describes the artist's attitude to his illness as follows: 'He accepted his illness as his fate, as Joyce did with his eye troubles. He never complained or allowed himself to dwell on it; he felt it was best overcome with stoicism, by continuing with his work and as far as possible with normal everyday life.'[499]

Ju Aichinger-Grosch characterized him thus during his illness: 'As a patient, Klee was extremely long-suffering, astute and perceptive. He told us with a smile that he really loved his doctor, a lovely old professor, because he always prescribed what he really liked, dried bilberries for example.'[500]

In April 1981, I had the opportunity to speak on the telephone with one of the nuns from Ingenbohl who nursed the painter during his final days in the Clinica Sant' Agnese in Locarno. **Sister Liobina Werlen** still remembers the 'polite, long-suffering and brave artist'[501], but she could not tell us any more about his illness.

I could only find one instance where Paul Klee mentions the pain caused by his illness. In 1938 he wrote: 'If only the enigma of death were not so ambiguous! No less so is the enigma of life, for one has to wonder what beauty and splendor can be found in the torments of recent times.'[502]

---

[498] Glaesemer 1976, p. 306.
[499] Giedion-Welcker 2000, p. 101.
[500] Aichinger-Grosch 1959, p. 52.
[501] Telephone conversation with Sister Liobina Werlen, Kloster Ingenbohl, CH–6440 Brunnen (Schwyz), April 29, 1981.
[502] Paul Klee, excerpt from letter, August 17, 1938, quoted in Klee 1960/1, p. 163.

Powers of Intuition, Conserving Energy, Concentrating on the Essentials

In 1901, when he was 22 years old, Klee wrote in a poem: 'But now I must suffer before I can achieve'[503]. Did the artist have a premonition of the harsh fate that awaited him? Perhaps he came to recognize this in 1935/36 when he became seriously ill. Once he had recovered a little from the first stage of the disease, which lasted five months, he was able to take up his creative work once again. Although he suffered regular relapses, it is likely that right up to his 60th birthday he clung on to the hope that he would see an improvement in his health, or even a cure. It is vitally important to keep such hope alive when serious illness strikes. But subsequently the artist was aware that 'the die is cast', to quote the Latin title of his multi-colored work on paper 'Alea jacta', 1940, 271[504], produced shortly before his death. Klee now sensed that his fate was sealed, he wrote to his friend Will Grohmann on January 2, 1940: 'Of course I did not just suddenly find myself on this tragic path, many of my works refer to it and declare: the time has come.'[505] But he did not share this foreboding with his wife and son. Right up to the day he died, Lily believed he would get over the latest crisis and make another recovery.[506] Jürgen Glaesemer thinks: 'Without a doubt Klee knew [in the last years of his life] that his condition was terminal.'[507] And Glaesemer believes: 'His drawing and painting [in 1940] became a battle of life and death, Klee had an unerring sense that he was working on his own requiem.'[508] Ju Aichinger-Grosch confirms this when she writes about her last visit to Bern, saying that Klee: '[was] keen and able, but with the constant awareness that he did not have much time left.'[509] The artist himself writes to that effect in a letter to the New York art historian J.B. Neumann on January 9, 1939: 'After all, I am an artist, and as such I work with concepts. I am not so young any more, but there are still things that I wish to achieve. This means that I always have to be ready to seize the moment. I have to be able to concentrate. My powers are dwindling, and today I feel they have deserted me.'[510]

Paul Klee is a prime example of how a person who intuitively senses he has a terminal illness can nevertheless harness his dwindling physical resources to complete his life's work. He

---

[503] Klee 1960/2, p. 30.

[504] The title refers to the well-known expression 'alea jacta est' (the die is cast), words supposedly spoken by Caesar when he crossed the Rubicon in 49 B.C.

[505] Letter from Paul Klee to Will Grohmann, Bern, January 2, 1940 (AWG), quoted in Gutbrod 1968, p. 84.

[506] Letter from Lily Klee to Will Grohmann, Bern, July 7, 1940 (AWG): 'Even the day before he died, the doctors were still hopeful. […] Everything had been done that was humanly possible (he had suffered greatly) but he was not thinking about death – nor was I, I still had hope.'

[507] Glaesemer 1979, p. 16.

[508] Ibid., p. 344.

[509] Aichinger-Grosch 1959, p. 54.

[510] Letter from Paul Klee to J. B. Neumann, Bern, January 9, 1939 (photocopy MoMAANY/NP), quoted in Frey 1990, p. 115.

kept the demands on his organism as low as possible so that he had the energy and discipline to concentrate on his work. Even when he was young, Klee understood that husbanding his energies was to be a basic principle for how he lived his life.[511] Josef Helfenstein writes: 'After the onset of his illness, this conservation of his energies was a prerequisite for working.'[512] In 1936, in order to protect his health and on the advice of his doctor, Paul Klee not only gave up smoking but also the violin-playing which he loved so much.[513] And, as already mentioned, he let his wife take over most of his correspondence for the same reason. He also tried to distance himself from anything which could weigh him down mentally or emotionally: this is why in 1938 he refused a request by a Bauhaus acquaintance to add his signature to a piece criticizing the National Socialists.[514] This was to be part of an artists' campaign, but Klee justified his refusal by pointing out that he had to take into consideration the position of various people who were close to him.[515] He was rightly afraid that if he signed, it could compromise his son Felix and wife Euphrosine, who lived in Germany, and also his friends Will and Gertrud Grohmann. He also did not want to jeopardize his planned attempt to gain Swiss citizenship. The Nazis knew who the Klees were in correspondence with in Germany, so many of their letters were censored.[516] For this reason Lily Klee never made political comments in her letters to Germany from the middle of 1934 until the end of the war, apart from a letter dated September 5, 1939, just after the outbreak of war.[517] But before[518] and after[519] this period she spoke out clearly and vehemently against the National Socialists. On January 30, 1933, the day that Adolf Hitler became Chancellor, Paul Klee took a far-sighted view of the political situation, fearing the worst. He wrote to his wife: 'But one still has one's own ideas and tries to give an opinion, as miserable as the whole theater of German domestic politics is and remains. The curious will soon find out what the effect will be on them personally. I think nothing can now be done about the overall situation. The people are unfit to deal with real things; in this respect they are stupid.'[520] The new ruling powers soon saw fit to make an example of him. After a smear campaign in the National Socialist newspapers, on April 21, 1933, Klee was one of the first teaching

[511] Cf. Helfenstein 2000, p. 144, also Klee Diaries, nos. 605, 824 and 958.

[512] Helfenstein 2000, p. 145.

[513] Cf. letter from Lily Klee to Emmy Scheyer, December 16, 1936 (NSMP), cf. Aichinger-Grosch 1959, pp. 48 and 54, cf. Klee 1989, p. 46 f, and cf. Klee 1960/1, p. 113.

[514] Cf. Glaesemer 1979, p. 18.

[515] Cf. letter from Paul Klee to Mrs. Freundlich, May 6, 1938 (ZPKB/SFK), quoted in Glaesemer 1979, p. 18. Mrs. Freundlich is unknown.

[516] A postcard from Lily Klee to Will Grohmann, March 7, 1941 (AWG) bears a stamp from the German Reich's censors, and a letter from Lily Klee to Gertrud Grohmann, October 13, 1943 (AWG) bears a stamp with the note: 'Letters which are short and to the point save time and prevent delays at the Censorship Office. Overseas Inspection Office.'

[517] Cf. letter from Lily Klee to Gertrud Grote, September 5, 1939 (ZPKB), quoted in Frey 1990, p. 118: 'On Friday [Sept. 1, 1939] there was a lot of commotion and we travelled here [to Faoug] feeling very downcast. What a mistake this war is.'

[518-519] See Appendices, Paul Klee and Lily Klee and the National Socialists (p. 268).

[520] Letter from Paul Klee to Lily Klee, January 30, 1933, quoted in Klee 1979, p. 1225.

Cryptic depictions of the National Socialists' reign of terror in Paul Klee's drawings and paintings (figs. 97, 127–139)

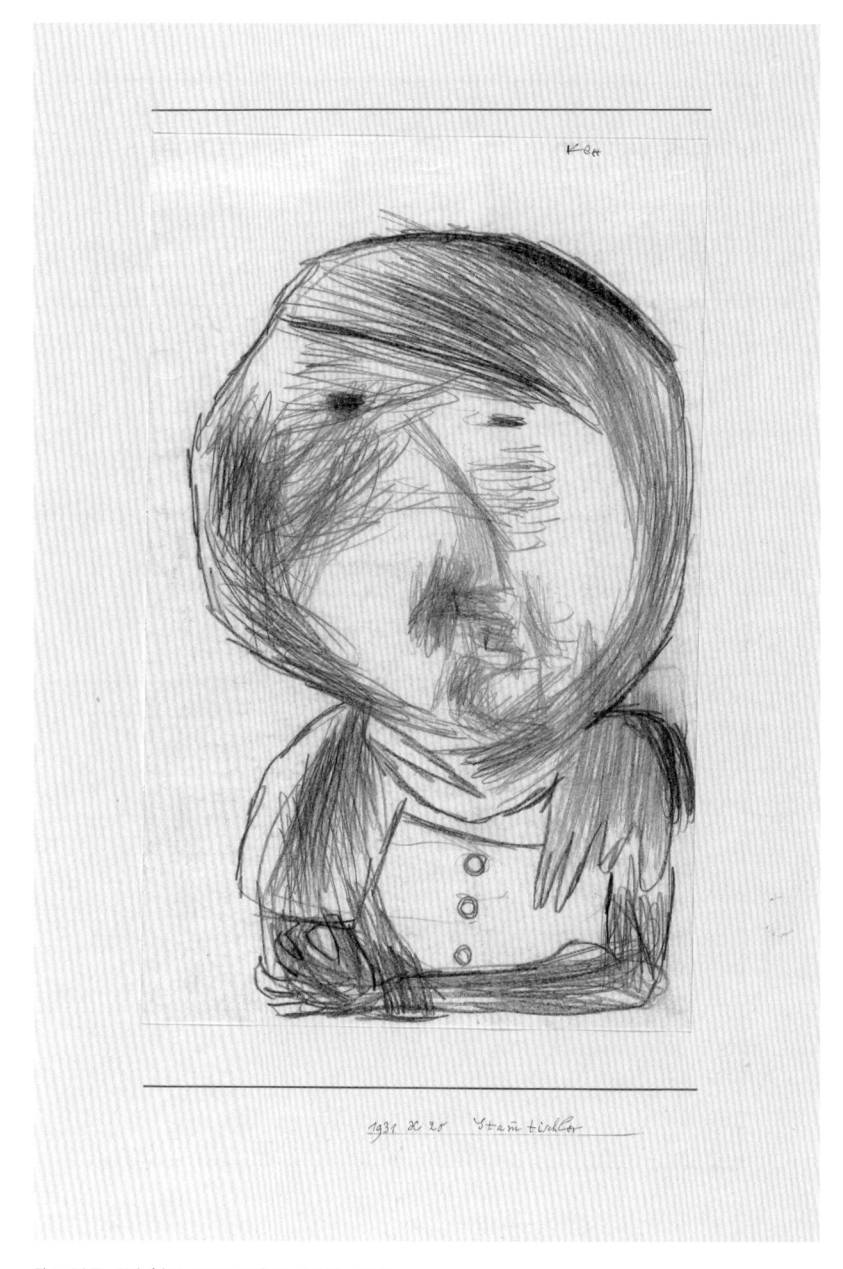

Fig. 127. Drinking companion, 1931, 280

Paul Klee had already created this character two years before Adolf Hitler came to power in Germany. He draws him – unmistakably – as a 'Drinking companion'.

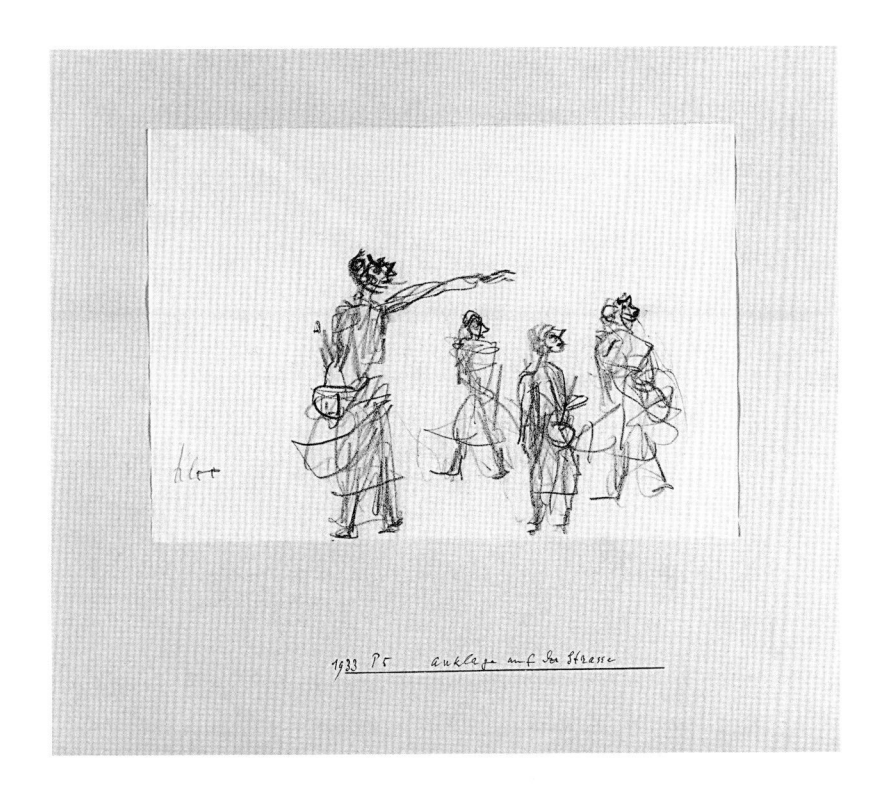

Fig. 128. Accusation in the street, 1933, 85

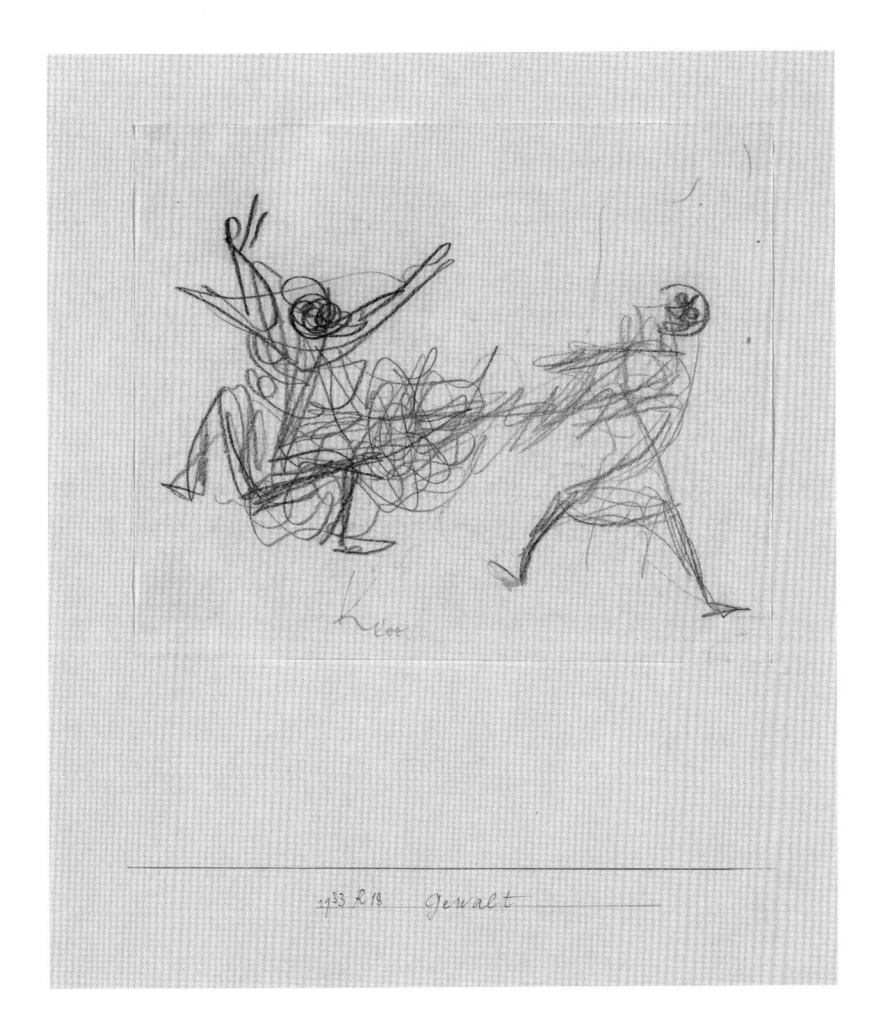

Fig. 129. Violence, 1933, 138

159

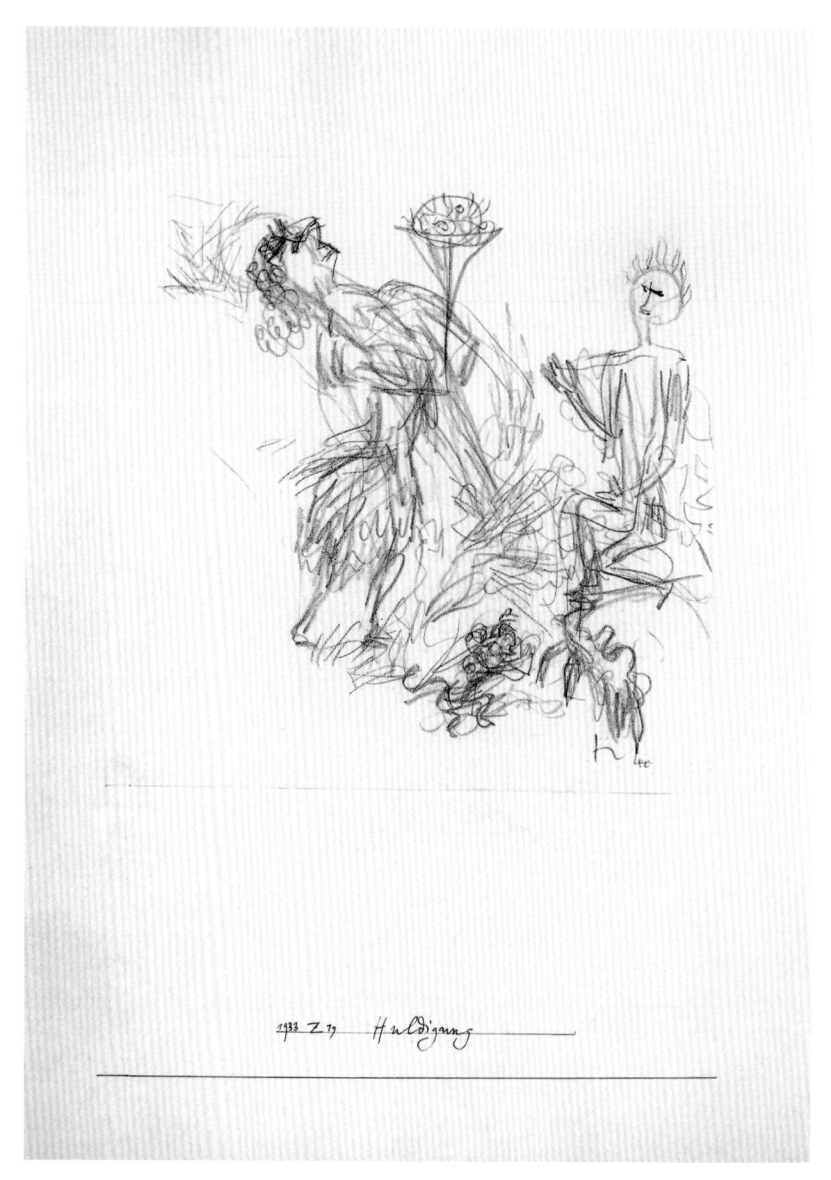

Fig. 130. Tribute, 1933, 299

artists to be suspended with immediate effect from his post, on the orders of the Prussian Ministry for Science, Art and Education, then on January 1, 1934, his employment contract at the Düsseldorf Academy of Fine Arts was revoked.[521]

Paul Klee had no desire to discuss politics with his friends and acquaintances.[522] However, he was outraged by the new government in Germany and he had a sense of foreboding that the political developments and the brutality of the Nazis would lead to catastrophe. He clearly expresses this in a ciphered, but unambiguous fashion in numerous paintings and

[521] Cf. Frey 1990, p. 112.
[522] Personal communication, Felix Klee to the author, Bern, September 20, 1983, and cf. Glaesemer 1979, p. 16, also cf. Helfenstein 1990, p. 61.

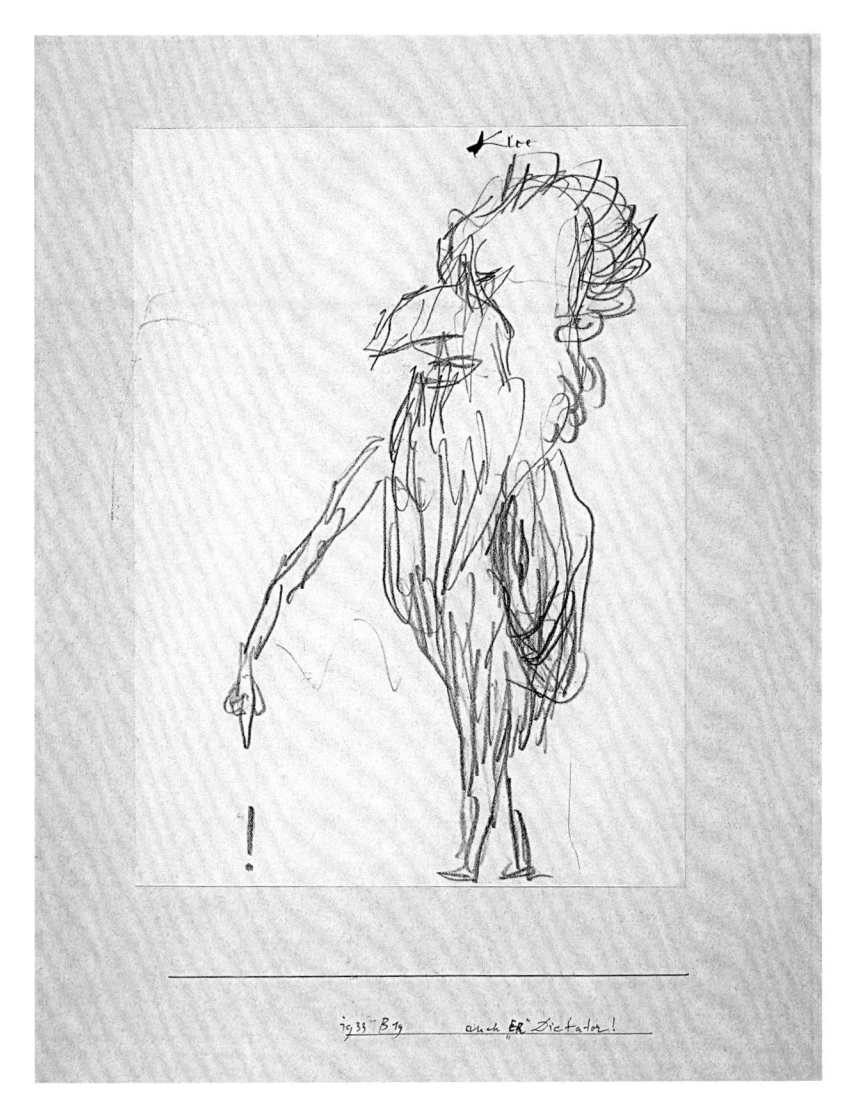

Fig. 131. 'He' a dictator too!, 1933, 339

drawings (such as those shown in figs. 97 and 127–139, among others).[523] Jürgen Glaesemer has carried out a detailed analysis of the artist's attitude towards the Nazis.[524] The Swiss sculptor Alexander Zschokke also shed light on this in a program he made for the Swiss radio station Beromünster on July 15, 1945, where he recounted his memories of an evening spent at Paul Klee's home in the summer of 1933.[525] At that time, Zschokke was, like Klee, a professor at the Düsseldorf Academy of Fine Arts. Klee showed him and the Director of the Academy, Walter Kaesbach, who was also visiting, the 200 drawings which took the National Socialist revolution as their central theme. For many years these drawings were thought to be lost, and it is thanks to Jürgen

[523] See Appendices: Paul Klee and Lily Klee and the National Socialists (p. 268).
[524] Cf. Glaesemer 1984, pp. 337–349.
[525] Cf. Zschokke 1948, p. 27, 28, 74, 76, more recently reprinted in Munich et al. 2003/2004, pp. 307–309.

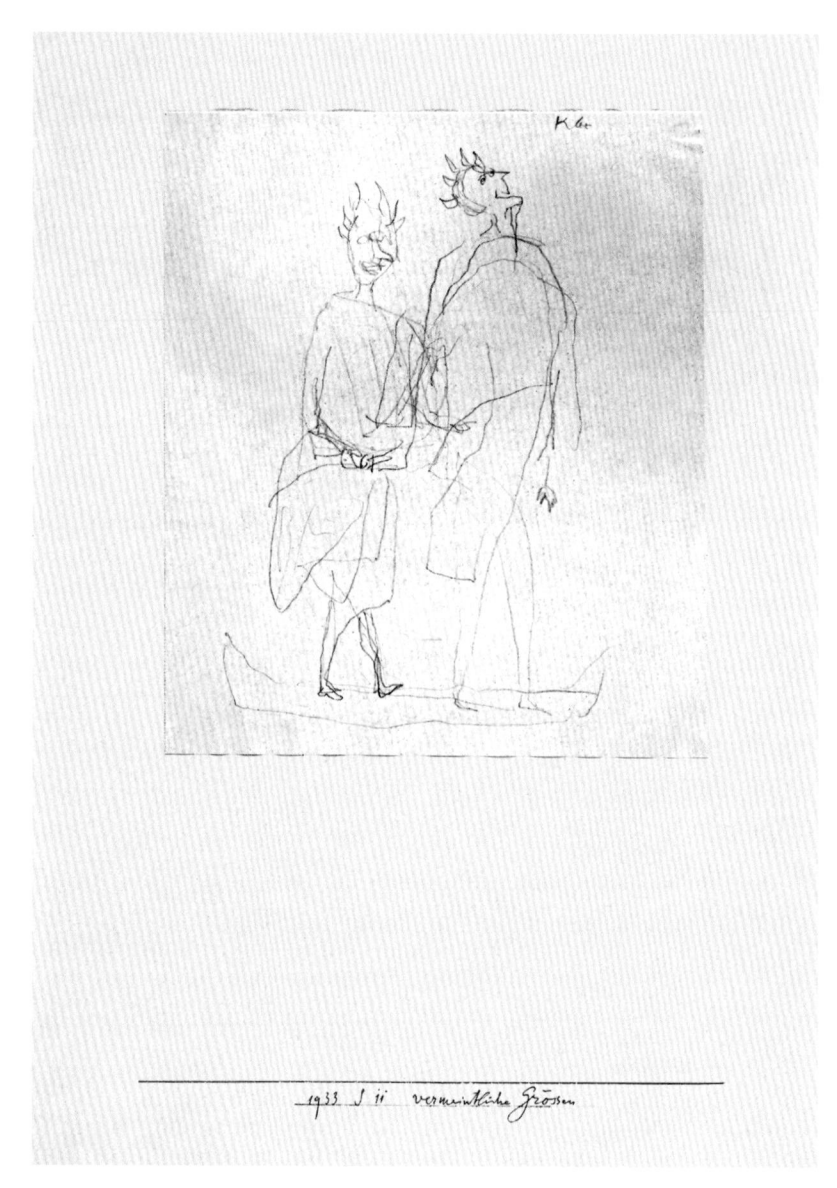

Fig. 132. Supposed celebrities, 1933, 151

Glaesemer's work in 1984 that most of the sheets held by the Paul-Klee-Stiftung have now been identified.[526] The American art historian Pamela Kort worked on this cycle and stresses that Klee '[…] used wit and parody in his attack on the NS cultural policies […]' and '[…] that for the first time since 1928 he had regained his inner composure, allowing him to freely and confidently assert his artistic identity.'[527] She characterizes '[…] the group of drawings which Klee produced in 1933 as one of the most far-reaching, albeit veiled, denunciations of National Socialist cultural policies that has ever been made through art.'[528]

[526] Cf. Glaesemer 1984, pp. 343–349.
[527] Kort 2003, p. 200 f.
[528] Ibid., p. 216.

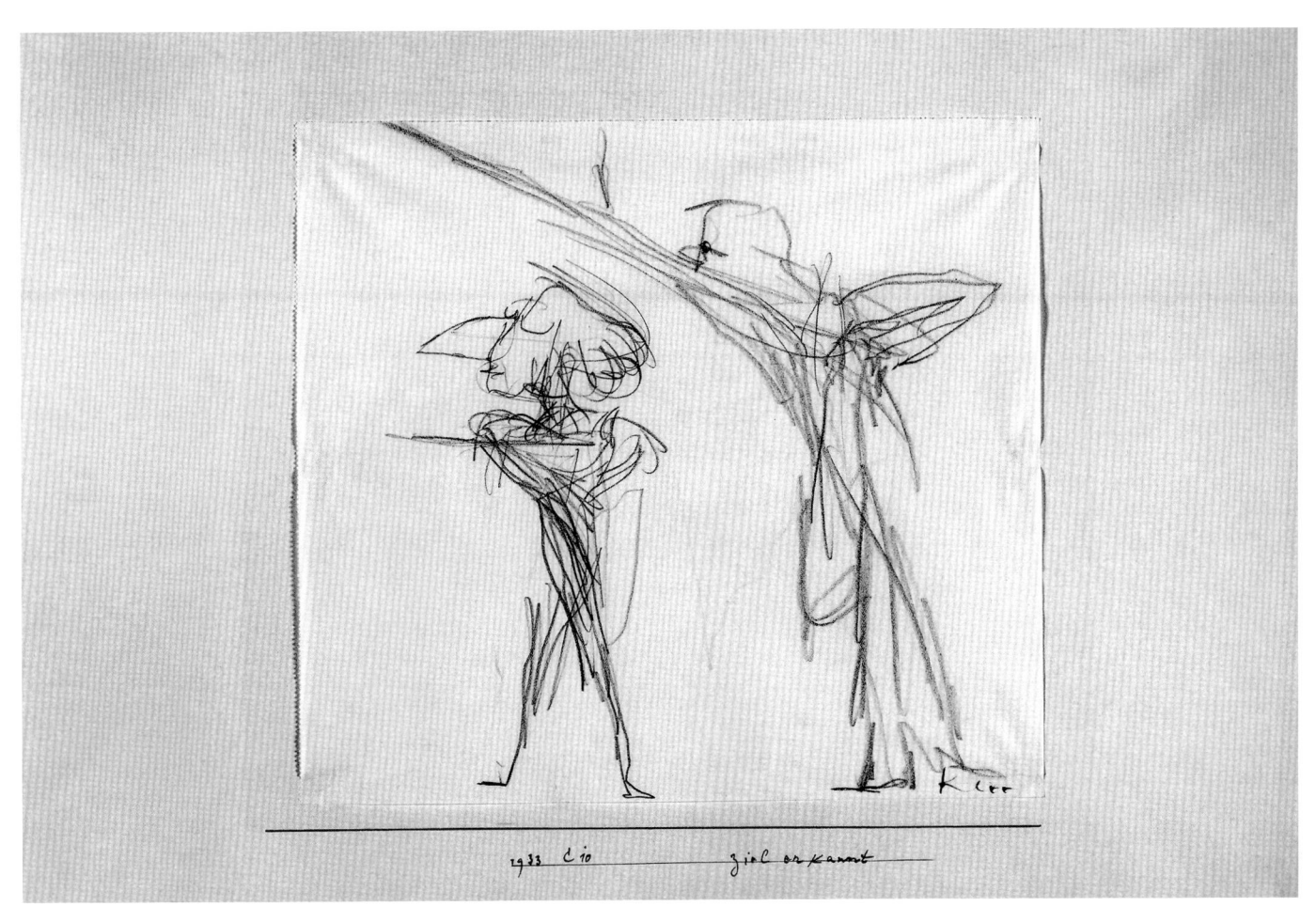

Fig. 133. Target recognized, 1933, 350

I would also like to mention Max Huggler's opinion that on May 10, 1940, just before he set off for the clinic in Locarno for the last time, the artist sensed that he would never return. Klee left on his easel a still life with strong colors on a black background (fig. 179, page 232), probably a farewell picture, because as Max Huggler writes: 'his great love of order makes [it] much more likely that he deliberately placed the picture there before his departure, knowing it would be his last [...]'[529].

Paul Klee himself talked about the role of intuition in artistic creation in the following terms: 'We construct and construct, but intuition is still a good thing. One can do a considerable amount without it, but not everything. One can work for a long time, create a variety of things, do important work, but not everything.'[530]

[529] Huggler 1969, pp. 212, 214.
[530] Klee, Paul, exakte versuche im bereich der kunst, quoted in Klee 1979, p. 130.

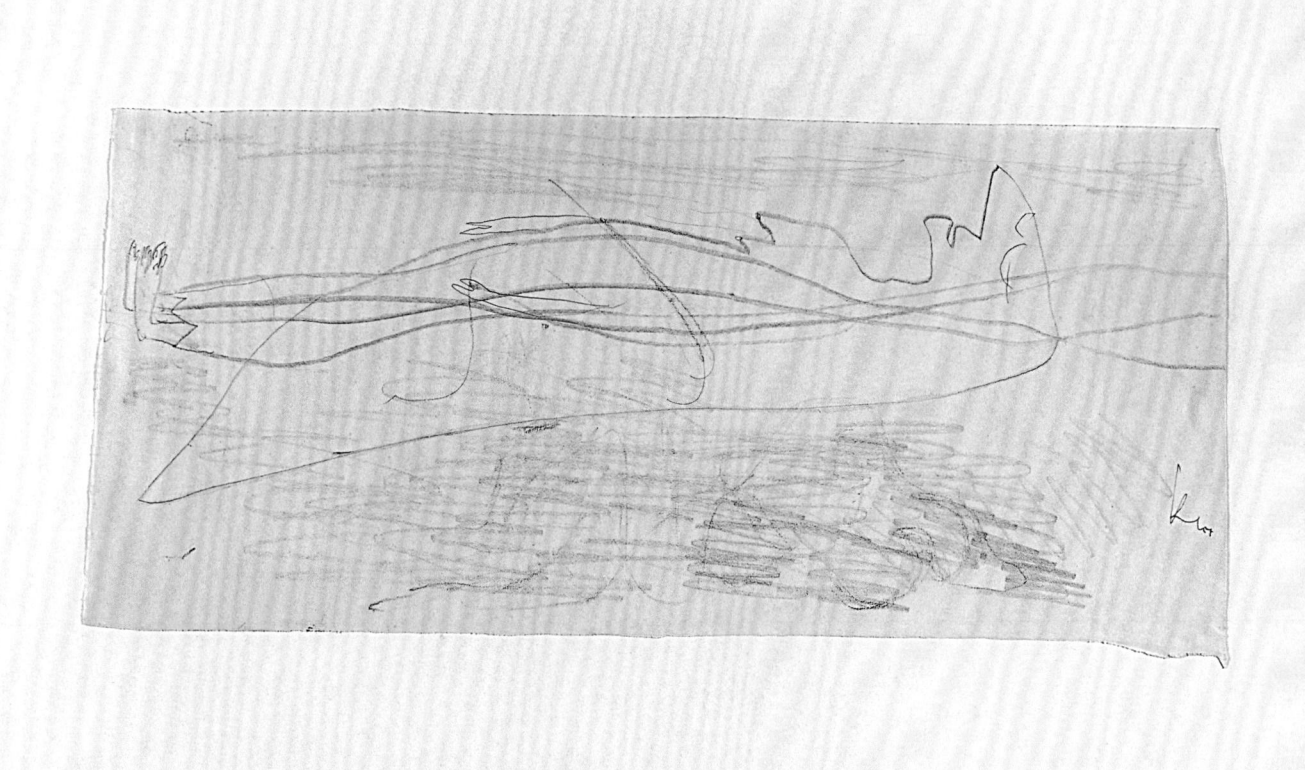

Fig. 134. Lonely end, 1934, 183

This depiction of death, created a year after Klee's emigration to Bern, a year before the onset of his illness, five years before the outbreak of war and six years before his death, could be evidence of his highly-developed intuition.

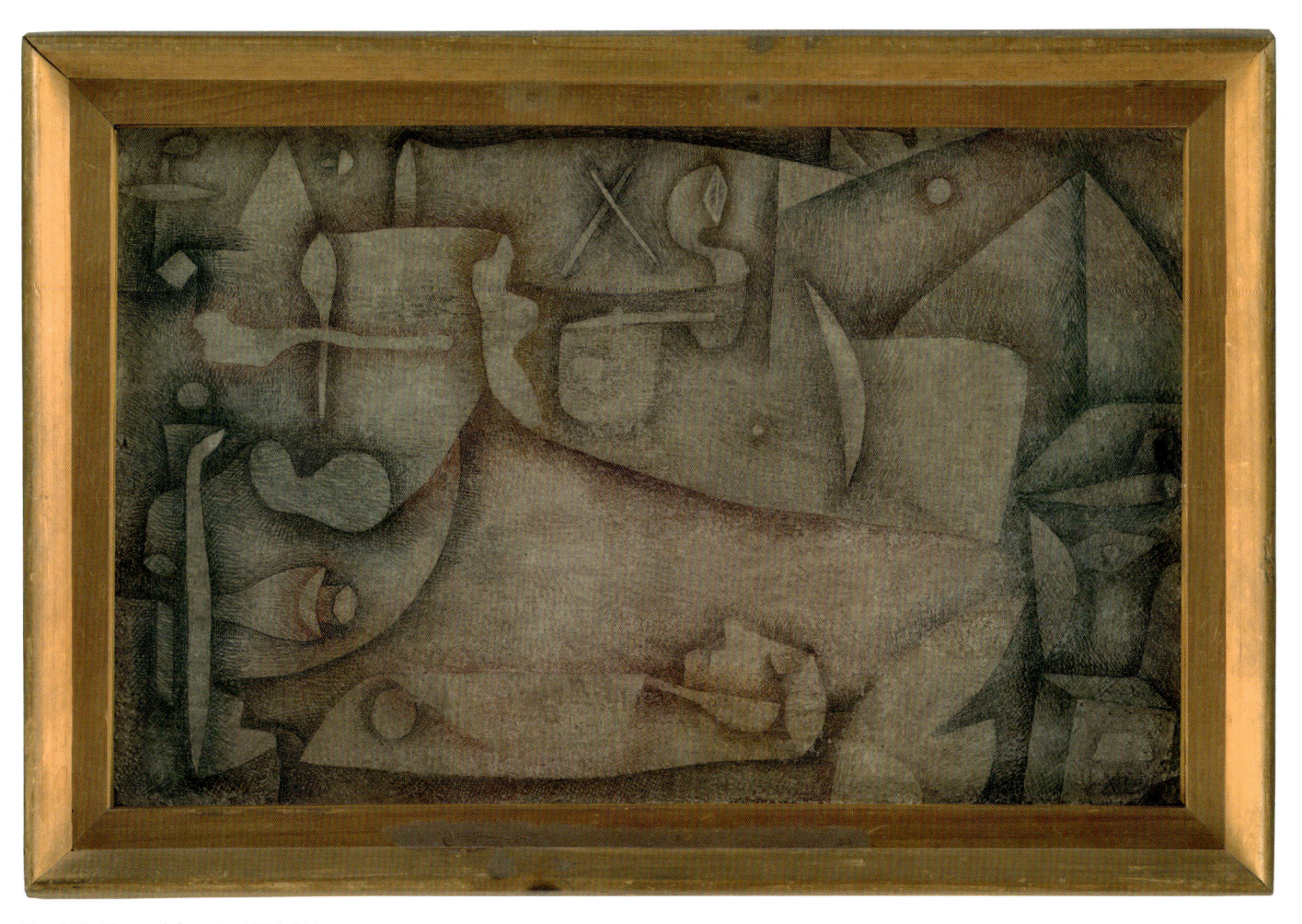

Fig. 135. The soul departs, 1934, 211

Klee painted this watercolor in the same year as the drawing 'Lonely end'. At the bottom of the picture, there is a similarly drawn corpse lying in a hollow, surrounded by plant motifs. At the top of the picture there is a cross directly above the deceased and next to it an S-bend with views beyond the burial chamber to the sun and the sickle moon. In the top right-hand corner we see a pyramid: perhaps a link to his beloved Egypt, to a pharaoh in his last resting place? 'Ent-Seelung' (the German title of the watercolor) means the splitting-away of the soul from the body in death. The artist emphasizes this meaning by splitting up the word in the title.

A bridge creates a link between two pieces of land or river banks. For structural reasons, long bridges tend to have more interconnected arches. In this painting the individual arches have broken away from each other. The pillars have become legs. The arches have 'broken ranks' (a military term[531], which Paul Klee used in the title of a watercolor with a similar image: 'Arches of the bridge stepping out of line', 1937, 11). There is an obvious association here with soldiers' legs brutally trampling people underfoot. The painting is another example of Klee's political foresight, presented in a cryptic way. Many bridges will be destroyed during the war, and many bonds will be broken.

'Revolution of the viaduct' is the second of five variations on a theme which was clearly of great interest to Klee.[532]

---

[531] Werckmeister 1987, p. 50.
[532] Ibid., and Klee, Felix 'Aufzeichnungen zum Bild "Revolution des Viaductes" von Paul Klee', in: Jahrbuch der Hamburger Kunstsammlungen, vol. 12, 1967, pp. 111–120 (quoted in Werckmeister, Otto, Karl, in: Werckmeister 1987, p. 55, note 123).

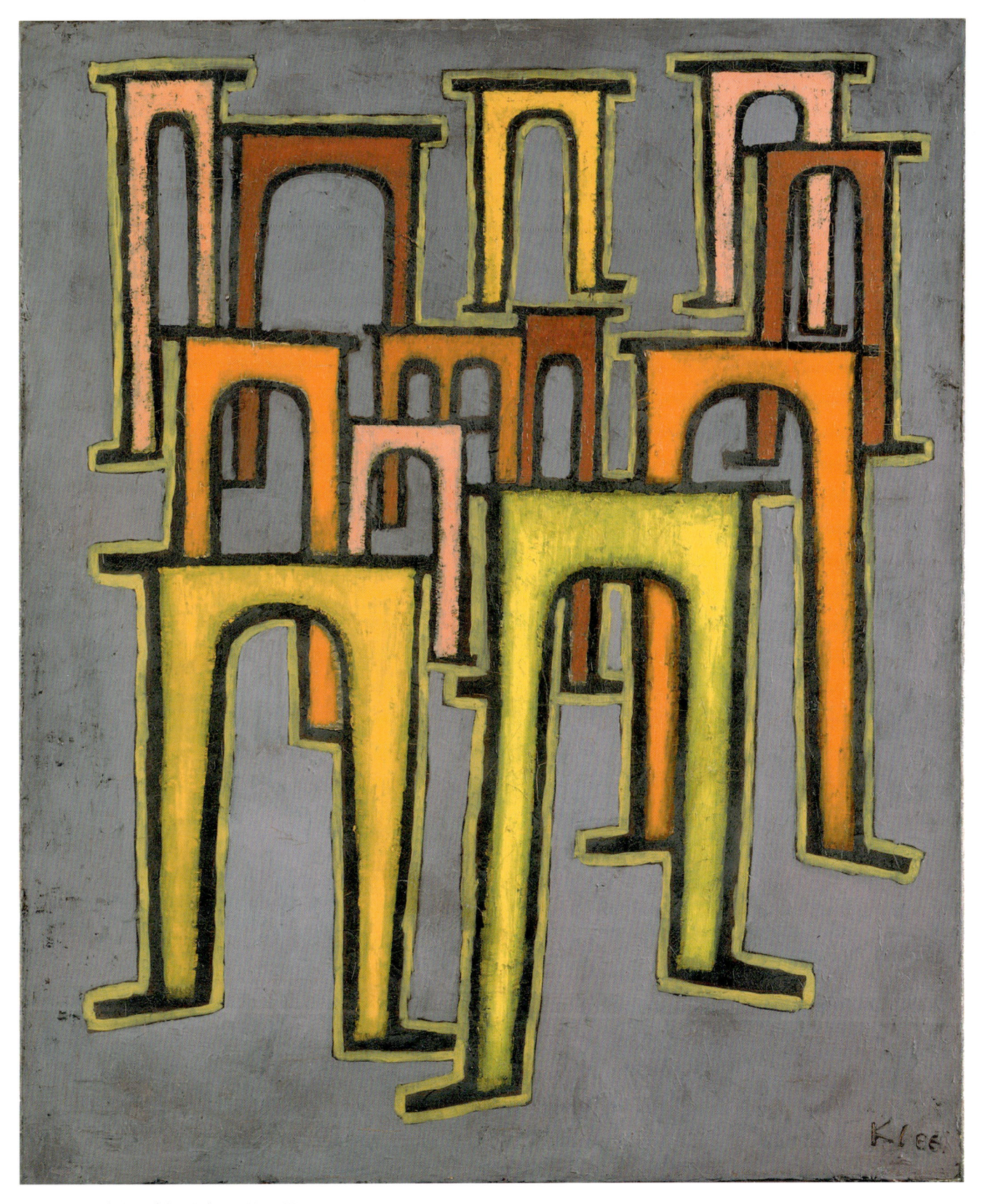

Fig. 136. Revolution of the viaduct, 1937, 153

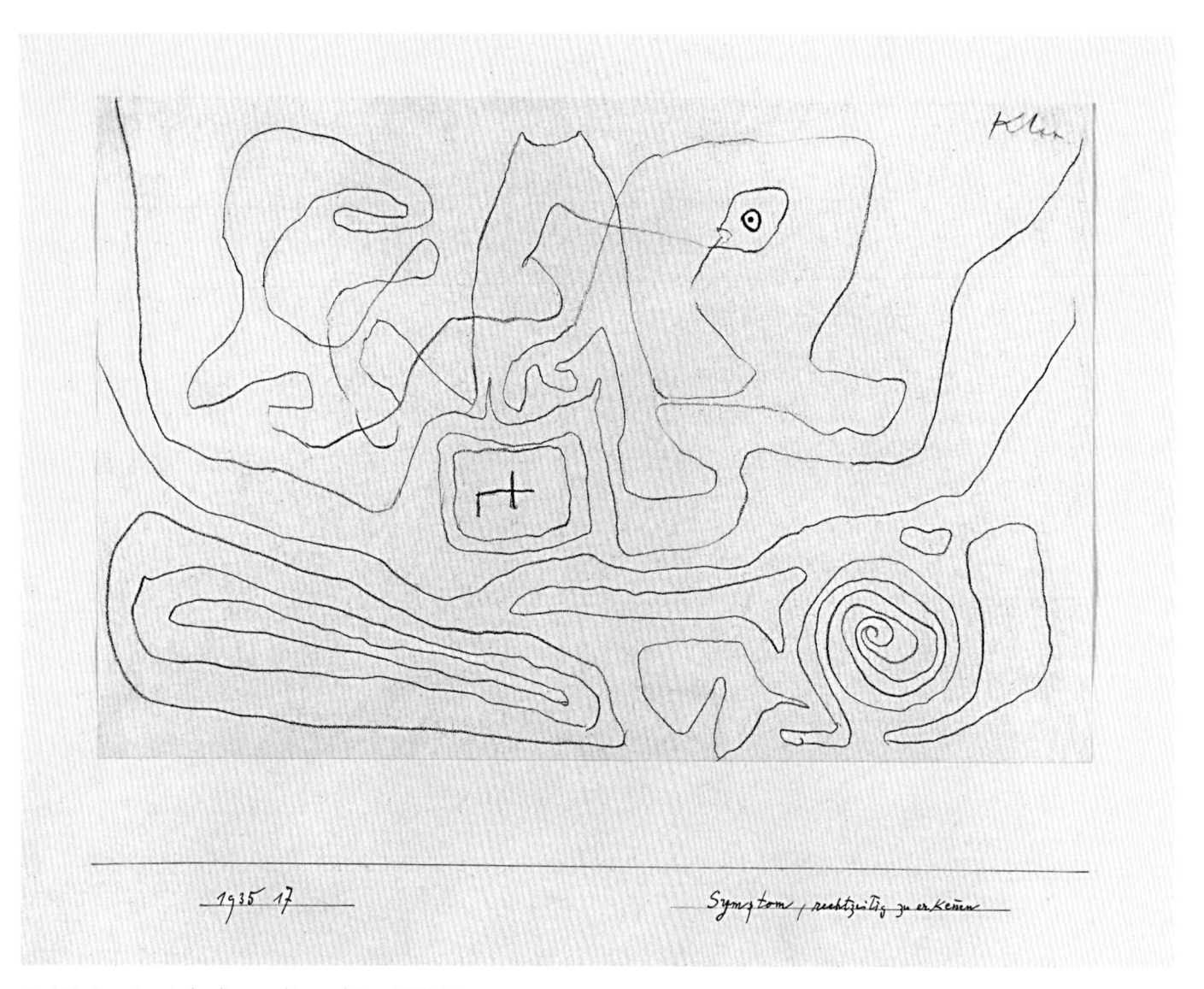

Fig. 137. Symptom, to be diagnosed in good time, 1935, 17

Paul Klee loves the language of symbols and coded messages. The 'symptom' – still not recognized by many people in 1935 – stands in the middle of the picture with a double box around it: the implied swastika is an omen of disaster. It is probably also a cross of death – a premonition of the many deaths in the Second World War. The message is reinforced by the finger of the hand above the cross which is quite clearly pointing at the 'symptom'. In the lower third of the drawing, clearly separated by a line from the animated scene above, there is a kind of stillness, like the stillness of the grave, and a suggestion of bones. Klee can intuitively see the terrible events that will overtake Germany. He has, as he wrote in the title, 'diagnosed' the signs 'in good time'.

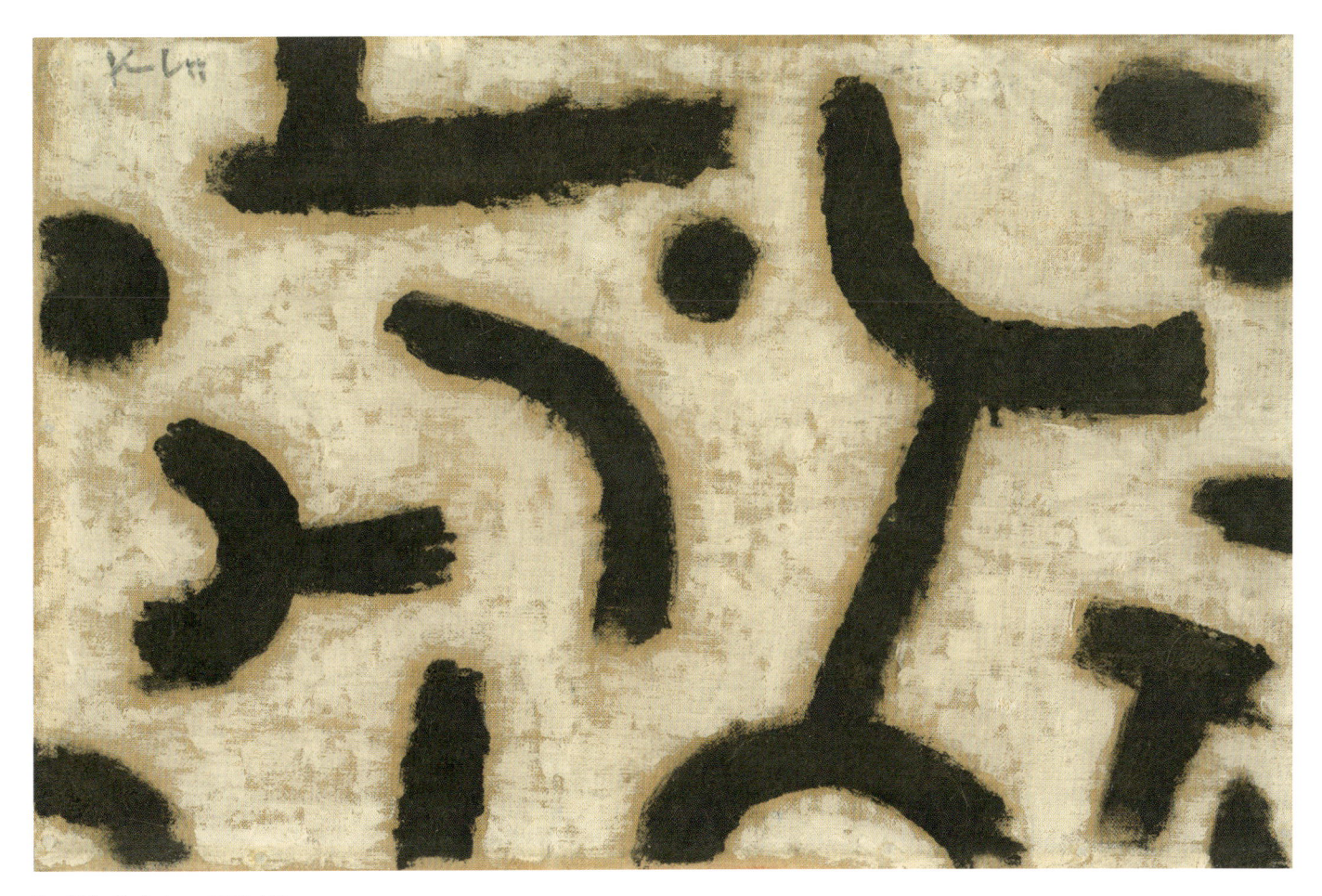

Fig. 138. Black signs, 1938, 114

The thick black bars clearly suggest that this is along the same lines as 'Symptom, to be diagnosed in good time' (fig 137). The bars seem to have broken away from some fixed structure and are now tumbling around each other in space. Some form of equilibrium has been broken. It seems likely that this is another reference to Germany.

In Europe the Second World War is looming. Paul Klee is aware that he is lucky to be living in Switzerland. Dulcis (Latin) means sweet, amarus, amara means bitter. He foresees that he will be able to live on a green island while the war brings horror, misery and death to those all around. He sees his privileged position as sweet and the inevitable war and his own fate as bitter. The death's head in the center bears eloquent witness to this. The art historian Carola Giedion-Welcker points to '[…] the auspicious harmony of herbal (solanum dulcamara) and maritime associations, of sweet and bitter flavors […].'[533] Her colleague Anna Schafroth alludes to the earlier use of this highly poisonous plant as a remedy for rheumatic diseases, which include scleroderma. The art historian also points to the scarlet fruits scattered around the painting, which are similar to the ripened fruits of solanum dulcamara.[534] The artist Bendicht Friedli suggests another association: the 'bittersweet' plant is a member of the nightshade family – the National Socialists are spreading their shadow over everything and have banished Paul Klee to a 'nightshade existence'.[535]

Paul Klee also commented on this in a letter to his daughter-in-law, written in the year he painted the picture: 'We should not be discouraged if there are some indigestible morsels in what comes our way; we can only hope that our strength remains equal to these harder things. Life is certainly more fascinating this way than if it were purely à la Biedermeier. Let everyone take what suits his taste from the two bowls of sweet and salt.'[536]

The painting is Klee's largest complete panel painting. Jürgen Glaesemer considers it one of the 'highlights of his later work'[537]: 'The antithesis of these two opposites (sweet-bitter) that Klee presents in "Insula dulcamara" serves as a key to understanding all of his later works, in terms of artistic form as well as content. This tension of opposites is an expression of the way his attitude to life swings between distanced composure and painful emotional turmoil.'[538]

[533] Giedion-Welcker 2000, p. 149.
[534] Cf. Schafroth, Anna, in: Zentrum Paul Klee 2005/2, p. 96.
[535] Communication from Bendicht Friedli to the author, CH–3800 Unterseen, August 14, 2001.
[536] Letter from Paul Klee to his daughter-in-law Euphrosine Klee, January 27, 1938 (quoted in Glaesemer 1976, p. 333).
[537] Glaesemer 1976, p. 133.
[538] Ibid.

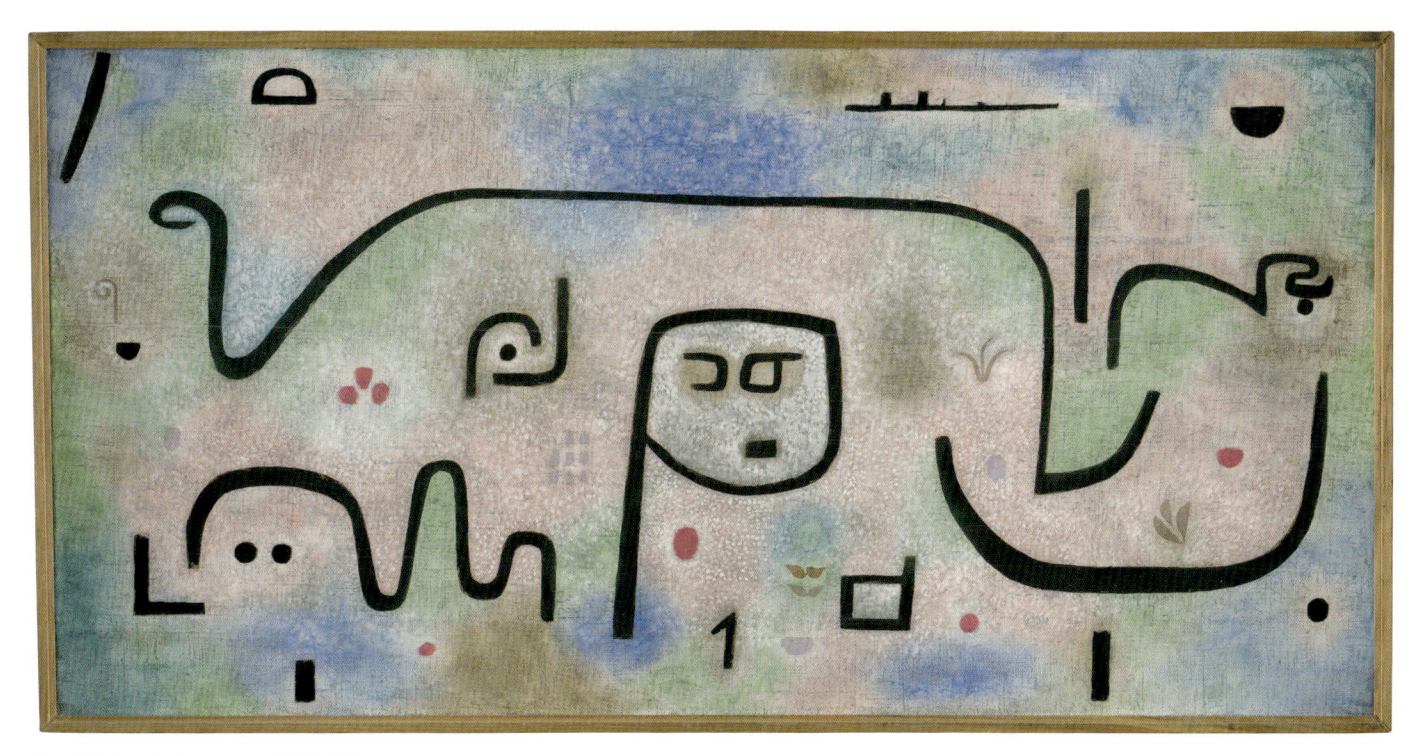

Fig. 139. Insula dulcamara, 1938, 481

The art historian Hans-Jürgen Bruderer defines an artist's intuition: 'Intuition is the ability to use one's clear knowledge of the artistic rules in order to bring to life the possibilities of form hidden within them.'[539] And indeed Klee was the master of this! His oft-quoted theory: 'Art does not reproduce the visible; rather, it makes visible,'[540] is heading in the same direction. Bruderer continues: 'Intuition is described as a realm in which the artist can create a new, autonomous order of potent artistic relationships, which are quite independent of natural form and inner structures. He does not feel compelled to create reproductions, but he is bound to follow the artistic rules. These rules are intrinsic to the artistic medium and cannot be created freely by the artist. In his first lessons, Klee made a rigorous analysis of their development and constructive interaction. After an initial creative activity they should then be reviewed by means of a receptive activity. Does the requirement for artistic freedom, which is led by intuition, in the end not call into question the constructive moments, and does the artist finally experience that romantic sense of elevation as a creator who transcends the rules and constraints of the world?'[541]

People with greater life experience normally have a more developed sense of intuition. This experience is gained through dealing with life's ups and downs, sickness and bereavement, and people with more varied life experience often find they have a better intuitive grasp of fundamental questions. They also are often more spiritually inclined. This was certainly true of Paul Klee.

Hans Christoph von Tavel thinks: 'His [Klee's] work, containing so many hidden layers of meaning, will increasingly be seen as an extraordinarily imaginative, sensitive and at the same time intuitive artistic interpretation of human existence.'[542] The poet Rainer Maria Rilke called Paul Klee 'a "truth-seer", a wise man who could see into the future and invoke it in his own way through drawing and painting.'[543]

Finally, Felix Klee mentioned an incident to me which also shows the artist's intuitive foresight. It was clear from a young age that Felix was also gifted artistically. After finishing school,

---

[539] Bruderer 1990, p. 21.
[540] Klee, Paul, contribution to the anthology 'Schöpferische Konfession', quoted in Klee 1979, p. 118.
[541] Bruderer 1990, p. 19.
[542] Von Tavel 1969, p. 156.
[543] Quoted in Pfeiffer-Belli 1978, p. 385.

he wanted to be a painter like his father. However Paul Klee advised him strongly against this. He was – quite rightly, in my opinion – convinced that his son would find it very difficult to establish his own identity as an artist. Felix would always be judged as 'Paul Klee's son' and would find himself standing forever in his shadow. At the time Felix did not accept this argument, but later he was to feel grateful for his father's advice.[544] Hans Christoph von Tavel assesses Felix Klee's choice of career as follows: 'When his father advised him [Felix] against becoming a painter, it was perhaps not so much because of the difficulty of making a living in this profession as the realization that his son's talent was more suited to outward expression, rather than to the internalization which he viewed as an artist's defining capability. Consequently, Felix was steered towards the theater.'[545]

[544] Personal communication, Felix Klee to the author, September 20, 1983.
[545] Von Tavel 1990, p. 18.

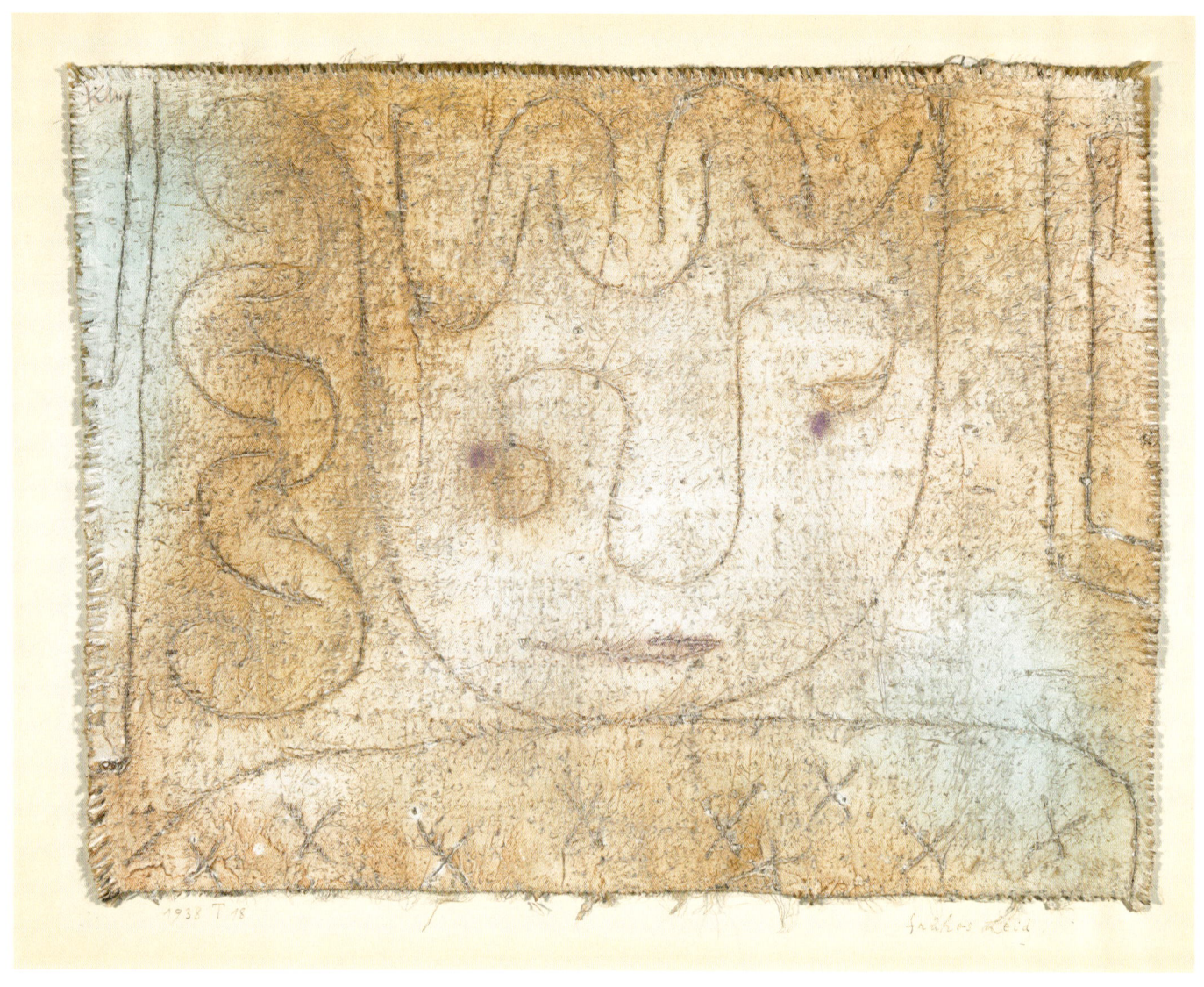

Fig. 140. Early sorrow, 1938, 318

Because so much of Klee's work in the final years is based on his personal experiences and feelings, this painting could be interpreted as follows: a teardrop falls from the eye of a grieving woman. The artist senses that he won't live much longer. His wife will experience 'Early sorrow'.

Fig. 141. Taking leave, 1938, 352

Even two years before his death, Paul Klee probably senses that his illness is incurable and that he will have to say goodbye prematurely. How moving is this simple image with the serious, sad eyes and the head hanging down in the narrow space. A space that will slowly get narrower and narrower until it finally disappears.

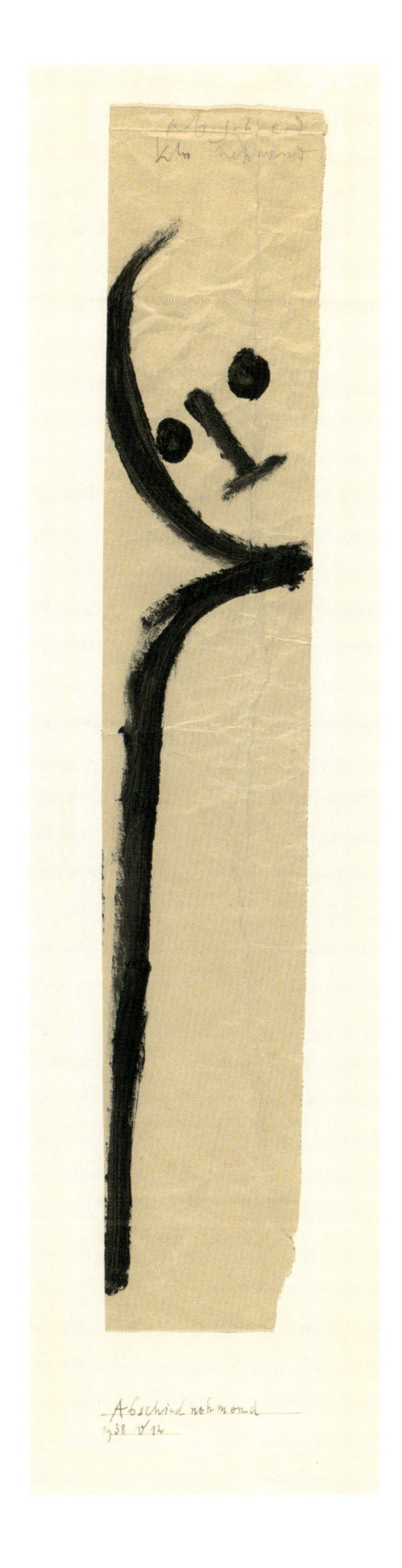

Belated Accolades

On December 18, 1939, Paul Klee turned 60. His wife relates: 'Klee has really been celebrated. The festivities lasted three days. But only with a few people each time. The first day on Dec. 16, he celebrated with his 90-year-old father. The afternoon and evening of Dec. 17, we went with a few friends to the castle at Bürgis near Bern, where the late Mrs. Bürgi had a collection of 50 Klees. This was really a memorable evening. It was just how he likes it, quiet and genteel. Then Dec. 18 was for ourselves, with [visits and] stacks of post, telegrams, gifts, books, flowers, gramophone records. A lot of affectionate letters arrived from Germany. But he is now also really respected and celebrated in Switzerland. All the newspapers carried notices or articles about him. […] It was very gratifying for him and he was so happy, reading all the letters and playing his records all day long. This day is now over, but we will always remember it fondly. Above all, it did him good to feel surrounded by such warmth and friendship.'[546]

Klee took great pleasure in these belated accolades, particularly those of the Swiss press, and they motivated him to carry on working. But first he personally replied to nearly one hundred letters of congratulations from home and abroad. As previously mentioned, he had to deal with this correspondence himself as his wife was in poor health at the time and not in a position to help him.[547] This put considerable strain on him, as did the subsequent final preparations for his anniversary exhibition at the Kunsthaus Zurich, an exhibition which he had personally conceived and which was to take place in mid-February 1940 with over 200 of his latest works.[548] His health deteriorated once more.[549] It was probably also exacerbated by emotional upheavals such as his father's death on January 12, 1940 and the long drawn-out process of being granted his Swiss citizenship.[550]

---

[546] Letter from Lily Klee to Curt Valentin, January 1, 1940 (MoMAA-NY/VP), quoted in Frey 1990, p. 120 f.

[547] Cf. letter from Lily Klee to Gertrud Grohmann, January 6, 1940, quoted in Frey 1990, p. 121.

[548] 'Paul Klee. Neue Werke', Kunsthaus Zurich, February 16 to March 25, 1940. It was the first comprehensive exhibition of his later work, and the only one which he personally set in motion. It total[led] 213 exhibits, most of them for sale – 76 panel paintings and 137 multi-colored works on paper – from the years 1935–1940 […] (Frey 1990, p. 122). And Giedion-Welcker 2000, p. 101: Carola Giedion-Welcker mentions a remark Klee made when she was visiting him in Bern a few weeks before his death: 'Klee told me that he would like to go to the South for a rest because all the problems of organizing the exhibition had tired him out.'

[549] Cf. letter from Paul Klee to Waldemar Jollos, Bern, February 18, 1940 (location unknown, photocopy: ZPKB), and cf. letter from Lily Klee to Josef and Hanni Albers, Bern, February 27, 1940 (Autograph Yale University Library, New Haven). It emerges from a letter from Wilhelm Wartmann, Director of the Kunsthaus Zurich, to Emil Friedrich, board member of the Zurich Kunstgesellschaft, February 7, 1940 (Kunsthaus Zurich) that the second meeting between Wartmann and the artist to discuss the anniversary exhibition could not take place until February 6, 1940, because of Klee's ill-health: 'We had previously been informed by telephone that Klee's condition was not good,' cf. also Frey 1990, p. 122. The two had met to discuss the exhibition for the first time on November 29, 1939, cf. Frey 1990, p. 120.

[550] On December 19, 1939 Klee finally received his federal citizenship permit. However he still had to apply for the so-called 'Landrecht' – the right to live in the canton of Bern – and for municipal citizenship of the City of Bern (see pp. 31–37 and notes 65–71, p. 265 and 266); cf. also Frey 1990, p. 121 f.

The Final Works

Despite the circumstances mentioned above, the artist continued to be extremely productive. In 1939 he produced on average 100 works per month, while in January 1940 he created an incredible 158 works, followed by 75 in February, 76 in March, 41 in April and another 16 during the first week of May.[551] Remarkably, in his last four productive months he changed his usual system of numbering his works. Since 1925 he had numbered them either on the card base or the frame, but not consecutively, instead he used a kind of code number which was a combination of a letter and a number. The letters stood for the tens and the hundreds, the numbers for the ones. For every 20 numbered works – 20 corresponded to one page in his catalogue of works – Klee used a letter, but he did not begin each year with 'A', for example 1937 began with 'K', 1938 with 'D' and 1939 with 'G'. The order of the letters followed the alphabet; from 1930 'Z' was followed by 'A', with some letters being omitted. He created a table which provided the key to this code.[552] But strangely, in January 1940 he gave the first code number the letter 'Z'; in this way the first work of the year of his death, 1940, 1, bears the code number 'Z 1' (fig. 142 [cat. of works 1940, first page, nos. 1–20]) and the last work registered in the catalogue of works, 1940, 366, bears the code number 'E 6' (fig. 143 [cat. of works 1940, last page, nos. 361–366]).[553] Josef Helfenstein interprets the alteration as follows: 'This numerical increase [in production] corresponds with diametrically-opposed symmetry to the "countdown" of the alphabet running backwards, which breaks off at letter "E" and number 366. It is as if Klee, by using the reverse alphabet, wants to point out that his race against time is intensifying.'[554]

This seems a very plausible argument. It is quite conceivable that at the beginning of January 1940 the artist felt that his end was drawing near; perhaps he would only be able to fill out one more page in his catalogue of works – the final page. Max Huggler was of the same opinion: '[…] knowing his end was near, he [Klee] wanted to gather together the fruit of his life's work.'[555] Marcel Franciscono describes this time as follows: 'Some of the paintings and drawings which he produced in his final months show that thoughts of death were

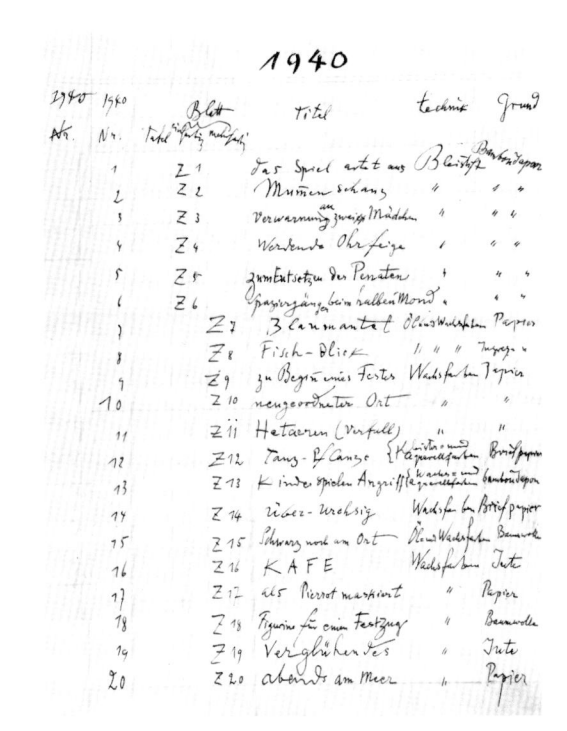

Fig. 142. Paul Klee's catalogue of works, 1940, first page

---

[551] Cf. Frey 1990, p. 122.
[552] For code numbers in general see Wiederkehr Sladeczek 2000, p. 148 f.
[553] Cf. Helfenstein 1990, p. 72.
[554] Ibid.
[555] Huggler 1969, p. 157.

at the forefront of his mind. And in 1940 Klee started noting down the months in his catalogue of works, something he had never done before.[556] He seems to have recognized the fact that he would not survive the year and started to treat every month as if it were a year, each one a period of time to which he allocated a group of finished works.'[557] Will Grohmann writes about the final works: 'Klee will have considered his final pictures as his most truthful and most complete, as they contain something of the inexorability and splendor of "death and rebirth". But this does not mean he devalued his earlier work, not even his very early attempts, for he built his work stone by stone, and each one was the necessary and right step which allowed his work to grow as he grew. Who can say whether he was finished by 1940; he had been through many metamorphoses in his life, but perhaps towards the end Klee skipped over some of these changes so that he could be in tune with death.'[558]

To begin with, terminally ill or very old people often go through a period of hope and have a strong desire to live. But when they suddenly sense that their end is near, they usually face death calmly, particularly if they can look back with satisfaction at their life and life's work. Once this point has been reached, death often follows within a matter of days or weeks. As a doctor I have seen this many times, not only in my patients but also in my family, friends and acquaintances, and it made a deep impression on me. Paul Klee was himself quite astonished that he got through the difficult month of January 1940 so well and that he lived for another six months. This is further proof of Klee's fundamentally robust constitution and of his desire to finish his life's work. He needed many pages to catalogue the works he produced between January and May 1940 – 19 in total – and rounded off his work with the note '1940, 366' and the code number 'E 6' (fig. 143).

The following observations are only idle speculation, but perhaps I can be allowed to muse a little on the letter 'E' which Klee used in recording his final works. For instance, the letter could have terminal overtones if we take it as an abbreviation for 'End' – the end of his work as an artist. Geographically,

[556] Marcel Franciscono overlooks the fact that Klee was already noting the months in 1939; Glaesemer 1979, p. 23: 'In September 1939, for the first time Klee noted details of the month in his catalogue of works. The entries for 1949 are noted exactly according to month. At that point he was obviously starting to take an interest in the number of works he produced per month.'
[557] Franciscono 1990, p. 20.
[558] Grohmann 1965, p. 382.

'E' means 'East'; and East also signifies 'Orient'. According to Will Grohmann, Paul Klee felt a strong bond with the Orient: 'His work is also infiltrated by the spirit of the Near East. This was not a result of his visits to Tunisia and Egypt; conversely these visits were a result of his interest in the lands of the Near East and in Islamic culture. Whether [on his mother's side] he had blood ties with the region is a moot point, but it is clear he felt a sense of kindredship with the Orient.'[559] 'e' is also an important symbol in mathematics and physics. In 1748 the Basel mathematician Leonhard Euler first used 'e' to signify 'the sum of an infinite series'. French mathematicians later termed this concept a 'transcendental number' and used it as a basis for natural logarithms.[560] In physics, 'e' signifies the smallest electric charge ('elementary charge') and the smallest quantity of energy.[561] 'Infinity', 'Transcendence' and 'Energy' are concepts which fit well with the personality and art of Paul Klee, along with other words beginning with 'E' that come to mind through free association, such as 'Ernte' (harvest), 'Engel' (angel) and 'Ewigkeit' (eternity).

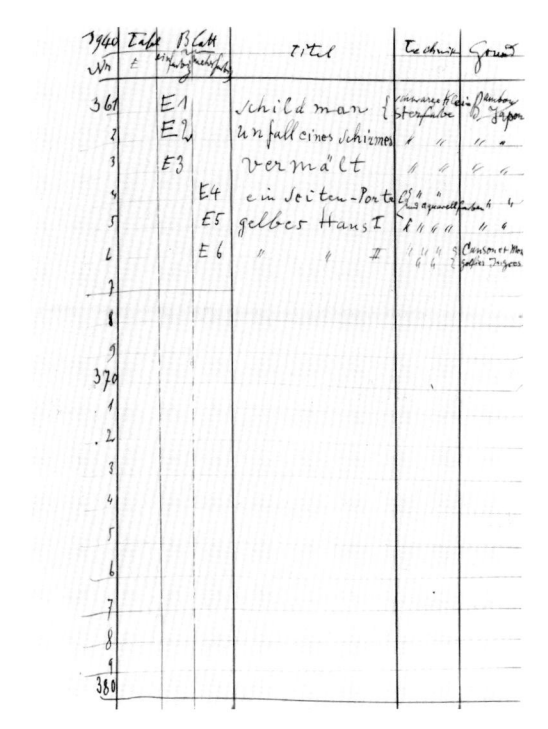

Fig. 143. Paul Klee's catalogue of works, 1940, last page

[559] Grohmann 1965, p. 380.
[560] Cf. Zürich 1945–1948, vol. 2, p. 1243, and vol. 3, p. 101.
[561] Cf. Luzern 1991–1993, vol. 2, p. 379, and vol. 5, p. 266 (keyword 'Quant').

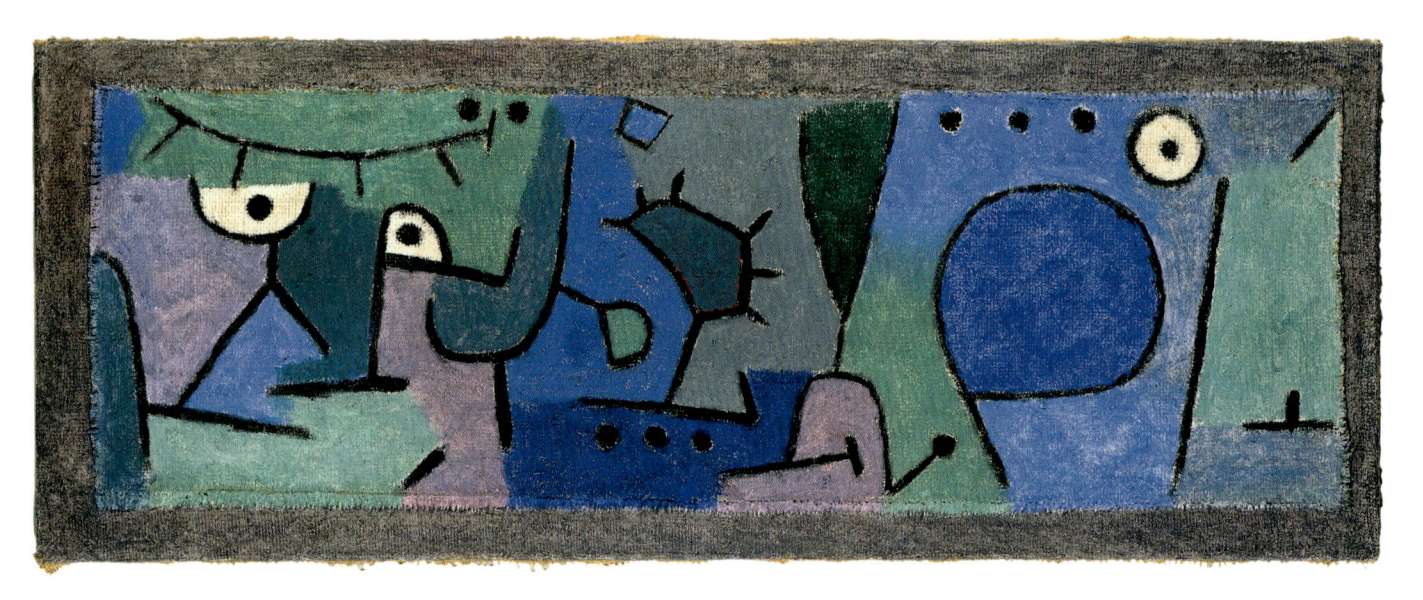

Fig. 144. Eyes in the landscape, 1940, 41

Sad eyes look from the landscape and out to the sea. The painting evokes boats at the jetty with portholes and rudders. In the distance, to the right, a ship sails out to sea. In the past, Klee loved to travel, but now his illness makes it no longer possible. These days he undertakes a different kind of beautiful journey: a journey into the world of color, and here he achieves a wonderfully harmonized and concentrated combination of colors.

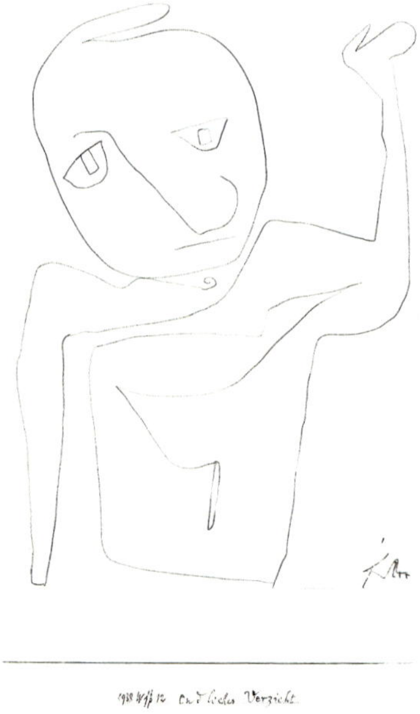

During his five years of illness, Paul Klee had to give up many things, such as his beloved violin and his visits to museums, concerts and theaters. He made these sacrifices with equanimity.

Fig. 145. Final renunciation, 1938, 372

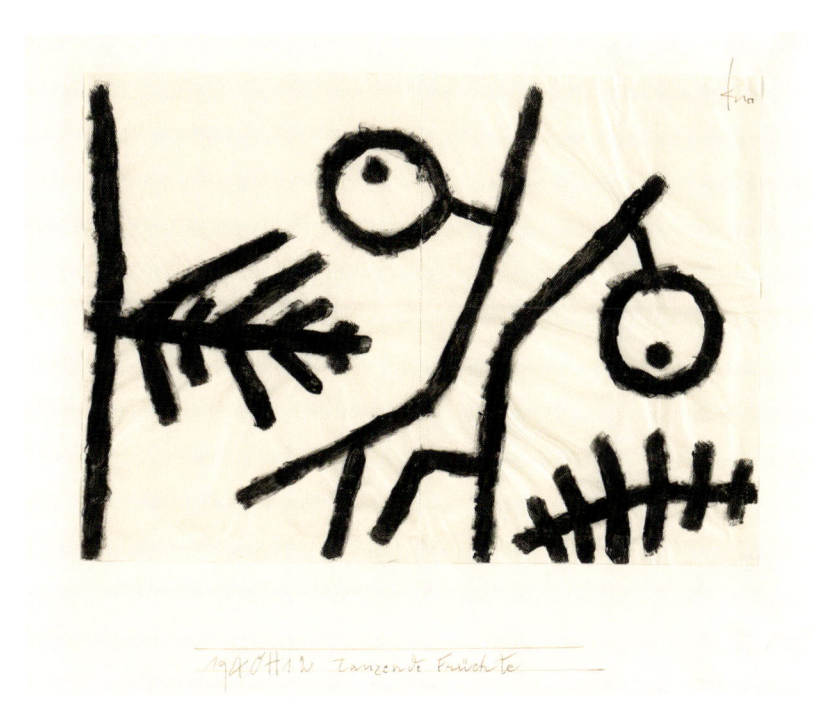

Fig. 146. Dancing fruits, 1940, 312

There is a fruit hanging on each of two branches; they could be apples. Using a wide brush Klee paints what looks like leaves next to them, with only their ribs visible. The fruit on the left does not hang vertically: it begins to swing, to dance, as though blown by a strong gust of wind. The other fruit does the same. A gust of wind could possibly soon cause the swinging fruit to fall. The drawing also looks like a face with staring eyes, full of fear. The leaves become fan-shaped spears that threaten the eyes. The figure is cornered and cannot fight back. Klee's life feels both trapped and threatened by his serious illness.

Scleroderma causes the skin to become thick, stiff and rigid and its suppleness is lost. In this drawing Klee depicts his own afflicted skin.

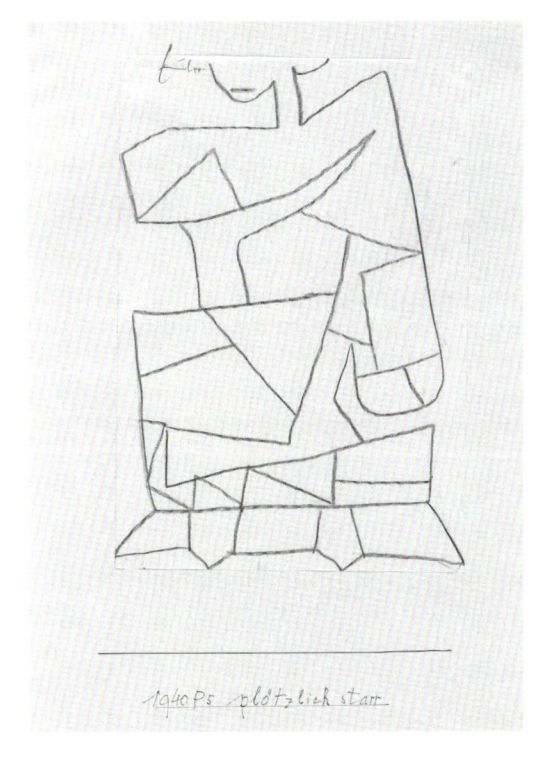

Fig. 147. Suddenly rigid, 1940, 205

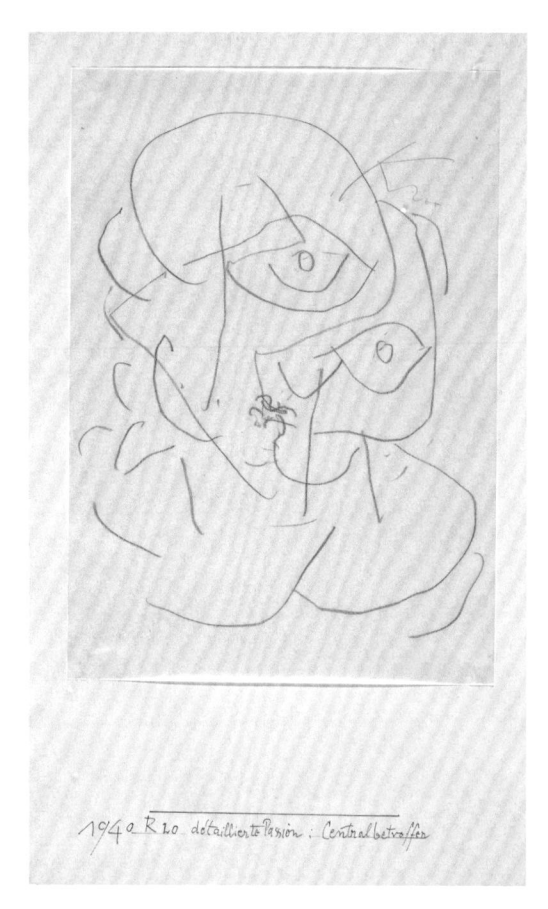

Fig. 148. Detailed passion: touched to the core, 1940, 180

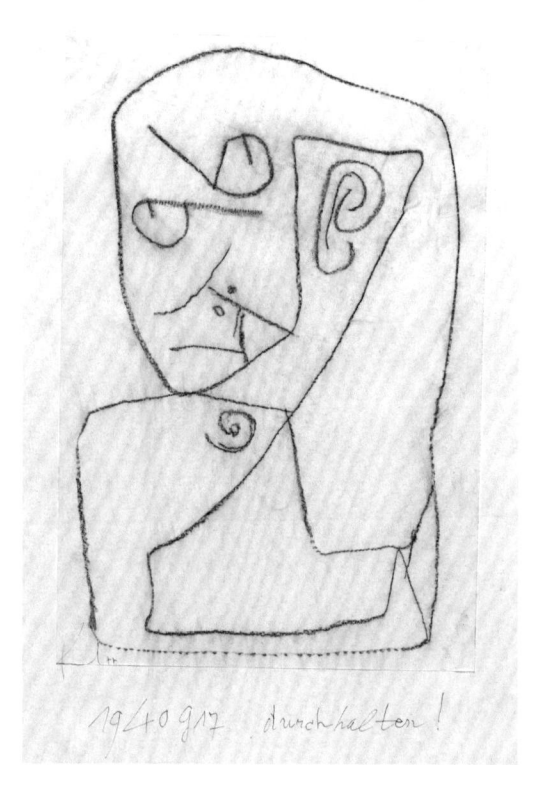

Fig. 149. Stick it out!, 1940, 337

Fate has dealt a harsh blow. A man suffers to his very core. This work belongs to a series of eight drawings from the artist's final year, all entitled 'Detailed passion'. By passion, Klee could mean either personal tales of woe or enthusiastic dedication. He bears his suffering patiently, but dedicates himself even more passionately to his art as death draws nearer. In contrast to most of his later drawings, which have decisive, joined-up lines, this series is characterized by shorter, broken and crossed lines. As a result the images appear disturbed and distorted: the person is 'Touched to the core', his face distorted with pain.

However, Paul Klee also draws a suffering figure that appears contemplative, looking defiantly inwards and resolutely telling himself 'Stick it out!'. Indeed, in the last few months of his life, the artist managed to defy his imminent death by producing a total of 366 complete works, with some others left incomplete. With 366 works registered in his catalogue of works, Klee was anticipating – no doubt consciously – that this would be his complete output for the leap year of 1940, in line with a saying he notes in his catalogue for the year 1938 (fig. 173, page 222).

In this drawing from January 1940, Klee alludes to the passage in the Bible where the Roman Governor Pontius Pilate parades Jesus before the people, proclaiming: 'Ecce homo' (Behold the man!), John, 19, 5. In the 15th century, Rogier van der Weyden introduced into art the theme of the Savior with the crown of thorns. Later, this Latin inscription was mainly to be found on wooden carvings and sculptures that depicted Jesus as the man of sorrows bearing the stigmata.[562] The link between Klee's drawing and the Bible passage is not only the crown of thorns, but also the four dots that follow 'Ecce', which represent the four letters of 'homo'. Is Klee depicting himself here as a victim who, like Jesus, has been subjected to injustice and suffering?

I tend to agree with Hannelore Mittag, who sees the face as a self-portrait of Paul Klee, showing the tight skin, pointed nose and narrow mouth brought on by scleroderma.[563]

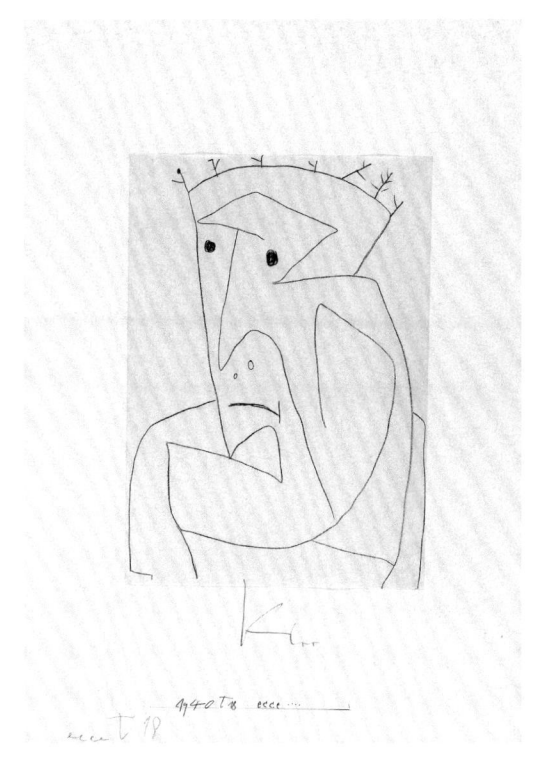

Fig. 150. Ecce ...., 1940, 138

[562] Zürich 1945–1948, vol. 2, p. 1251.
[563] Mittag/ML 2001, p. 203.

184

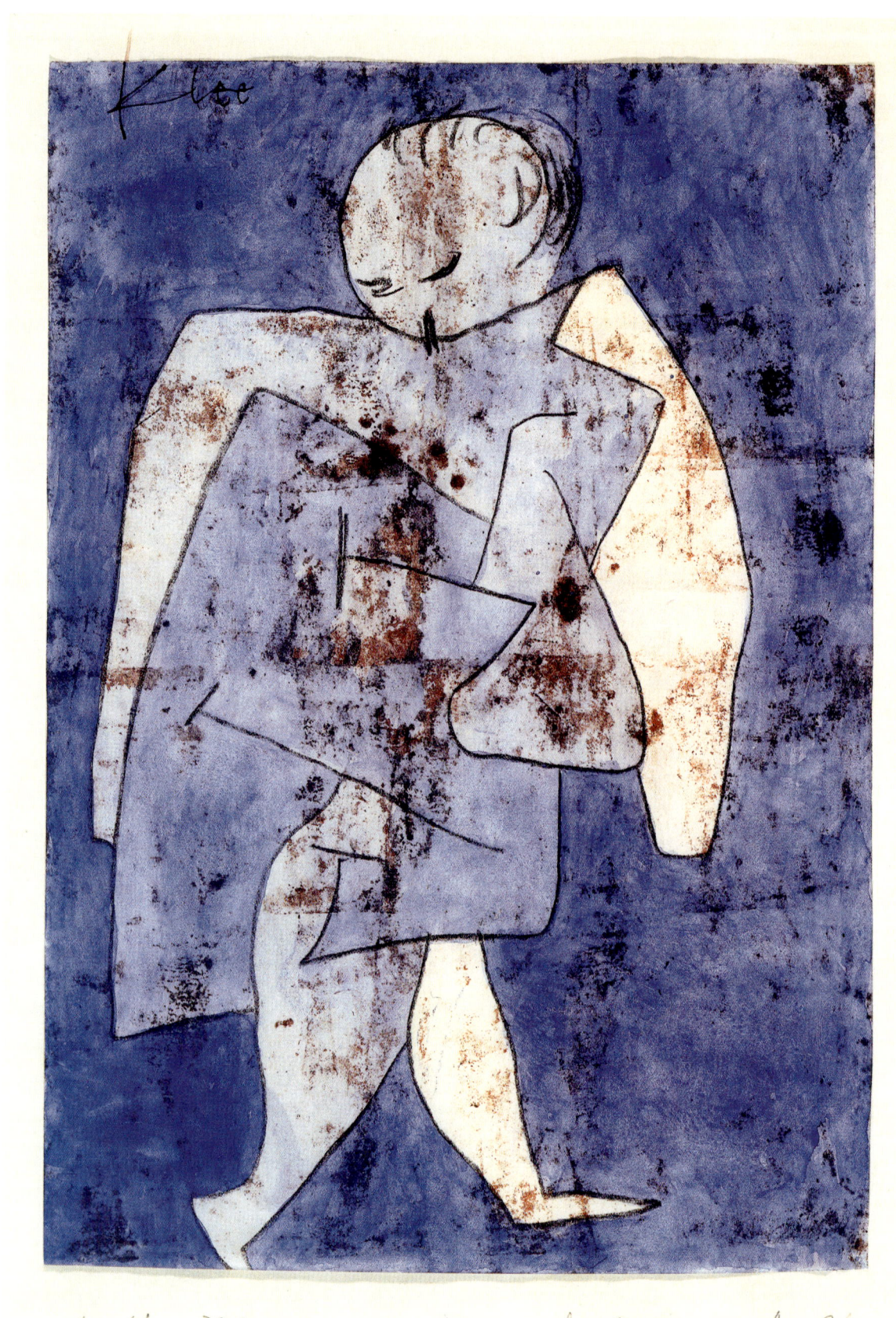

5. Klee's Late Work as a Reflection of His Personality, Social Environment, Illness and Proximity to Death

Isolation and Solitary Internalization

Paul Klee's late works are clearly distinguishable from those of his earlier period. In subject and composition they are quite new. Jürgen Glaesemer writes in this respect: 'The emigration marked a tragic reversal in his [Klee's] personal and artistic fortunes. One feels in his later works that his life has been totally overtaken by the threats of "physical reality". He faced the chaos of the external sphere, the onset of his terminal illness with its attendant chronic suffering, his fears and the shadow of death with a total lack of self-pity. This is what gives his later works their particularly poignant intensity.'[564]

Surprisingly, his involuntary isolation bore ripe and luscious fruit. Glaesemer later states: 'His work was created in isolation from his external surroundings as an expression of his state of solitary internalization, which even those closest to Klee could barely penetrate.'[565] Josef Helfenstein adds: 'During his Bern years, Klee was forced by circumstance but also by private determination to make a radical retreat into his personal cosmos. He not only suffered geographic, intellectual and artistic isolation, but he was also set apart by his illness and by his ascetic lifestyle with its narrow focus on work. The fact that, even in 1940, his relationship towards his own work was once again transformed, is perhaps not only linked to the shadow of death which was clearly hanging over him,

Fig. 151. Whence? where? whither?, 1940, 60

[564] Glaesemer 1976, p. 306.
[565] Glaesemer 1979, p. 12.

but also to the historical fact that modern artists in Europe were forced into isolation during that period.'[566] Jürgen Glaesemer also believes the political storm clouds which were gathering over Europe at that time had an effect on the artist's work: 'Along with his illness, the pressures of the contemporary historical situation had a decisive effect on the development and expression of his later works.'[567]

'Death Is Nothing Bad'

Even in his youth, the artist regarded death – and the possibility of an afterlife – with equanimity.[568] As a 21-year-old student in Munich he mused on death: 'Then I reflect on death, which completes those things that are left unfinished in life. A longing for death not as oblivion but as the pursuit of perfection.'[569] Awareness of the finiteness of (earthly) life leads the young Klee to discover that, for him, 'the pursuit of perfection' constitutes the meaning of life. He wants to use and develop to the utmost every ounce of his creative abilities. This desire for perfection may be a clue to understanding why Klee was able to race to finish his life's work despite his later severe illness and foreseeably shortened lifespan. Looked at this way, his involuntary isolation and his intuition early on that he was suffering from a terminal illness were perhaps a prerequisite for him to be able to reach the ambitious goals he set for his life.

In 1914 the artist wrote in his diary: 'I am forearmed, I am not here, I am in the depths, far away … I am glowing among the dead.'[570] Here he anticipates two of his very last works: 'Dying down', 1940, 19 and 'Death and fire', 1940, 332 (fig. 152, page 191).

In 1918 Klee described his position in his famous words: 'In the here and now I cannot be understood, for I live as well with the dead as with the unborn. Somewhat nearer the heart of creation than normal – and yet not nearly close enough.'[571] These words were carved on his gravestone in 1941 / 1942.[572]

---

[566] Helfenstein 1990, p. 68.
[567] Glaesemer 1979, p. 16.
[568] See notes 468 and 470.
[569] Klee Diaries, no. 143.
[570] Ibid., no. 931.
[571] From Paul Klee's diary in: Zahn 1920, p. 5. Contrary to the caption in Zahn 1920, this 'diary' entry does not appear in the diary. Klee probably wrote the words especially for Leopold Zahn (as told by Stefan Frey to the author, Bern, July 14, 2006).
[572] Cf. Frey 1990, p. 128.

In 1930 the artist once again spoke about death: 'Death is nothing bad; I long ago reconciled myself to it. How do we know what is more important, our present life or what comes after? […] I won't mind dying if I have done a few more good paintings.'[573] In 1930 Paul Klee was at his peak – he had achieved a great deal and was respected as a man, teacher and artist. He was already close to fulfilling the goals he had set for his life. Death was not to be feared. He would just like first to round off his work with 'a few more good paintings'. Nothing stood in his way; he was (still) in good health and at the height of his powers.

But then fate took a cruel and unexpected twist, striking like a lightning bolt from a cloudless sky. At first Klee felt artistically paralyzed by his illness, but then he once again gathered his energies, for he still wanted to produce 'a few more good paintings'. In 1938, two years before his death, and after three years of wearisome illness, Klee ponders his fate in the following words (as previously quoted): 'If only the enigma of death were not so ambiguous! No less so is the enigma of life, for one has to wonder what beauty and splendor can be found in the torments of recent times.'[574] Suddenly death, with all its mysteries, was knocking at his door. And the artist now also had to face the enigma of life, as his previously untroubled existence turned into one of pain and affliction. Paul Klee thought back to the goals he had set for his life when he was young, and characteristically continued to strive unerringly for perfection. He writes to Will Grohmann: 'One's enjoyment of life is a little hampered these days, but perhaps it is possible to reconstruct it to some degree through one's work? It seems so to me, and I think one can derive a certain amount of happiness from it. When work is going well, one feels a kind of happiness. New paths – a simile for creation.'[575]

The art historian Wieland Schmied thinks the themes of dying and death are interwoven in Klee's art: 'His [Klee's] pictures are parallels to nature; the painter creates them through a process of organic growth. Growth is a crucial word for understanding Paul Klee's work. Klee shows us the stages, the phases of a constantly evolving transformation, the metamorphosis of forms, the changing aspect of shapes.

[573] Quoted in Petitpierre 1957, p. 65. Grohmann 1965, p. 358, dated the quote to the year 1930. See also note 468.

[574] Paul Klee, extract from letter, August 17, 1938, quoted in Klee 1960/1, p. 163.

[575] Letter from Paul Klee to Will Grohmann, November 1939, quoted in Gutbrod 1968, pp. 81 and 84.

Outwardly, there is no dynamic movement, but movement is the essence of his paintings. Movement signifies growth, transition and ultimately also decay – what we could term the cycle of existence. Death always appeared in his pictures, as death is everywhere in life. Now death steps forward and calls a halt. Klee feels this long before his own demise. He reflects the fact of death in a way which had never been seen before in the visual arts. This is what gives these seemingly small and modest works their greatness and meaning.'[576]

In the same way that change is part of life, Klee's art was in a state of constant flux. I believe this element of change is an essential criterion for all great art. Standing still is the same as going backwards; real progress comes from looking ahead, developing new concepts and bringing them to fruition. I would repeat Klee's words: 'new paths – a simile for creation.' An innovative and autonomous artist will always be involved in a slow but steady process of transformation.

Marcel Franciscono also sees death as an integral part of Klee's art: 'Death is the overriding theme of Klee's work during his last months, but for the most part he expresses it in different forms: its presence is mainly felt through the reactions and behavior of the human figures depicted. In 1940 Klee produced two series of drawings on the theme of death, "Eidola" and "Detailed passion". […] the pictures in the "Detailed passion" cycle do not deny the existence of death and the fear it instills; but by depicting death as a constant and familiar part of life, Klee takes away some of its terror.'[577]

It is worth noting that Vincent van Gogh, who had much in common with Paul Klee in the way he dealt with his suffering, also had a similarly positive attitude towards death. Herbert Frank quotes the painter from Arles as follows: 'His credo was: "The difference between good luck and bad luck! Both are valuable, death – which is basically evanescence – and life. I hold firm to this belief, despite my bewildering and disturbing illness". In this way he makes death a part of life, and does not conceive of it as an end.'[578] Van

[576] Schmied 1986, p. 53.
[577] Franciscono 1990, p. 21 f.
[578] Frank 1999, p. 113 f, letter T 607.

Gogh spoke about his painting 'Wheat Field with Reaper' from June 1889: '[…] that he sees in the "reaper" a symbol of death and the crop he is cutting represents humankind. But there is nothing sad about this death, it is happening in broad daylight, in beautiful golden sunshine.'[579]

[579] Frank 1999, p. 112, letter T 604.

A man is leaving this world. He raises his right arm to wave goodbye. In his palm he proudly presents us with a golden ball set against a fiery red background. The face is ashen. The mouth, nose and eyes are made up of highly significant letters: 'Tod' (death). The head is drawn in the same way as the death's head in the painting 'Insula dulcamara' from 1938 (fig. 139, page 171). The man's body will burn in Hell, but not the golden ball, which is boldly delineated in black. We can take this to be the artist's life's work, his legacy to us all. On the right, a thin, shadowy figure approaches the fire with hesitant steps. The organic body will leave this world and with it the pale, familiar face with its large black eyes full of composure, resignation and hope. Paul Klee has resigned himself to the inevitable. He salutes us for the last time, full of expectation, conscious of the valuable legacy contained in the golden ball, which he holds proudly aloft. In the left and lower parts of the picture a soft sky blue, a cerulean blue, spreads gently out from the slowly-dissolving body. Despite its sad message the picture is somehow comforting.

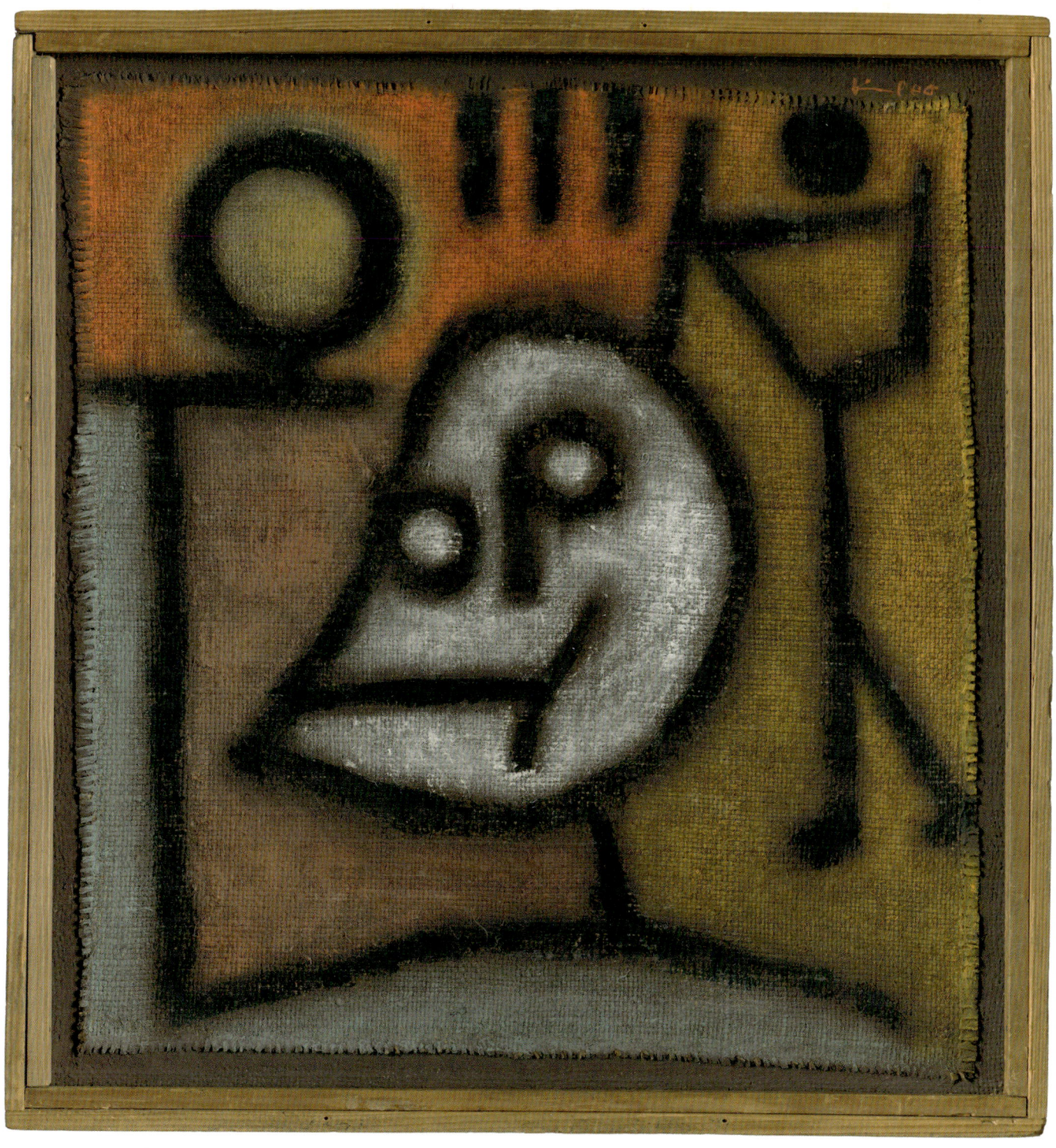

Fig. 152. Death and fire, 1940, 332

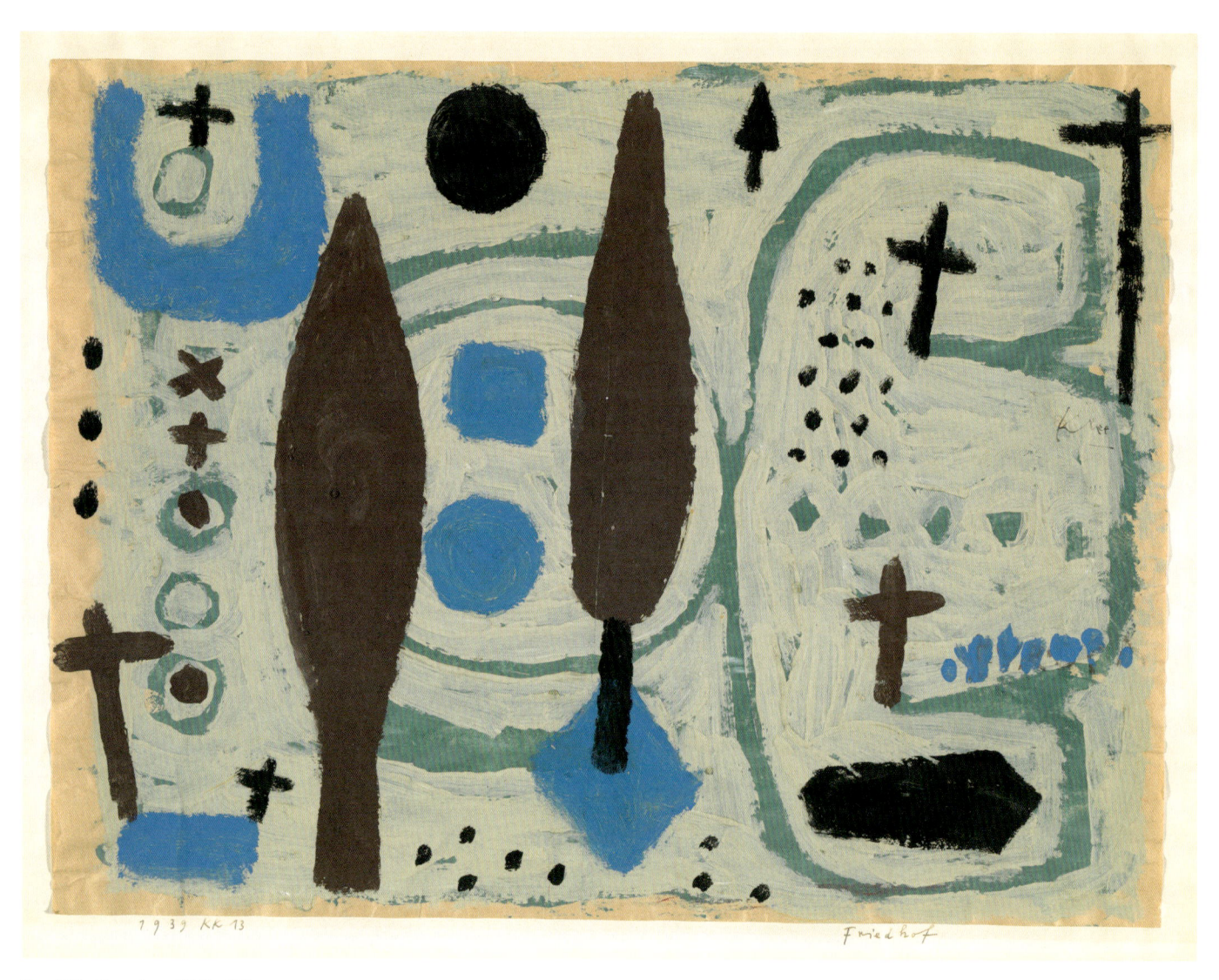

Fig. 153. Cemetery, 1939, 693

The cemetery is identified by seven crosses, two dark sepia-colored cypress trees and a black coffin awaiting burial. An arrow points upwards. Jürgen Glaesemer considers these elements to be 'symbols of [Klee's] own death'.[580] The art historian points out that if you turn the painting through 90° to the right, the corpse appears: pale-faced, with wide open blue eyes and a creamy-white burial gown (fig. 154).

[580] Glaesemer 1976, S. 341.

Work Full of Spirituality

Paul Klee worked in silence, in isolation, alone with his thoughts and dreams in his little studio in Bern. By nature he was quiet and thoughtful, and he possessed a vivid imagination. He loved to withdraw into himself and his work, letting himself roam in the world of his imagination, but at the same time always keeping one foot on the ground. He understood how important this dreaming was for his work. Karl Jaspers says something similar: 'Allowing the mind to move freely in the realms of fantasy brings forth the impulses which prevent work from being interminable, unimportant and empty. It seems to me that a person should take the time each day to dream, otherwise he blocks out the light of that star which can guide him in his work and his life.'[581]

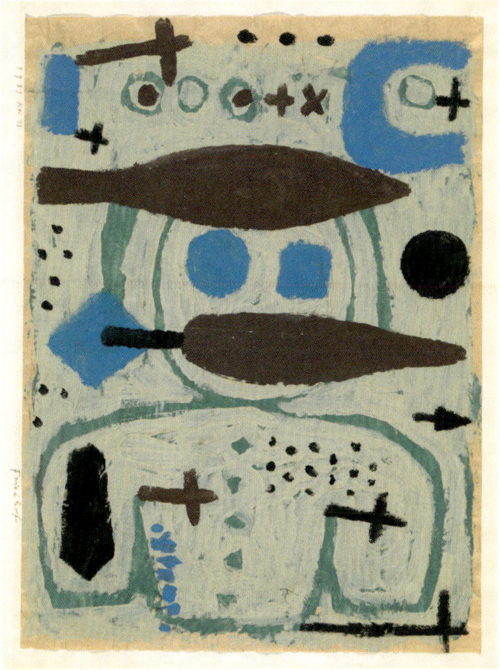

For Klee, drawing and painting were his personal form of meditation. It seems to me that this ability to sink into deep thought while working provided an excellent opportunity to get anxiety and distress out of his system. Paul Klee was a drawing, painting philosopher. His metaphysical ideas were in the main very similar to those of Immanuel Kant. Karl Jaspers comments: 'In contrast to the stalled positions of the ontologists [those who deal with the nature of being] and other philosophers, Kant achieves a state where he can look at the world more freely. He asserts that the world of experiences stretches ahead into infinity. The world is neither closed nor closable. Kant opens up this experientiality, but believes these experiences must then be used in order to gain real awareness.'[582] Jasper continues: 'For as long as man can raise himself above his existence, the process of philosophizing will drive metaphysics onward. Beings communicate with each other in the world and metaphysics sheds a light which can help them gain transcendence. Then at this point it depends on the individual. He can either decide to deceive himself or he can act as a rational thinker and find deep certainty within himself.'[583]

Without a doubt, Klee found this 'deep certainty within himself', perhaps particularly because of the way he was unexpectedly forced into isolation. As a result he was largely thrown back onto his own resources. He overcame the diffi-

Fig. 154. Cemetery, 1939, 693 [turned through 90° to the right]

[581] Quoted in Gottschalk 1966, p. 57.
[582] Jaspers 1957, p. 244.
[583] Jaspers 1973, p. 32 f.

culties in his life caused by circumstance and illness and through his meditations he entered a spiritual realm, where he was weightless and could 'float', where he could 'spread his wings as an earthly angel' and touch transcendence. He concentrated all his efforts on his creativity and in his art he created for himself visions which, despite his physical frailty, must have filled him with strength, energy, stamina, joy and happiness.

Paul Klee's late work is filled with spirituality. The artist often lived in an 'intermediate world',[584] a world between this life and the hereafter, between existence in this life and existence in the before and after. Here he concurs with Novalis, who states in fragment 59: 'If there should be a higher sphere, then it is that which lies between being and not-being, the hovering between the two – the nameless; and here we have the concept of life.'[585] Klee loves to be at the limits, where the cosmic laws can be perceived. But he has no desire to try to fathom these mysteries. 'Should we know everything? I don't think so!'[586], he noted in pencil in the corner of one of his compositions[587], which remained unfinished in 1940 when he traveled to Locarno. He just freely abandons himself to the cosmic laws.

Many of Klee's pictures exude this sense of abandon and inspire his viewers to experience a similar feeling. Those viewers who give themselves up to peace and tranquility are afforded a very special feeling of happiness. For example, I clearly remember visiting an exhibition at the Kunsthaus Zurich in 1967/68, where the collection held by Sir Edward and Lady Nika Hulton of London was being shown.[588] I spent a long time looking at the painting 'Spiral flowers', 1926, 82, with its wonderful spiraling flowers before a kind of closed window at the end of a flight of steps with raised 'theater curtains'. Suddenly in my imagination the window opened and behind was revealed a paradise, a flower garden blazing with color. This is an image which stays with me to this day. After visiting an uplifting exhibition, we find our experience of nature is more intense and more beautiful than before.

[584] Cf. for example Haftmann 1961, p. 166, cf. Rotzler, Willy, Engelbilder bei Paul Klee, in: du 1986, p. 52, and 'Im Zwischenreich', Klee 1957/2.
[585] Quoted in Huggler 1969, p. 240 f.
[586] Quoted in Glaesemer 1979, p. 50.
[587] Frey/Helfenstein 1991, no. 1940, N 7. There is no note of when the composition was begun (Stefan Frey).
[588] Exhibition from December 3, 1967 to January 7, 1968 (including 48 of Paul Klee's works).

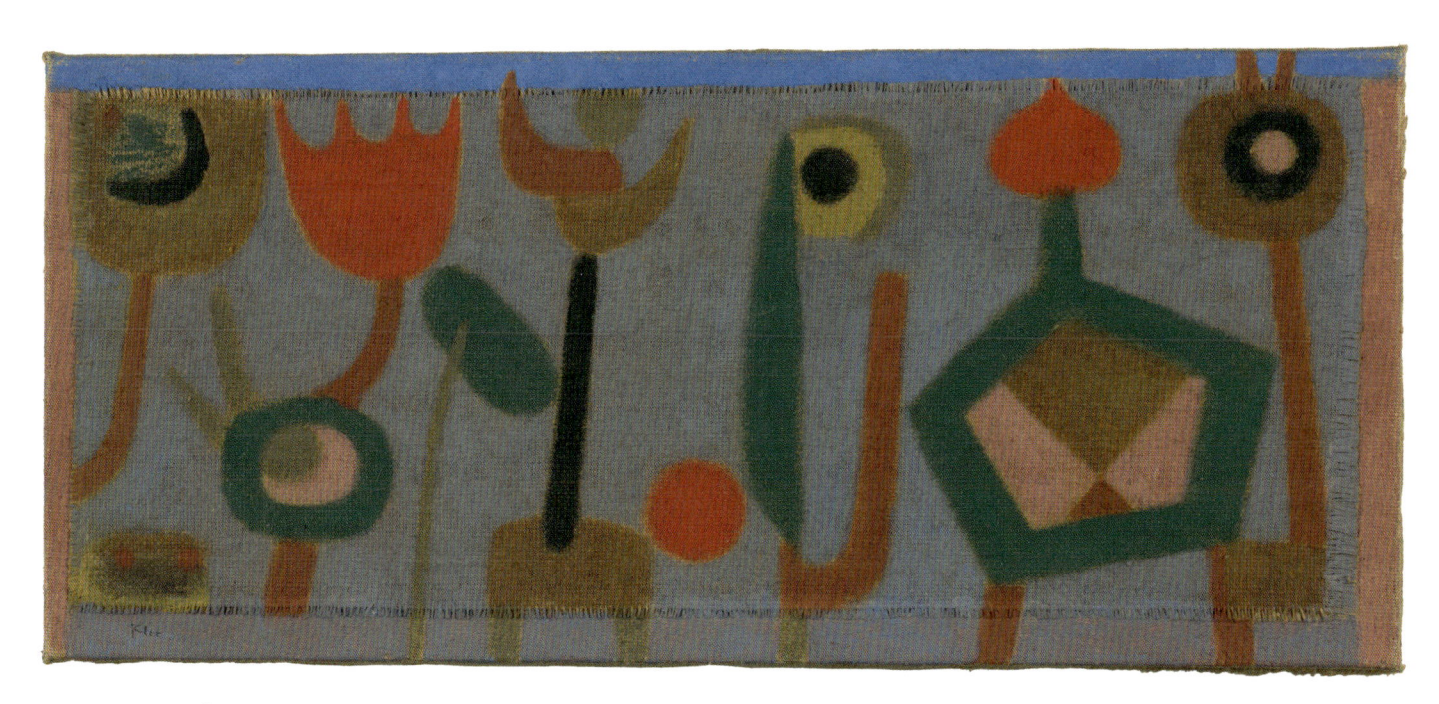

Fig. 155. Twilight flowers, 1940, 42

A painting from the year the artist died. The watercolor shows vermillion and orange flowers in the shape of goblets, hearts and discs, painted on mouse-grey burlap. Red-brown plant stems and dark green leaves add to the geometric balance of the picture. A mystical, violet sky glows above the flowers. It is twilight. The day will soon turn into night; the flower heads will close up: a parallel to the end of Klee's life in the somber second year of the Second World War. And yet what a blossoming is happening within!

> Klee is dealing with death, with pure spirituality; where angels, as the highest, supernatural level of creation, are the links and intermediaries between this world and the afterlife. But here he still sees himself as 'In the antechamber of angelhood'. Somewhat afraid and uncertain, he hides his head in his wings, seeking sanctuary. An unusual depiction of an angel drawn with typical Klee humor!

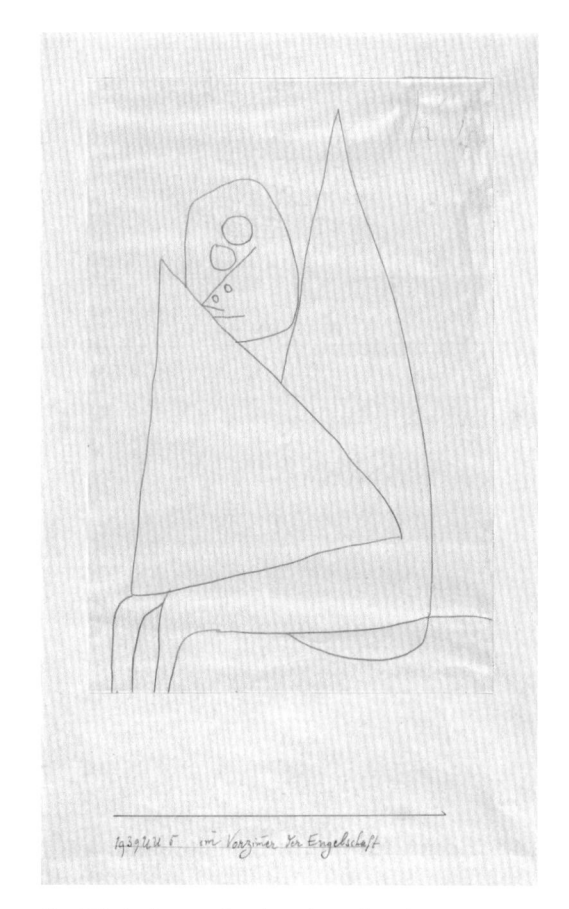

Fig. 156. In the antechamber of angelhood, 1939, 845

Klee exquisitely portrays this 'intermediate world' through his half-earthly angels. The word 'angels' comes from the Latin 'angeli', literally messengers of God. They bring mankind messages from the afterlife or bestow divine protection. Willy Rotzler says: 'There is no other artist in the 20th century who portrays angels so often, in so many different guises and with so many interpretations as Paul Klee. Christian Geelhaar believes Klee's angel symbolizes proximity to Creation, which can also mean proximity to God or to death. The angels in the paintings and drawings do not represent perfect, ideal creatures which are elevated above mankind. Klee's angels are also part-human and suffer from human weaknesses. They are in the process of becoming angels.'[589] This would seem to be a new way of portraying angels. Jürgen Glaesemer comments: 'Even in his early works, Klee thought of angels as being creatures who possessed extraordinary humanity and contrasted them with the "lowness of earth". "The angels are not sitting together drinking beer"[590], he wrote in 1915, a time when he started to produce his first images of angels. However, they do not appear in his work in large numbers until 1939 – for this year alone, his catalogue of works includes 29 angel-related titles.'[591]

As a young man, Paul Klee finished his poem 'Zurufe' (Cheers) with the last two lines:

> 'Einst werd ich liegen im Nirgend
> bei einem Engel irgend.'[592]
> (One of these days I shall lie in nothingness
> beside an angel of some kind.)

---

[589] Quoted in Rotzler 1986, p. 52, without reference to the origin of Christian Geelhaar's words.
[590] Letter from Paul Klee to Franz Marc, February 3, 1915 (Germanisches Nationalmuseum, Nürnberg, visual arts archive, Marc estate).
[591] Glaesemer 1976, p. 341.
[592] Klee 1960/2, p. 9.

Werner Haftmann discusses Klee's portrayal of angels as follows (also with reference to the above quotation): 'His allegiance to these angels now grows stronger and provides him with companionship on the last part of his journey. Klee always felt at ease in the intermediate realms and loved the transformations from one to the other. He regarded colored forms as the most direct means of effecting these transformations, and by virtue of their magic he was able to pass from things earth-bound to those moving in the cosmos, from things inorganic to things organic, from things growing to things moving, from plants to animals and so on to man. Change was the root of all being, and every sort of possibility was latent in reality. On the religious plane, the greatest possibility for earthly metamorphosis still lay with the angels, and in his final meditations Klee sought to penetrate that intermediate realm – to find his angel of some kind.'[593] It is also enchanting how Klee's subtle humor shines through in these later angel drawings (for example in figs. 156, 158 and 159).

Jürgen Glaesemer writes in this respect: 'According to Klee's own definition, they [the angels] are figures in "the angels' antechamber"; human beings who are taking their "last steps on earth" in order to become new "fully-fledged" angels. He describes this process of transformation not with pathos but with humor, in an attempt to make it understandable from an earthly perspective.'[594]

And Will Grohmann: 'Klee's angels also live in a great unity which encompasses life and death, and they discern in the indiscernible a higher level of reality. But for Klee, particularly towards the end of his life, this was also true of man; this life and the afterlife are intertwined and man has a part in both. Klee lived "somewhat nearer the heart of creation than normal".'[595]

Some of the angels Paul Klee draws for us are: a guardian angel (fig. 157), a contemplative angel ('Sits and ponders', 1939, 1018), a sad angel ('It weeps', 1939, 959), but also an 'Angel full of hope', 1939, 892.

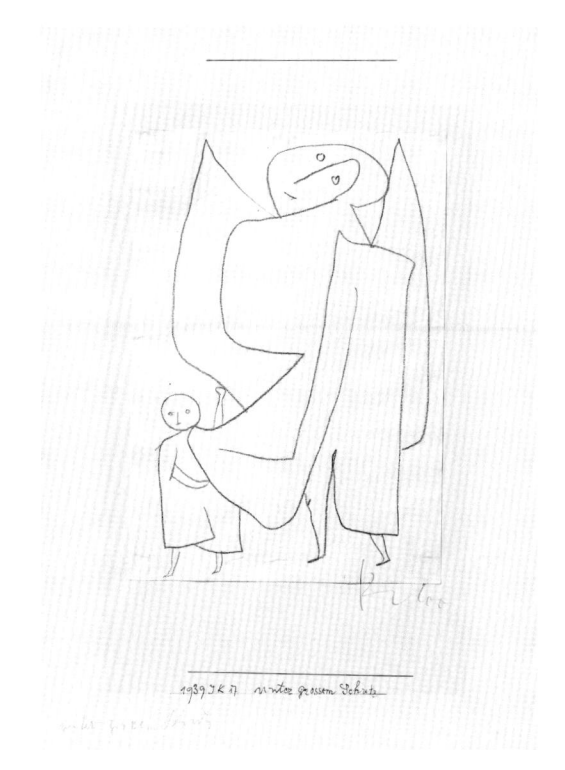

Fig. 157. Under grand protection, 1939, 1137

[593] Haftmann 1961, p. 166.
[594] Glaesemer 1979, p. 40.
[595] Grohmann 1965, p. 349.

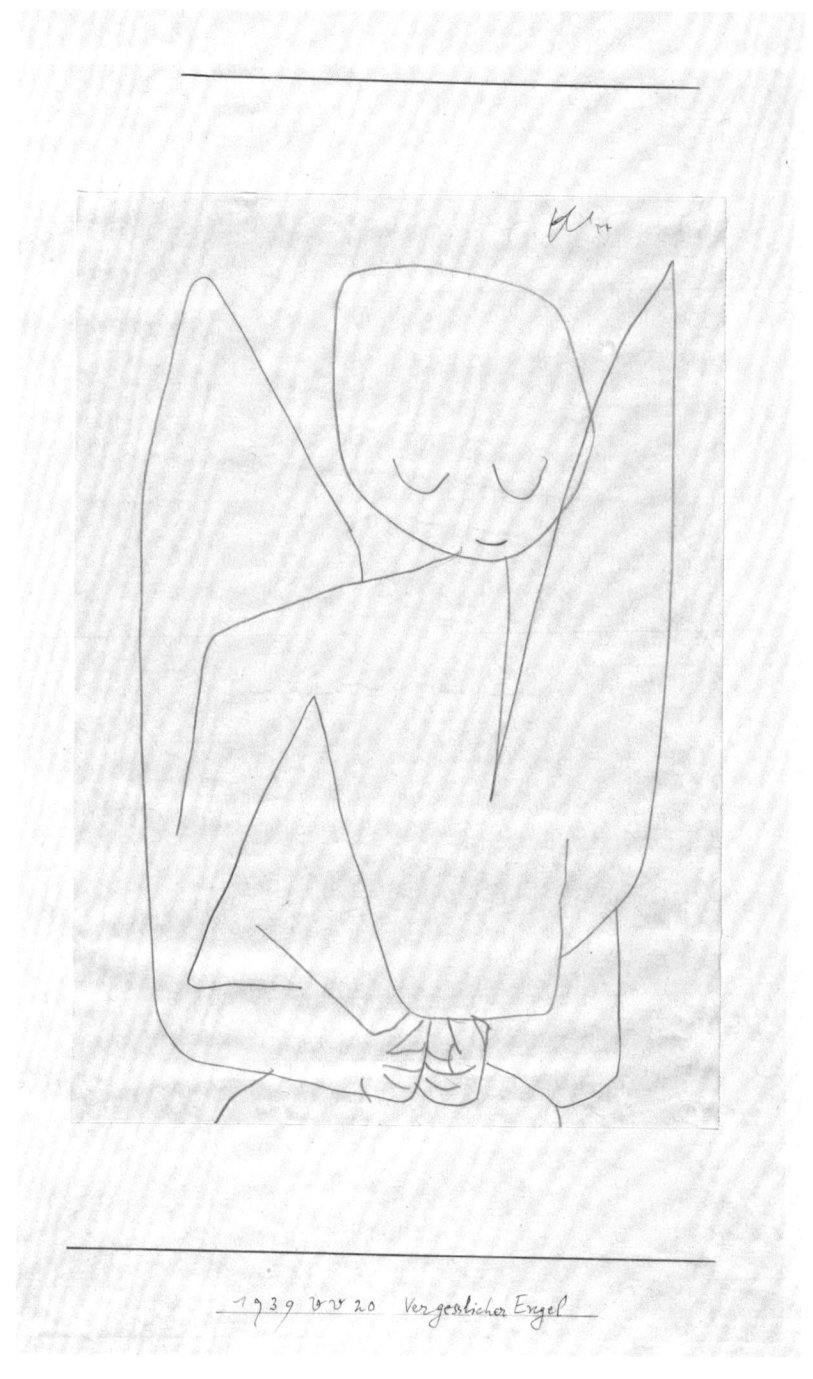

Fig. 158. Forgetful angel, 1939, 880

Forgetfulness is a typically human characteristic. This likeable angel is desperately wringing his hands and trying hard to remember something he has forgotten. In effect, he is still waiting 'In the antechamber of angelhood' (fig. 156, page 196).

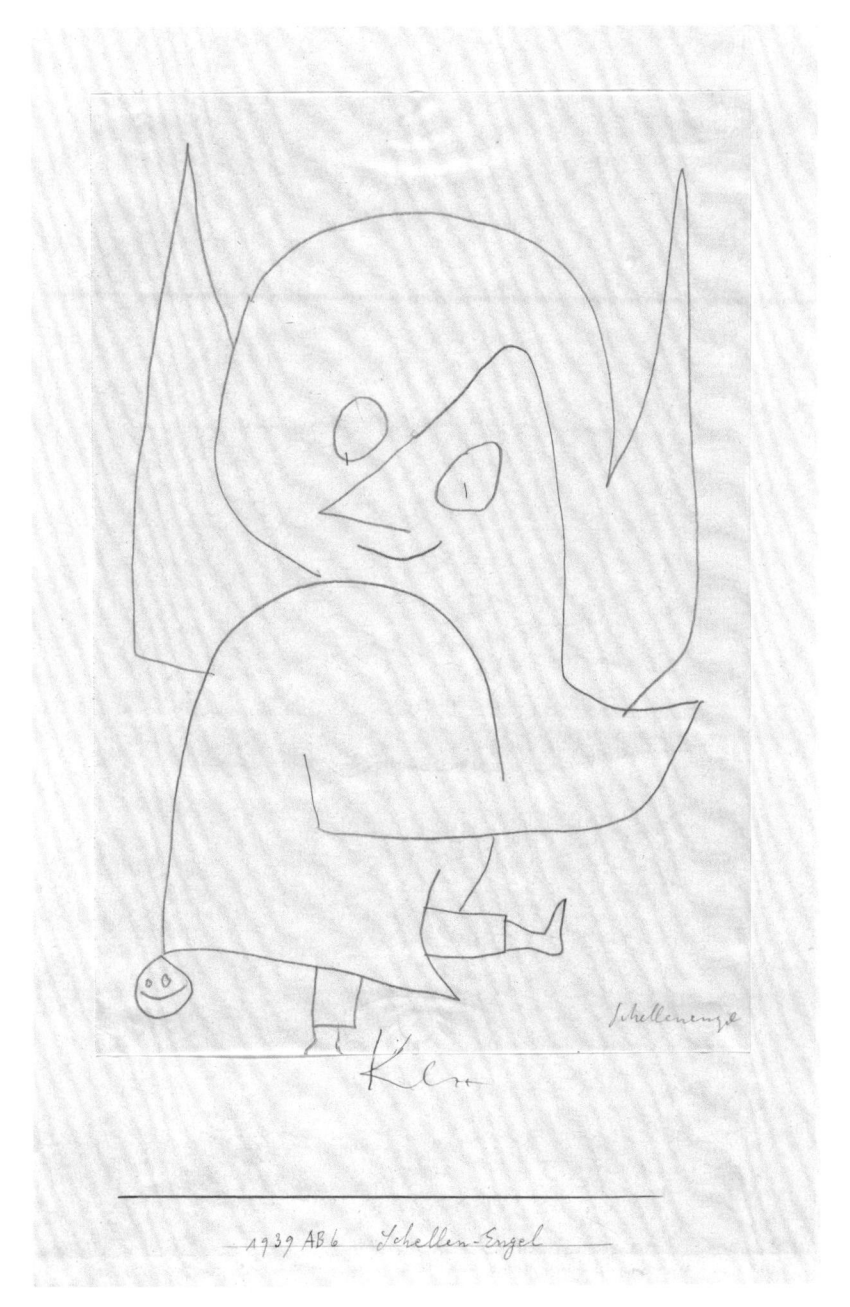

Fig. 159. Bell angel, 1939, 966

In 'Bell angel' an angel is overjoyed by a small merrily tinkling bell hanging from the hem of his robe. Despite his illness, Klee retained his keen sense of humor right up to the end of his life.

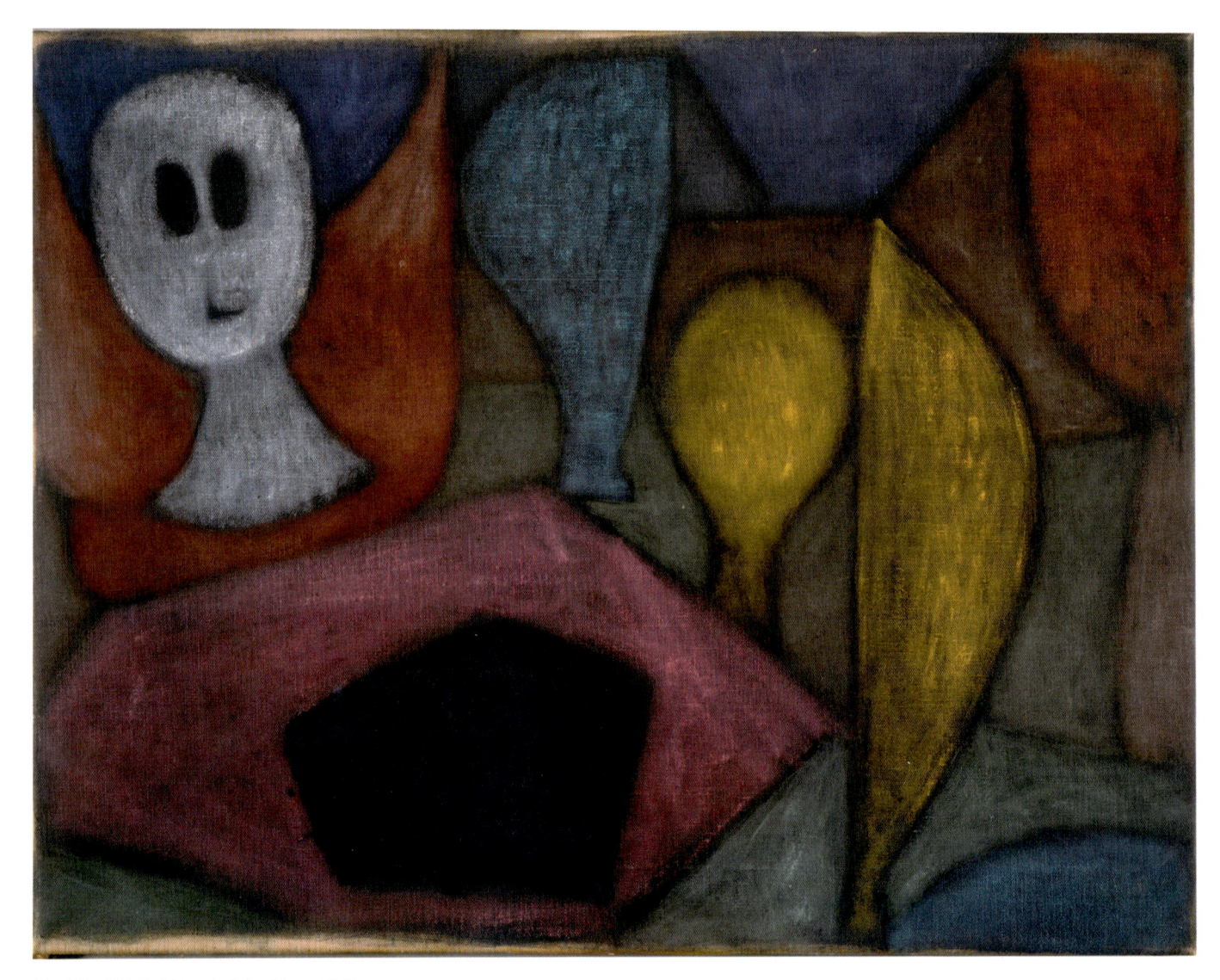

Fig. 160. Untitled (Angel of death), ca. 1940

Klee did not give a title to this painting, nor did he include it in his catalogue of works. It was only given a title after his death. Inge Herold: 'In the upper left- hand corner we can see the head of an angel with red wings, floating above a landscape of trees and hills. Below the colorful but muted shapes we notice a dark hexagonal area, which seems to open up like a hole into the depths. Taken in conjunction with the angel, whose empty black eyes and white face suggest it is the angel of death, this hole can be interpreted as a "The gate to the depth" (cf. the painting of the same name 1936, 25) that leads to the afterlife.'[596]

[596] Herold, Inge, in: Klee 1996, p. 157.

'Art Is a Parable of Creation'

In 1920 Kasimir Edschmid published an anthology entitled 'Schöpferische Konfession', and Paul Klee was a contributor.[597] In his piece he contends: 'First and foremost, art is genesis, it is never just a product.'[598] What counts is the creative process, not the work of art as a commercial item. With his theses 'art is a parable of Creation'[599] and 'art does not reproduce the visible; rather, it makes visible'[600], Klee has formulated some key elements of 20th century art theory. He continues: 'A formal cosmos should be created, one so closely resembling the Creation that a breath is sufficient to turn an expression of religion or religious feelings into reality.'[601]

Klee was a Protestant, but he was not religious in a dogmatic, doctrinal sense. His sense of religion was supra-denominational; it could perhaps be described as a 'cosmic religiousness'.

Every living thing is a microcosm, a particle of the universe and the world order, and as such it also produces energy in its own right. Artists transmit energy through their works, which become to some extent energy carriers. But this energy is then used in different ways. Some works remain dull, cool and distanced, while others virtually leap out at the viewer. Paul Klee totally understood how to imbue his works with an 'elemental energy' which shone through with a mystical intensity.

Paul Klee left behind a body of work that cannot be pigeonholed into one particular movement.[602] In his work he was always uniquely himself – an icon as a person and an artist. He created his very own cosmos within the universe. He was a mystic through his surrender to and immersion in his art, and he was a metaphysicist through his 'cosmic religiousness'. The art historian Oskar Bätschmann writes: 'Klee generally required an artist to have "an ability to move". He should take a searching and penetrating look at the existing forms of nature, so that instead of carrying the imprint of the present shapes of nature in his mind, he can see that the "single essential image of creation is genesis". This "movement along the natural paths of creation" teaches the artist

[597] Klee 1920.
[598] Ibid., quoted in Klee 1976, p. 120.
[599] Ibid., p. 122.
[600] Ibid., p. 118.
[601] Ibid., p. 121.
[602] Cf. Wedekind 2000, p. 230.

about form and is also the freedom "to move in the way that nature in her grandeur moves". An artist who soon comes to a halt en route is one who has pretensions, nothing more. Klee says the artists with real vocations travel to "within fair distance" of that hidden, fundamental origin, the bosom of nature, the primordial source of creation, "where the primal law feeds evolution". Klee wishes that all artists could live here, in the center of cosmic movement: "There, where the central organ of all temporal and spatial movement – we may call it the brain or the heart of creation – makes everything happen. What artist would not wish to dwell there?" From the mystical image of a primal source, an arc is once again drawn to the pictorial elements, as the dreams, ideas or fantasies which emerge only become "realities of art" when they are combined with the "proper pictorial elements and given form".'[603]

---

[603] Bätschmann 2000, p. 123 f. The author refers here to a lecture given by Paul Klee at an exhibition at the Kunstverein in Jena on January 26, 1924; cf. Klee 1924.

His Illness as a Constant Companion

Jürgen Glaesemer comments on the effect of Paul Klee's illness on his art as follows: 'It is not easy to tell from the works themselves how much his later production was affected by his illness. His illness became a constant companion which he [Klee] never spoke about but which was a determining factor in his thought and work.'[604]

In his paintings and drawings Klee deals with his illness and the themes of dying, death and the afterlife with an intuitive, almost playful touch. But it must again be emphasized that he also gives creative expression to many thoughts and ideas which are not related to his illness. As in the past, he let his imagination have free rein, and his innate sense of humor[605] always shone through, a further proof of his well-developed personality. He never let his suffering grind him down. His characteristic love of color runs through many of his works, even the later ones which were overshadowed by his illness.

Klee's artistic activity during the course of his illness is largely linked to his feelings at each stage: suffering, fear, doubt, resistance, hope, and finally despondency and resignation. Many of Klee's drawings reflect his mood at the time, just as a seismograph day after day records the tremors in the earth's interior. This 'recording' of his feelings will have been an important way for him to work through his anxiety and distress, helping him to banish his fears. In the end it all leads to a quiet acceptance of his condition: Klee has to accept that 'the rower will lose his battle with death'[606]. On January 2, 1940, he wrote to Will Grohmann: 'Of course I did not just suddenly find myself on this tragic path, many of my works refer to it and declare: the time has come.'[607]

Paul Klee was very well-read. He liked to read French and Greek Classics in the original language and he was interested in Greek theater[608], where masks played an important role, a motif which he picked up on and often used in his own work. Examples of these are the drawings: 'Mask of an angry woman', 1912, 62, 'Row of masks', 1923, 254, 'Masked man resting', 1933, 79, 'Group of masks', 1933, 133, 'Activity of masks', 1933, 43, and the paintings: '(Youth) Actor's mask',

[604] Glaesemer 1979, p. 14.
[605] Paul Klee probably inherited his sense of humor from his father Hans Klee (see note 34, p. 265), and it was also passed on to Felix Klee. He loved the Bernese dialect, which he never quite mastered, as he naturally spoke High German, but he loved to use it in a humorous and sometimes exaggerated way (the author).
[606] Idea linked to Klee's drawing 'Rowing competition', 1940, 172 (fig. 123, p. 150).
[607] Letter from Paul Klee to Will Grohmann, Bern, January 2, 1940 (AWG), quoted in Gutbrod 1968, p. 84.
[608] Klee (Felix) 1948, p. 14: 'Every evening he went to bed at ten o'clock and lay for hours reading French and Greek Classics in the original language (it was his favorite reading).' In addition, Felix Klee told the author: 'Paul Klee was also particularly interested in Greek theater', Bern, September 20, 1983.

Fig. 161. Chronometric dance, 1940, 133

Josef Helfenstein writes of this drawing: 'The metrically orchestrated dance, the synchronization of the physical movement with the mechanical ticking of the clock are reminiscent of Klee's motif of the puppet, of a "mechanism", directed by outside forces, controlled by strings. The motif of the two figures, moving to the beat like automatons, is an extreme illustration of Klee's antithetical concept of life and death, of the physical and the mechanical. The title of the drawing suggests that the predefined rhythm of the clock as it ticks away the remaining time – the small clock at the bottom of the clock face shows 12 o'clock – has become the metronomic beat for his artistic output (the "dance"). In an almost exemplary fashion, this drawing reveals how Klee's artistic activity is influenced by and apparently subordinated to his existential situation and to other external, objective factors. The drawing "Chronometric dance" is like an illustrated commentary on the famous passage in Klee's letter to Will Grohmann at the beginning of 1940, where he wrote – alluding to the precarious state of his health – that many of this works were telling him "the time has come"[609].'[610] The clock has become the clock of Klee's life, and it will soon stop ticking.

1924, 252, 'Woman's mask', 1933, 482, 'Masks at twilight', 1938, 486 (fig 162, page 207). Sometimes actors are wearing these masks. Obviously, a face is characterized by its physiognomy and its expression. An actor can express inner feelings through his facial expressions, whether the feelings are his own or those of the character he is playing. When he dons a mask, he no longer has this means of expression. Masks are fixed, so the actor has to portray the essence of the character through voice, language, gesture and behavior. This is analogous to the Latin word for mask: 'persona' – literally where 'the sound comes through' – from 'personare', to sound through, to proclaim (speaking through the gap for the mouth in the mask).[611]

[609] See note 607.
[610] Helfenstein, Joseph, in: Klee 1990/2, p. 71.
[611] Thanks to the artist Bendicht Friedli for the reference and explanation of the word. The word originally denoted the actor's mask, and then also came to mean his role.

1940 L 13 chronometrischer Tanz

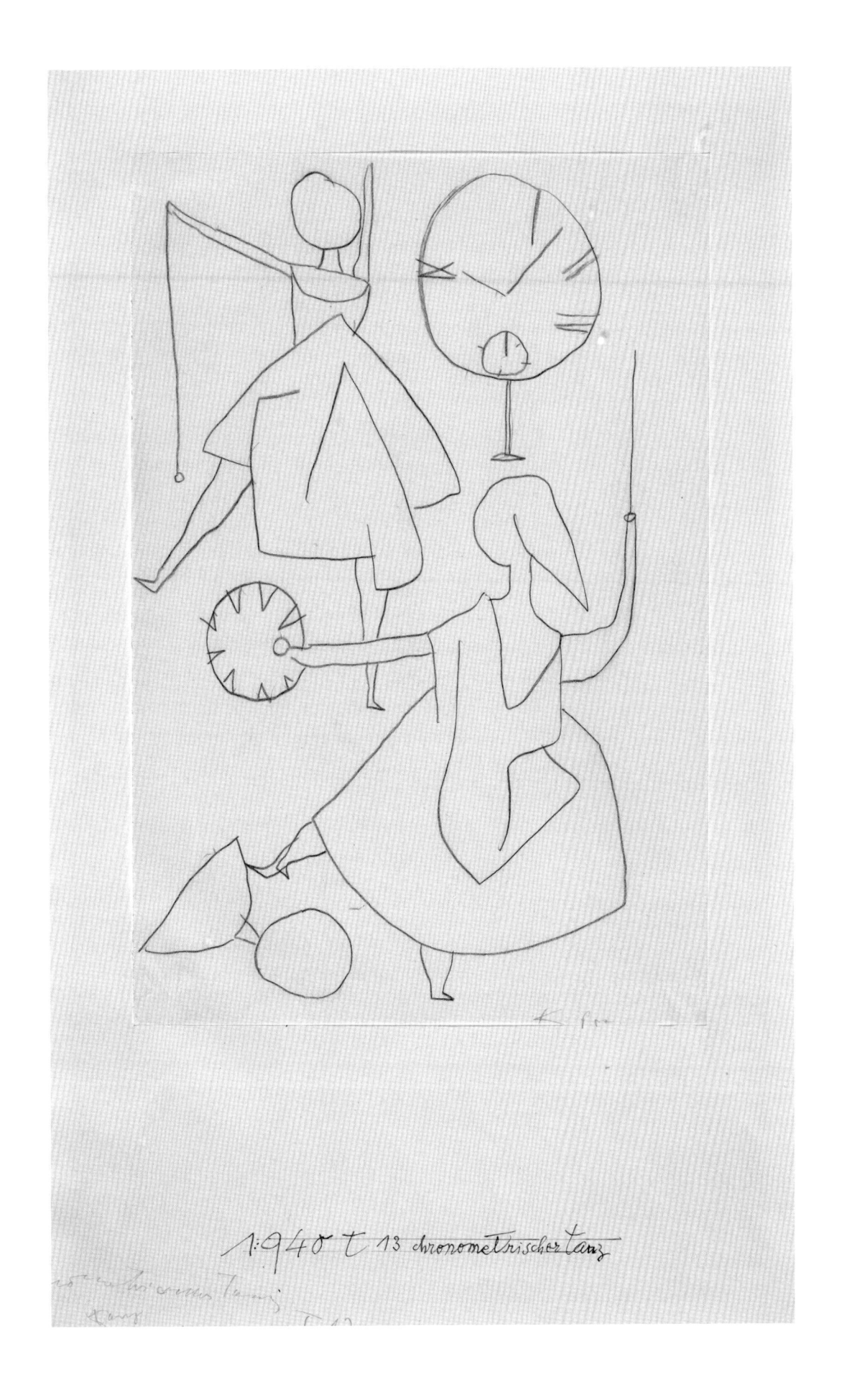

Fig. 162. Masks at twilight, 1938, 486

Carola Giedion-Welcker notes that, particularly in his later works, Paul Klee was greatly preoccupied with the world of the human psyche.[612] Even at the very beginning of his development as an artist, he formulated the following 'thoughts on the art of portrait painting': 'Some people will think I have not reflected reality. But they should bear in mind that it is not my purpose to mirror surface reality (this can be done by photographic plates) [,] it is my task to penetrate beneath the surface, right to the heart. I write words on the brow and around the corners of the mouth. The faces that I draw are truer than the real ones.'[613] And in 1905 he adds: 'If I were to paint a realistic self-portrait, I would paint a curious shell. And I would make it clear that I am sitting inside this shell, like the kernel of a nut. This work could also be called an allegory of encrustation.'[614] Klee drew a 'realistic self-portrait' in 1938, when his face had stiffened and become mask-like as a result of the disease. He entitled this touching drawing 'Mask: pain' (fig. 48, page 57).[615] The face is like an 'encrusted shell' because of the physical changes brought on by the illness. The eyes reflect the psyche, the inner soul, the 'kernel' – they express his inner pain. It is interesting to note that 19 years previously Klee had produced two drawings of a stiff face which he entitled 'Mask'.[616]

---

[612] Cf. Giedion-Welcker 2000, p. 138.
[613] Klee Diaries, no. 136.
[614] Ibid., no. 675.
[615] Klee depicted a similar facial expression in the drawing 'Mask: after the loss', 1938, 212.
[616] 'Mask', 1919, 76, and 'Mask', 1919, 77.

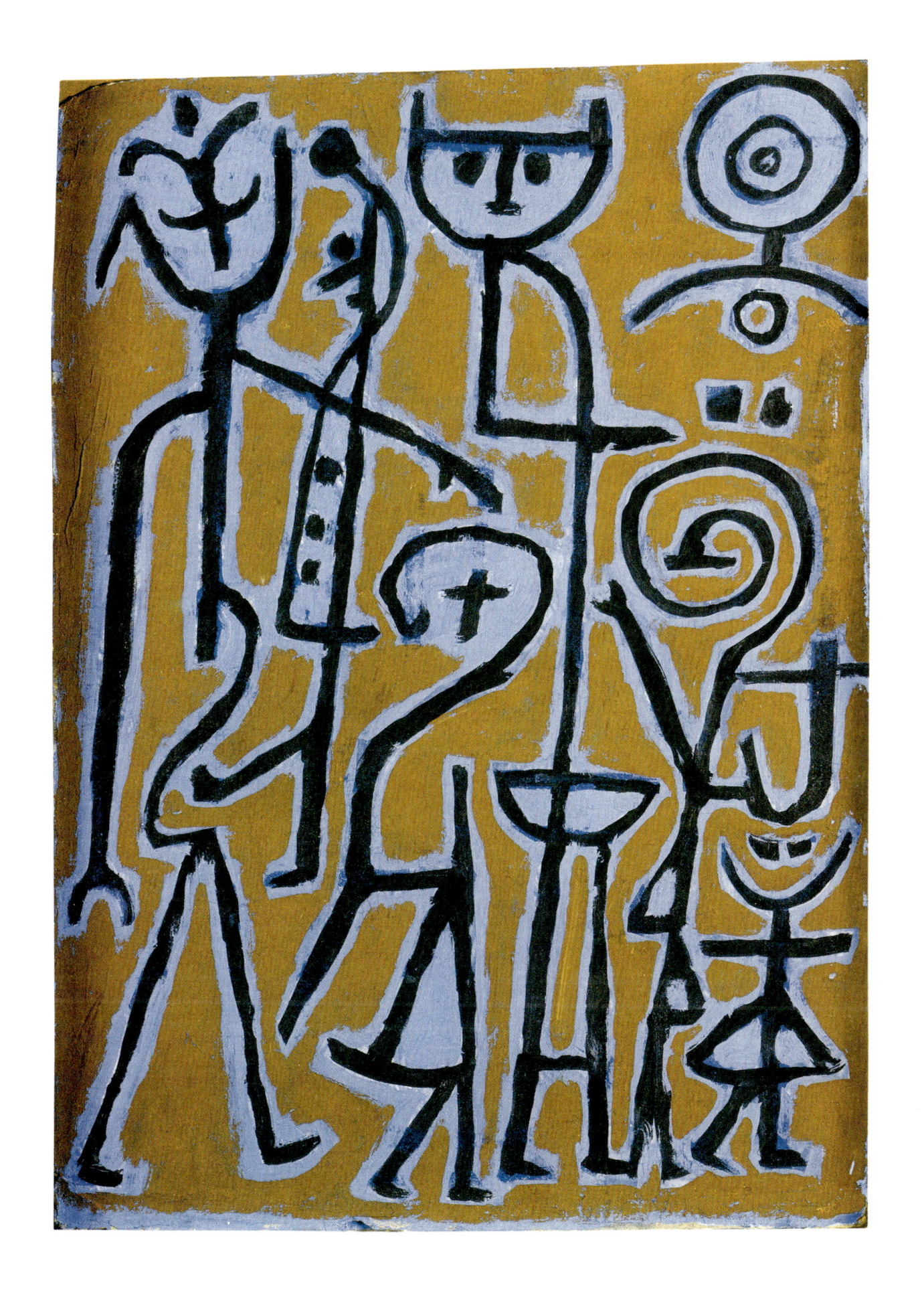

Humorous drawings
Paul Klee, like his father, was a humorous man. This can be seen in many of his works, especially in his drawings, for instance figures 156, 158, 159 and 163–166.

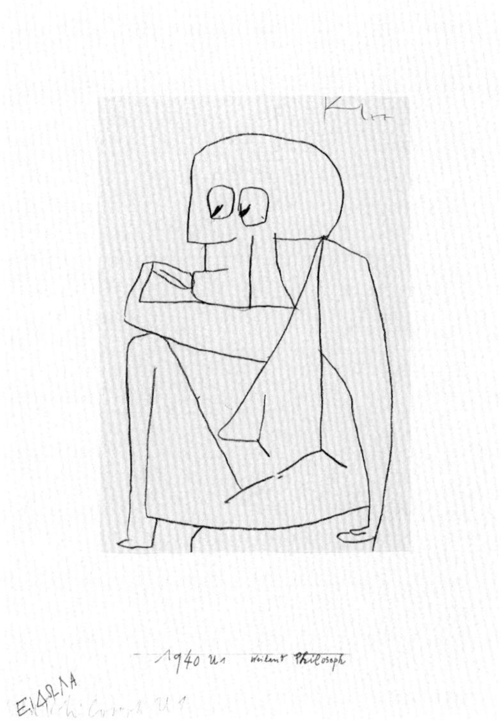

Fig. 163. Eidola: erstwhile philosopher, 1940, 101

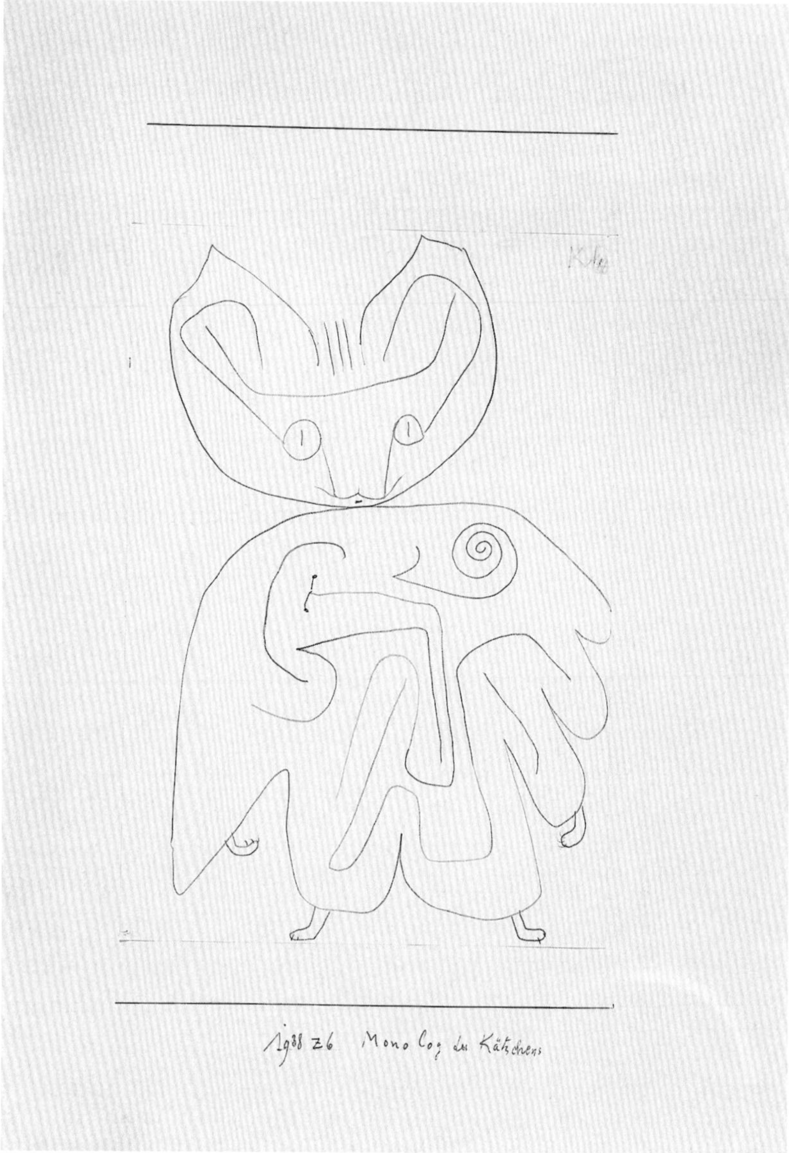

Fig. 164. Monologue of the kitten, 1938, 426

The drawing in figure 163 is part of a series of 26 drawings, all entitled 'Eidola'. The name is Greek and means 'apparition', 'reflection', or 'phantom'.[617] According to Jürgen Glaesemer the term describes a group of shadowy beings who have been carried away from life into a transitional state between life and death.[618]

---

[617] Duden, Fremdwörterbuch, 3rd ed., vol. 5, Bibliographisches Institut, Dudenverlag, Mannheim/Wien/Zürich 1974, p. 198.
[618] Glaesemer 1979, p. 39.

In the 'Eidola'-series, Klee adds the word 'weiland' (erstwhile) when he portrays figures. In doing so, he is suggesting that these people are in a place somewhere between this world and the afterlife – just like his angels. Jürgen Glaesemer is of the opinion that all these 'Eidola' figures 'are beings, like Klee himself, who are going through a metamorphosis, in which they still retain a vestige of those characteristics which "erstwhile" defined them.'[619] It may also be possible to make the following distinction: the 'Eidola'-people are looking back from a place just this side of the threshold to the afterlife. The angels have already stepped over that threshold, but still have not cast off their human traits.

Paul Klee often created works in series, depicting subjects in different ways and creating imaginative variations on chosen themes. He could complete a whole series of images in a short space of time, finishing one drawing and letting it fall to the floor as he immediately started on the next one.[620] A passage in one of his wife Lily's letters in 1937 gives a good illustration of this: 'He sits until 11 o'clock every evening letting sheet after sheet fall to the floor, just as he used to'.[621]

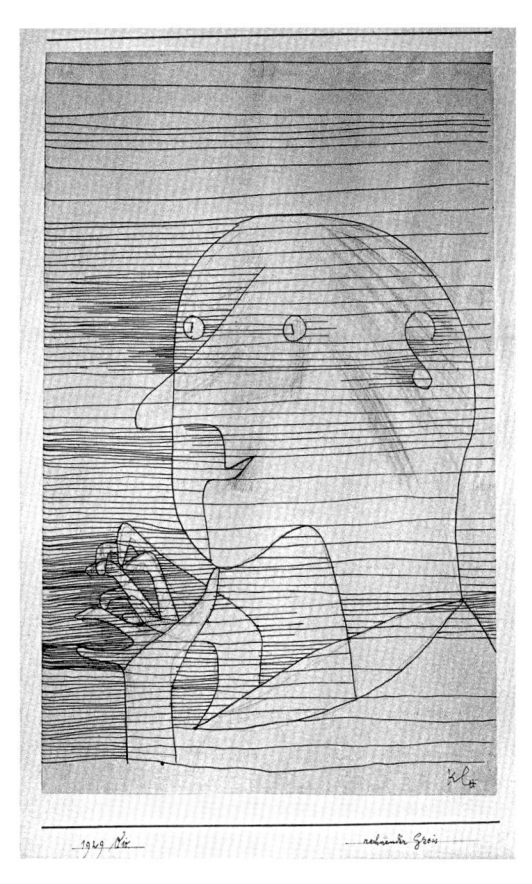

Fig. 165. Old man counting, 1929, 60

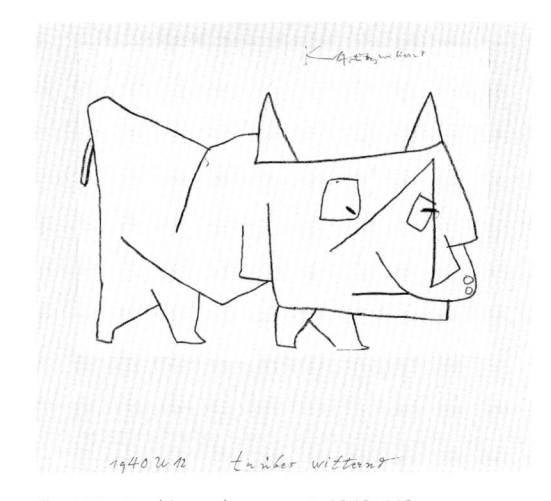

Fig. 166. Catching a dreary scent, 1940, 112

[619] Glaesemer 1979, p. 39.
[620] Personal communication, Felix Klee to the author, Bern, September 20, 1983.
[621] Letter from Lily Klee to Will Grohmann, Bern, July 8, 1937.

A New Style of Extraordinary Intensity and Spontaneity

An artist's style often changes as he gets older. What was important to him in his youth and as he reached maturity comes to be viewed with a certain distance as he grows older. He tends to take a more panoramic view rather than focusing on the details, and his work often becomes more simplified, with broad strokes taking the place of fine lines. Approaching death brings with it the wisdom and serenity which stems from knowing what is important in life. An artist's late works often reflect this preoccupation with the metaphysical and transcendent.

Paul Klee's later works also display stylistic changes; indeed these changes are more obvious and pronounced than in most other artists. Jürgen Glaesemer claims that the drawings he produced in the last years of his life appear 'in a new style of extraordinary intensity'[622]. They somehow pour out of his hand. It seems that the artist captures his soul on paper. One is always particularly moved by works which are born of adverse circumstances, something Glaesemer also feels when he writes: 'These drawings are no longer isolated, self-contained works. Every sheet is part of a series, one phrase in a longer text. Klee's work has never before expressed so completely his state of health and his personal needs. In his later drawings he is only striving for one thing: to give form to the images which were thronging his mind. He no longer "wrote" his pictorial symbols for anybody to read – the writing came from within.'[623]

Between the ages of 19 and 39, so from 1898 to 1918, Paul Klee kept his diary assiduously. From 1921 onwards he was teaching at the Bauhaus in Weimar and Dessau and then at the Academy of Fine Arts in Düsseldorf, so his time was spent on thoroughly preparing his lessons and also on concentrating as much as possible on his own artistic endeavors. He probably had little time to write in his diary, and perhaps he no longer felt the need. Interestingly, his isolation in Bern in the later years of his life aroused a desire in him to begin a diary-like record once more. But this time he did not write his everyday thoughts in a notebook, instead he noted them in the most succinct form possible, as outlines, by drawing

---

[622] Glaesemer 1984, p. 429.
[623] Glaesemer 1979, p. 26.

them on paper. Jürgen Glaesemer remarks on this: 'In his later drawings, Klee was not really producing complete works of art; he was rather having an uninterrupted dialogue with himself. The drawings were similar to entries in a diary.'[624] The outline drawings could also be compared with the movement of a seismograph needle, which precisely records on paper all the oscillations of Klee's inner life.

Glaesemer continues on the theme of Paul Klee's later style: 'His new and spontaneous style of drawing meant that, even on large panels, Klee could sketch freehand, i.e. without using a template, the basic framework of the composition in pencil or charcoal directly onto the material. In the later panels and colored sheets this new way of working is reflected in the strong linear shapes, the broad bars, and the outlines of the forms which are always balanced within the overall surface of the picture.'[625] Elsewhere he adds: 'The heavy lines are always an expression of a tragic earthly burden.'[626] Doris Wild compares the outlines with the lead frames in glass windows.[627] And Will Grohmann remarks on Klee's later style as follows: '[…] as he grew older, he [Klee] used a particular, incontrovertible form of "bar-writing", which confined itself to the absolute essentials and discarded everything superfluous.'[628] However, this 'bar-writing' can also be misinterpreted to mean that Klee could no longer do fine drawings and paintings because his hand was affected by his illness. In fact it has been shown that he had unrestricted movement in his hands right to the end of his life.[629]

Klee's late work is also characterized by a new way of portraying bodies. The bodies of the figures are falling to pieces, heads, trunks and limbs are detaching themselves. The organism is in the process of dismantling itself (for example in figs. 98, 99 and 102, pages 130, 131 and 136; see also page 132). This is of course characteristic of everything organic and the basic principle of Creation: be born and die, flower and fade, take shape and disintegrate.

The spontaneity and impulsiveness of Klee's drawings during the years of his illness stand in stark contrast to his earlier well thought-out, deliberate and reflective designs done in

[624] Glaesemer 1979, p. 25.
[625] Ibid., p. 27.
[626] Glaesemer 1976, p. 342.
[627] Cf. Wild 1950, p. 219.
[628] Grohmann 1966, p. 38.
[629] Personal communication, Felix Klee to Prof. Alfred Krebs and the author, Bern, November 9, 1979, and Felix Klee to the author, Bern, September 20, 1983, also Max Huggler to the author, CH–7554 Sent, August 15, 1981.

pen and pencil. Klee knew intuitively that his time was short, leading him to increase his production by improving his efficiency and work rate. In his final years he developed great creative ability, which came close to that of Pablo Picasso, an artist whom Klee greatly admired for his spontaneous and precise linear compositions.[630] Picasso was also impressed by Paul Klee as an artist and as a person.[631] He remarked that Klee's pictures seemed to have 'an inner light shining through'[632], and in memory of his visit to Klee in Bern on November 28, 1937, he called his colleague 'Pascal-Napoléon'[633]. Will Grohmann took this to mean that the Spaniard 'was obviously thinking of his mixture of wisdom and energy, fierce asceticism and single-minded intensity, but also of his Mediterranean appearance.'[634]

These two luminaries of 20th century art not only had totally different characters, but they were also at opposite ends of the scale in their work. Picasso's art is material, physical, sensual, bound to the earth, while Klee's art is dematerialized, metaphysical, reflective and cosmic. In 1941, the Director of the Museum of Modern Art in New York, Alfred H. Barr, described the of both artists as follows: 'Picasso's pictures often roar or stamp or pound; Klee's whisper a soliloquy – lyrical, intimate, incalculably sensitive.'[635] And Emil Nolde hit the mark when he described Paul Klee as 'a butterfly floating in the vastness of the stars.'[636]

[630-631] See Appendices: The Mutual Appreciation between Paul Klee and Pablo Picasso (pp. 268 and 269).

[632] Pfeiffer-Belli 1978, p. 394.

[633] Grohmann 1965, p. 87: 'When François Lachenal reminded Picasso in 1951 about his visit he immediately remembered the face of the great solitary artist. "Pascal-Napoléon" were the words he used to describe the overall impression he had of Klee at that time […]' Detailed descriptions of the visit are given on pp. 214–216, in: Geiser 1961, pp. 53, 88 and 90, and Bhattacharya-Stettler 2001, pp. 81–84.

[634] Grohmann 1965, p. 87.

[635] Barr 1941, p. 6.

[636] Quoted in Pfeiffer-Belli 1978, p. 394.

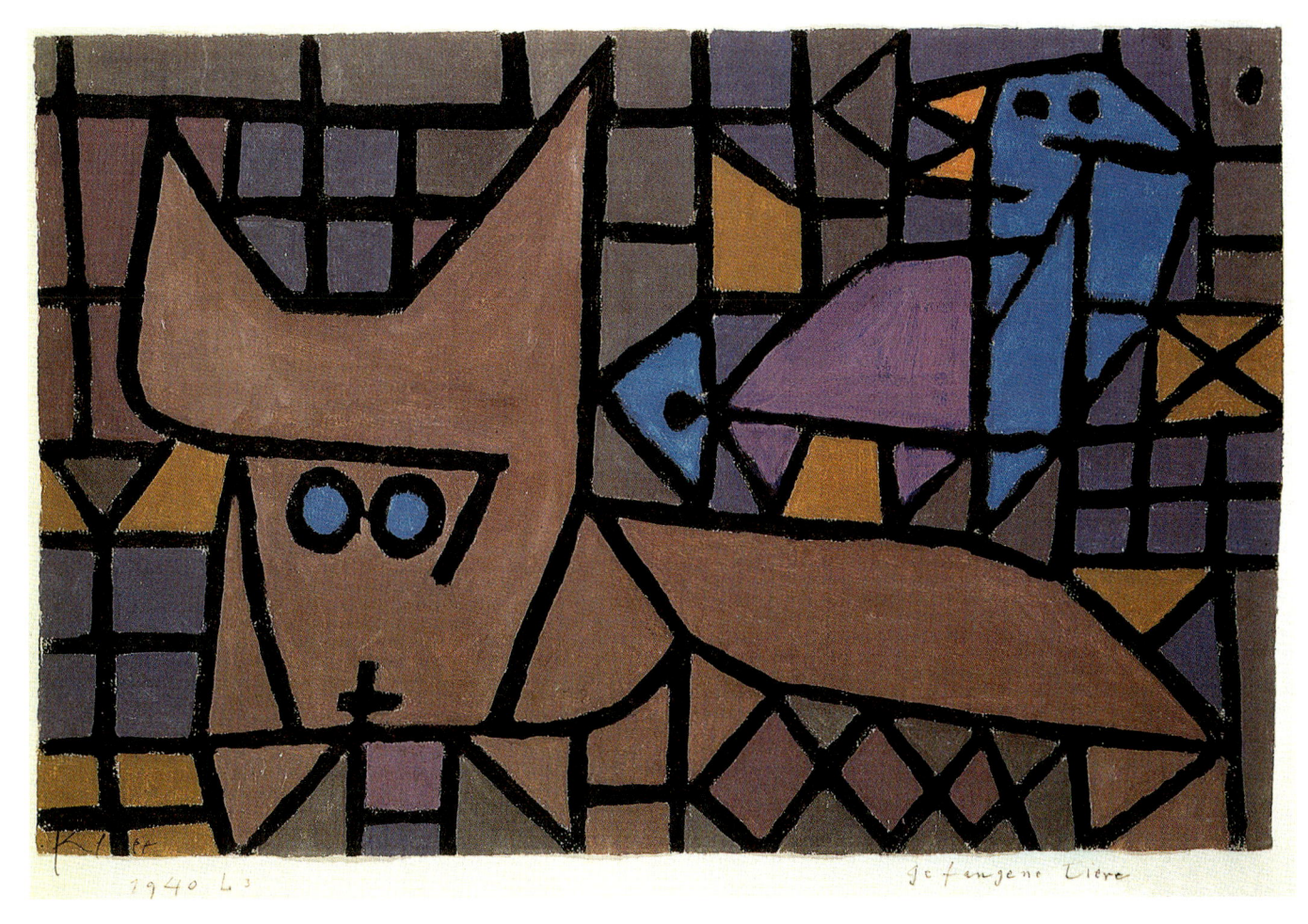

Fig. 167. Animals in captivity, 1940, 263

Two animals, a fox and a bird, are caught in an enclosure. They are aware of their hopeless situation. They look at us sadly. The mood is gloomy. Klee could identify with captive animals. He felt imprisoned by his own body and by his isolation in Bern. Brown colors dominate. There are different shades of brown, in contrast to the monochrome blue in the eyes of the fox and on the head, breast and tail of the bird. A blue which links their fates.

This wonderful painting displays a stylistic idiosyncrasy which is often apparent in Klee's later works: the delineation of surfaces using thick black lines. These 'bar lines' can be interpreted as a reduction to the bare essentials as part of the artistic simplification which became typical of his work. We can also see this in the simple outlines of his later drawings.

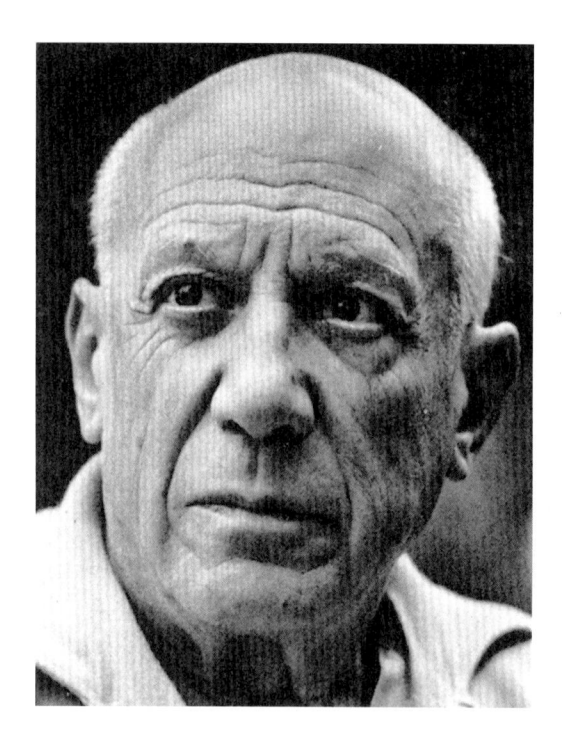

Fig. 168. Pablo Picasso, 1963

Meeting with Pablo Picasso

On November 28, 1937, Pablo Picasso visited Paul Klee, who already at that time was seriously ill, in Bern.[637] The Bern art historian Bernhard Geiser gives an amusing account of this, the only time the two artists met (author's own abridged version below).[638]

Picasso brought his sick seventeen-year-old son Paolo to consult a doctor at the Lindenhofspital in Bern. The art dealer Daniel-Henry Kahnweiler suggested to Picasso that he should look up Paul Klee and the collectors Hermann and Margrit Rupf while he was in Bern. On November 27, 1937, Bernhard Geiser met Picasso and his son at the railway station in Bern (in 1933 Geiser had published a collection of Picasso's graphic work from 1899 to 1931). Paul Klee was told to expect a visit on the following day at four in the afternoon. On the morning of November 28, Picasso visited his son at the clinic and then was invited by Hermann Rupf to enjoy a hearty lunch at a country inn. When they got back to Bern, Geiser suggested a visit to the Bern History Museum, as it was still too early to visit the Klees. The museum was on the way to their home, so Picasso agreed and once there he was fascinated by the many historical treasures on display. Geiser reminded him: 'Now it's time to go and visit the Klees', but Picasso was going from room to room, immersed in the exhibits, and he was not to be dragged away. Geiser knew that Paul Klee was expecting his visitor to be on time, so in the end he took his guest's arm and led him to the exit. Here Picasso discovered a flight of stairs going down to the basement. 'Un moment' (just a moment), he said – and disappeared down the stairs. Once again he could not be persuaded to leave, and it was only when the alarm sounded at five o'clock to signal that the museum was closing that they finally exited the museum. Picasso wanted to take a taxi because he was tired from spending so long in the museum, but these could only be hailed at the station. Geiser told him it was as far to walk back to the station as to walk to the Klees' house. But Picasso was adamant, so they walked over the Kirchenfeld bridge and through the arcades of the old town of Bern to the station. On the way the illustrious visitor disappeared into a confiserie. Geiser thought he wanted to

[637] Cf. Geiser 1987, p. 77.
[638] Cf ibid., pp. 76–82, and cf. Stettler, Michael, Georges Bloch und Picasso, in: Lehrer und Freunde, 1997, pp. 159–163; also published in: Bhattacharya-Stettler 2001, pp. 81–83. Bernhard Geiser's personal account was also published in: Haldi/Schindler 1920, pp. 41–46, und du 1961, pp. 53, 88, 90 and 92.

buy a sweet gift for the Klees, but in fact he emerged with a bag of 'marrons glacés' which he had already opened. 'C'est bon, je vous jure, c'est bon' (it's good, really, it's good) – and before he knew it, Geiser had a candied chestnut in his mouth! Picasso was thirsty and suggested they should eat the 'marrons' in the station buffet so that they could also get a drink. Geiser felt his temperature rising and begged the artist to remember they were late for the appointment. 'But we can take a taxi!', he replied, and the next minute they were in the restaurant. When the waitress came, Picasso immediately offered her a chestnut. She recommended a strong red wine from the Valais, which she said would go wonderfully with the chestnuts. In a flash half a liter of Dôle was on the table. But unlike Picasso, Geiser could take little enjoyment from the wine and chestnuts. By the time they were finally on their way to the Klees in a taxi it was already getting dark. Klee opened the door in his woolen dressing gown and felt slippers – he had obviously given up on his visitors. Geiser tried to explain why they were so late, but with little success. Klee took his belated guest into his studio. On a small table in the corner was a half-eaten cake. Klee offered his guest something to drink, but this was politely declined, for he had already quenched his thirst in the station buffet … Without waiting to be asked, Picasso sank into a chair, and when Klee asked him if he would like to see some of his latest work, he replied 'Avec plaisir!' (with pleasure!). Picasso carefully studied the watercolors and drawings which Klee showed him, but said nothing. Bernhard Geiser: 'Suddenly Picasso held a picture away from him and turned it upside down. Following a long artists' tradition, he wanted to view it this way round. But Klee retained his aplomb, just smiling and saying: "You can turn everything upside down, and a lot of things are already upside down!" He was obviously referring to the situation in Germany at the time.' But they did not have a real conversation. Picasso merely asked: 'avec la plume?' (in pen?), to which Klee replied: 'avec la plume.' They looked through whole portfolios with barely a word being exchanged, Picasso just said thank you very politely as he handed back each final sheet. It was clear that he was enjoying himself; he just did not want to show it, as though this was somehow inappropriate. Suddenly the doorbell

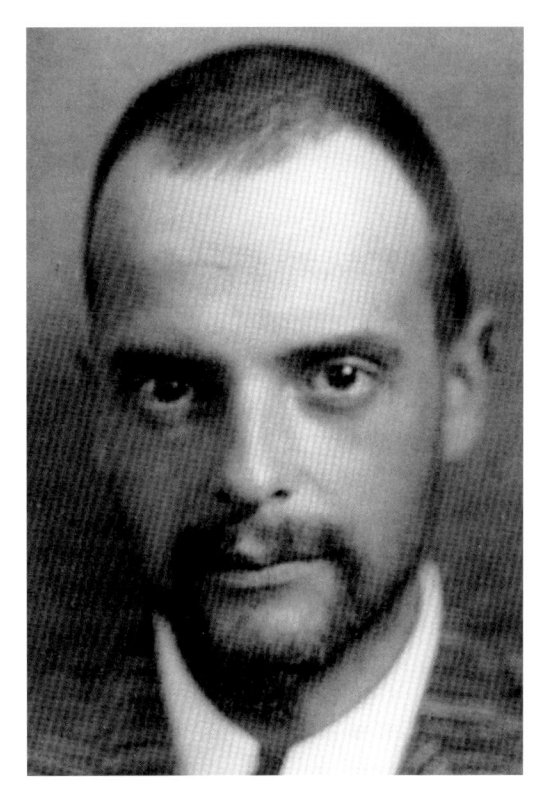

Fig. 169. Paul Klee, 1912

rang. It was Hermann Rupf, who had come in his car to collect the visitor at seven o'clock, as arranged, in order to take him to his home for dinner. Their parting was cordial; Klee's initial ill-humor had melted away.

This one short, historic meeting highlights the fundamentally different personalities of these two artists. First of all, the brilliant bon vivant: an extroverted, lively, spontaneous, rather chaotic character who never worried about appointments but who was charming and jovial. Then there was the equally brilliant thinker: introverted, retiring, orderly, rather perfectionist, an amiable person who always stood above things and never bore a grudge.

Roland Penrose quotes Pablo Picasso after this visit to Paul Klee: 'He [Klee] was marvelous, a very dignified man who garners respect through both his bearing and his work.'[639]

'His Creation Breathes Lightness and Grace'

Doris Wild characterizes Paul Klee and his work as follows: 'Klee's being is a triumph of the spirit over time and circumstance; it cannot be shaken by personal misfortune or the chaos of external events. He transforms cruel realities and carries the viewer to a higher world, illuminating pain and distress with light and joy. Although he was critically ill and knew that his end was near, he worked with a lightness of touch. He understood the forces which were driving and creating turmoil in the world at that time, and often recorded them in his pictures years before they impinged on the public awareness.'[640] [...] 'Like a gift from the gods, Klee was bestowed with something which was perhaps not to be found in Kandinsky. His creation breathes lightness and grace, a free use of line; it is swept along by an imagination which is grace.'[641] Hans Christoph von Tavel says something similar: 'Klee's late work has nothing in common with the work of his generation. It is one individual's incredible achievement which towers above his time and becomes ageless.'[642]

Leading up to his death, Klee produced many drawings which were spontaneous, spare, diary-like recordings of his condi-

[639] Penrose 1981, p. 361.
[640] Wild 1950, p. 218.
[641] Ibid., p. 217.
[642] Von Tavel 1969, p. 159.

tion. But it is also fascinating to note that at the same time he was painting fresh, richly-colored works, despite his pain and personal setbacks. Werner Haftmann describes his later work as being reduced to the simplest formula, possessing a pictorial asceticism and a 'light from within'[643]. 'Yet despite this asceticism the colors shine out with a mystic glow. Indeed on the formal plane the most sensational development in Klee's work during the last years of his life is the new force which his colors acquired through simplification. And because the mystic dimension is attained through color, all that has to be read is contained in these carved black hieroglyphics. Like lead frames in a stained glass window these magic black signs bring out the maximum of luminosity in the colors and give them a similar mystic significance'[644] (fig. 171, page 219).

This brings us to another aspect of Klee's work: the wonderful combination of colors in his paintings is always harmonious and has a musical effect. This is not surprising in an artist who as a young man was a talented and keen violinist. Carola Giedion-Welcker mentions this in connection with Klee's shift towards small-format oil paintings after the end of the First World War: 'This is the beginning of Klee's infinitely delicate and vibrating chamber music in colors. […] These small oil paintings seem like tropical flowers which are animated by an inner light; they have an element of festive solemnity and a deep sense of reconciliation, like the music of Bach and Mozart, whose compositions he so loved and often played'[645] (fig. 170, page 218).

[643] Haftmann 1961, p. 168.
[644] Ibid.
[645] Giedion-Welcker 2000, p. 52 f.

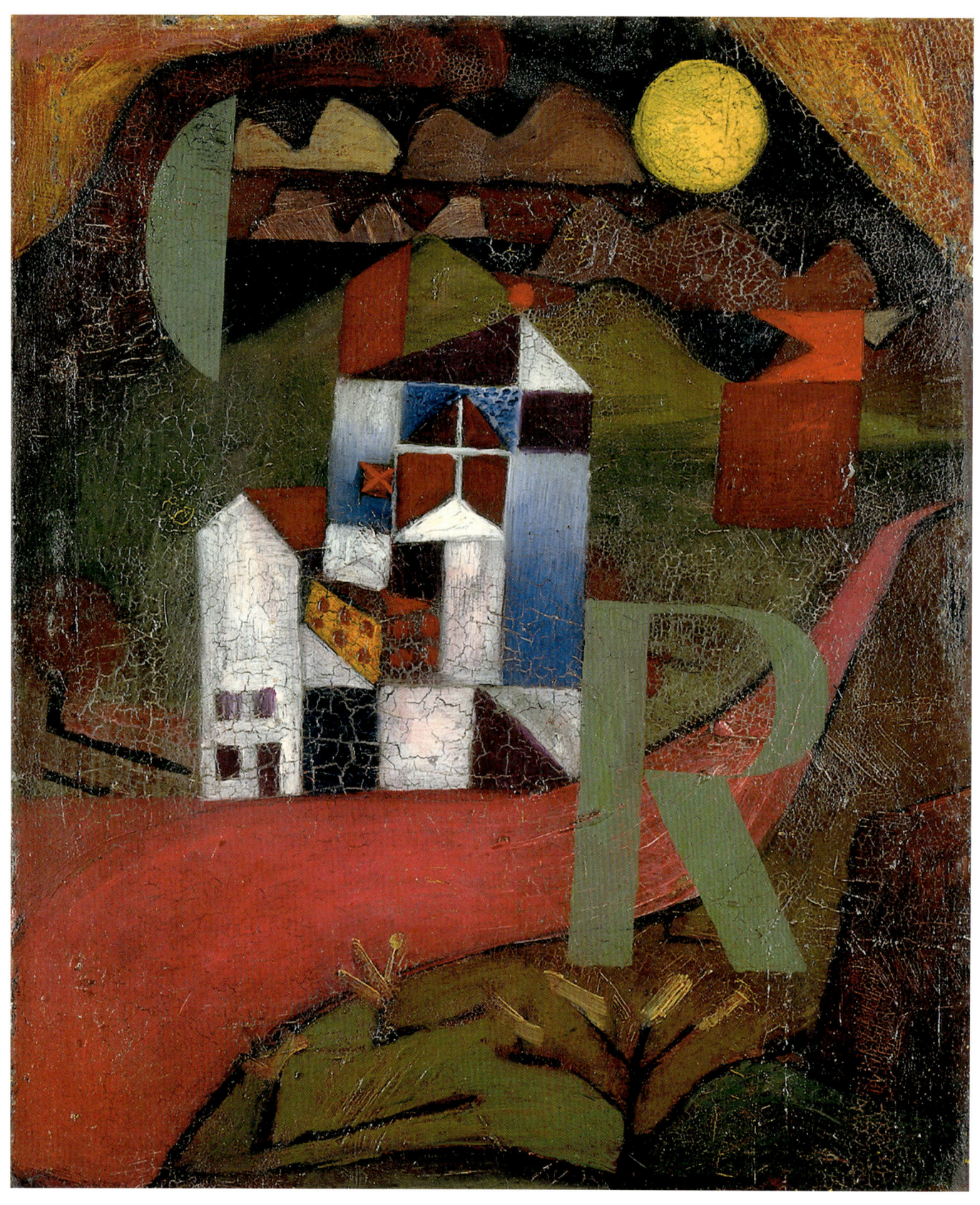

Fig. 170. Villa R, 1919, 153

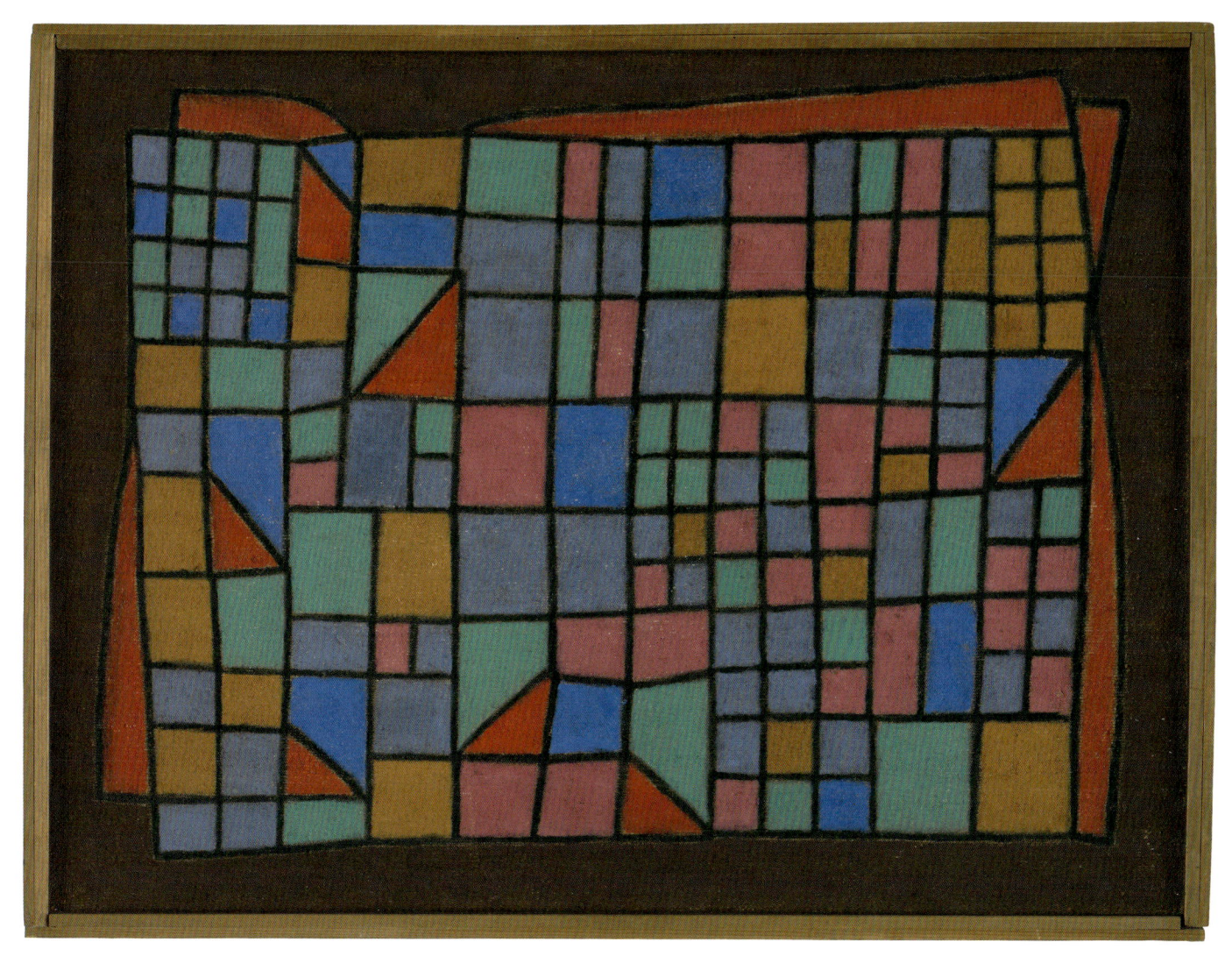

Fig. 171. Glass façade, 1940, 288

This superb painting of a stained glass window is full of clearly-defined red, blue, green and ocher tones. A luminous light shines from behind (as if from the hereafter), illuminating our earthly world with mystery and promise. (see page 217).

◁ Re. Fig. 170
After the First World War, Paul Klee painted small-format oil paintings that could be compared to chamber music (see also page 217).

'Productivity Is Increasing and the Tempo Is Accelerating'

Paul Klee kept an accurate, handwritten catalogue of works which sheds light on his artistic productivity.[646] In 1935, the year when his illness began, he still recorded 148 works – one third fewer than the previous year – but in 1936 his production suddenly fell to 25 works. The artist found it almost impossible to work because of his illness, his confinement to bed and the total exhaustion which he felt after the long and difficult first stage of his illness. Despite his trips to the mountains to convalesce (to Tarasp in the Unterengadin and Montana in Valais), Klee's recovery was very slow. The following year things improved: in 1937 he produced a total of 264 works, which was about the same as before he fell ill. In 1938 the number increased to 489, and then in 1939 Klee produced the incredible total of 1,253 works, mainly drawings[647] (the 'outline drawings' of the last year of his life took relatively little time and work to complete). Klee writes: 'Productivity is increasing and the tempo is accelerating, and I can no longer quite keep up with these children of mine. They run away with me.'[648] The fact that he calls his works his 'children' shows how important they were to him. Early in 1940 Klee writes to Will Grohmann, looking back at the previous year: 'It was a prolific year for me. I have never drawn so much, never worked more intensively.'[649] His wife also tells us: 'At such times, Klee sits at his work like Jerome in his study and forgets about the world.'[650] Here she is comparing her husband with the Christian priest and apologist from Dalmatia who in the 4th century AD translated the Old Testament from Hebrew to Latin and the New Testament from Greek to Latin; Albrecht Dürer depicted him as a recluse working alone 'in his study' (fig. 172).[651]

The artist used the four productive months that remained to him in 1940 to create and record a further 366 works, despite his previously mentioned physical debility.[652] 1940 was a leap year, and it is highly likely that Paul Klee consciously aimed to complete this number of works.[653] He noted in his catalogue of works for 1938, between numbers 365 and 366 – as an allusion to the number of days in the year – the quotation from Pliny: 'nulla dies sine linea' (no day without a

---

[646] Jürgen Glaesemer comments on the detailed entries in the catalogue of works: 'There is no doubt that he [Klee] took pleasure in his system. At no point does he lose concentration during his final years; he records every work, right up to the last, with the same thorough attention to detail.' (Glaesemer 1979, p. 23).

[647] Cf. Glaesemer 1976, p. 319, also see table 2, p. 222.

[648] Letter from Paul Klee to Felix and Euphrosine Klee, Bern, December 29, 1939, quoted in Klee 1979, p. 1295.

[649] Letter from Paul Klee to Will Grohmann, Bern, January 2, 1940, quoted in Gutbrod 1968, p. 84.

[650] Letter from Lily Klee to Curt Valentin, Bern, January 1, 1940 (MOMAANY/VP).

[651] Thanks to Prof. Hans Bietenhard, Th.D., CH–3612 Steffisburg for information on Saint Jerome.

[652] Cf. Glaesemer 1976, p. 344.

[653] Personal communication, Felix Klee to the author, Bern, September 20, 1983. And Helfenstein 1990, pp. 72 and 73: 'The symbolic number of 366 works in 1940 leads us to believe that Klee's convalescence in Locarno was already planned in early April. So it was definitely not a last-minute trip to Ticino […] Klee's accelerated rate of artistic production in his final year can be compared to a symbolic victory over external time. For the significant figure 366 also indicates that the internal time of the artist, who was terminally ill but at the same time working with great intensity, should be independent from that real, external time, which Klee refers to in his numbering system. The number of works recorded in 1940 leaves no doubt that in the last year of his life Klee deliberately created this total number of works which had a personal symbolic significance for him.'

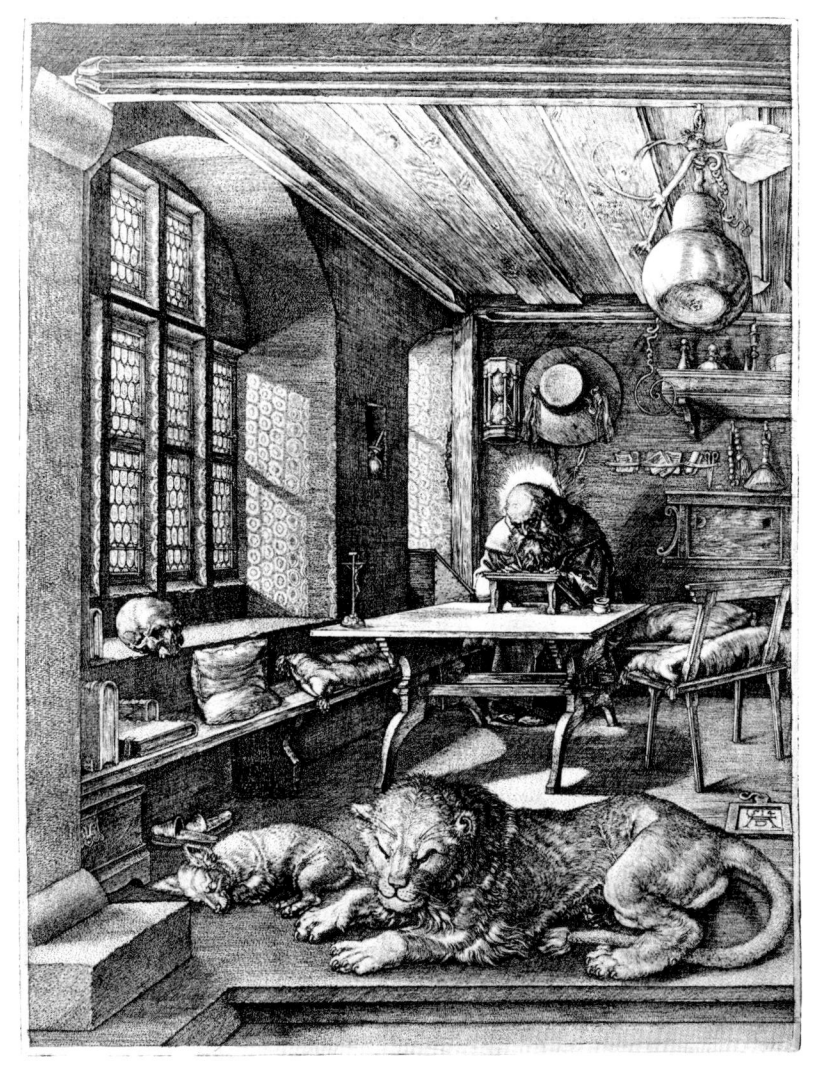

Fig. 172. Albrecht Dürer, 'Saint Jerome in his study', 1514, copper engraving (from: Bodmer, Heinrich, Dürer, Wilhelm Goldmann Verlag, Leipzig 1944, p. 83)

line, without a drawing; fig. 173, page 222).[654] Klee will have felt a certain sense of satisfaction once he reached this target of 366 works within the first few months of the leap year 1940. He could then record the final finished works in his catalogue before leaving for the sanatorium in Ticino on May 10, 1940 (his studio contained several works[655] which he did not record in this list, either because they were not finished or, perhaps more likely, because he consciously wanted to round off the catalogue for 1940 with a total of 366 works). This provides another striking parallel with Vincent van Gogh, who created 70 works in the last 70 days of his life.[656] Van Gogh suffered from a totally different illness but, like Klee,

[654] Glaesemer 1979, p. 25: 'Working on the drawings was similar to writing in a diary. The motto "nulla dies sine linea" is very clear in this sense. […] It is characteristic that he [Klee] chose a quotation which had previously mainly been used by writers to allude to his constantly increasing production of drawings.' According to Glaesemer 1976, p. 25, note 47, the quotation 'nulla dies sine linea' comes from chapter 35 of the 'Historia naturalis' by the Roman author Pliny the Elder (Gaius Plinius Secundus).

[655] 33 pictures which are not recorded in the catalogue of works are listed in: Klee 1998–2004, p. 233 f.

[656] Cf. Frank 1999, p. 121.

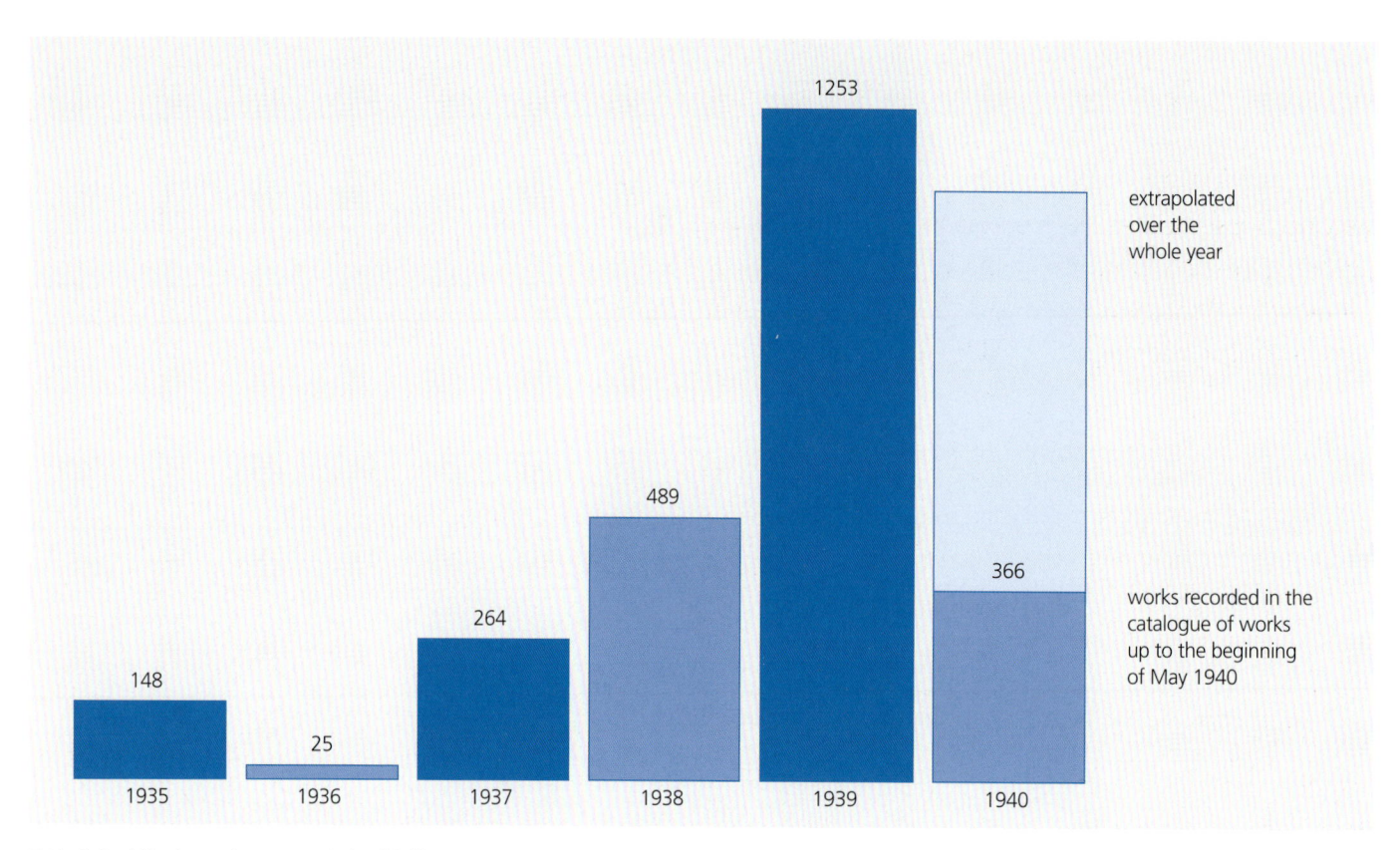

Table 2. Paul Klee's creative output during his illness

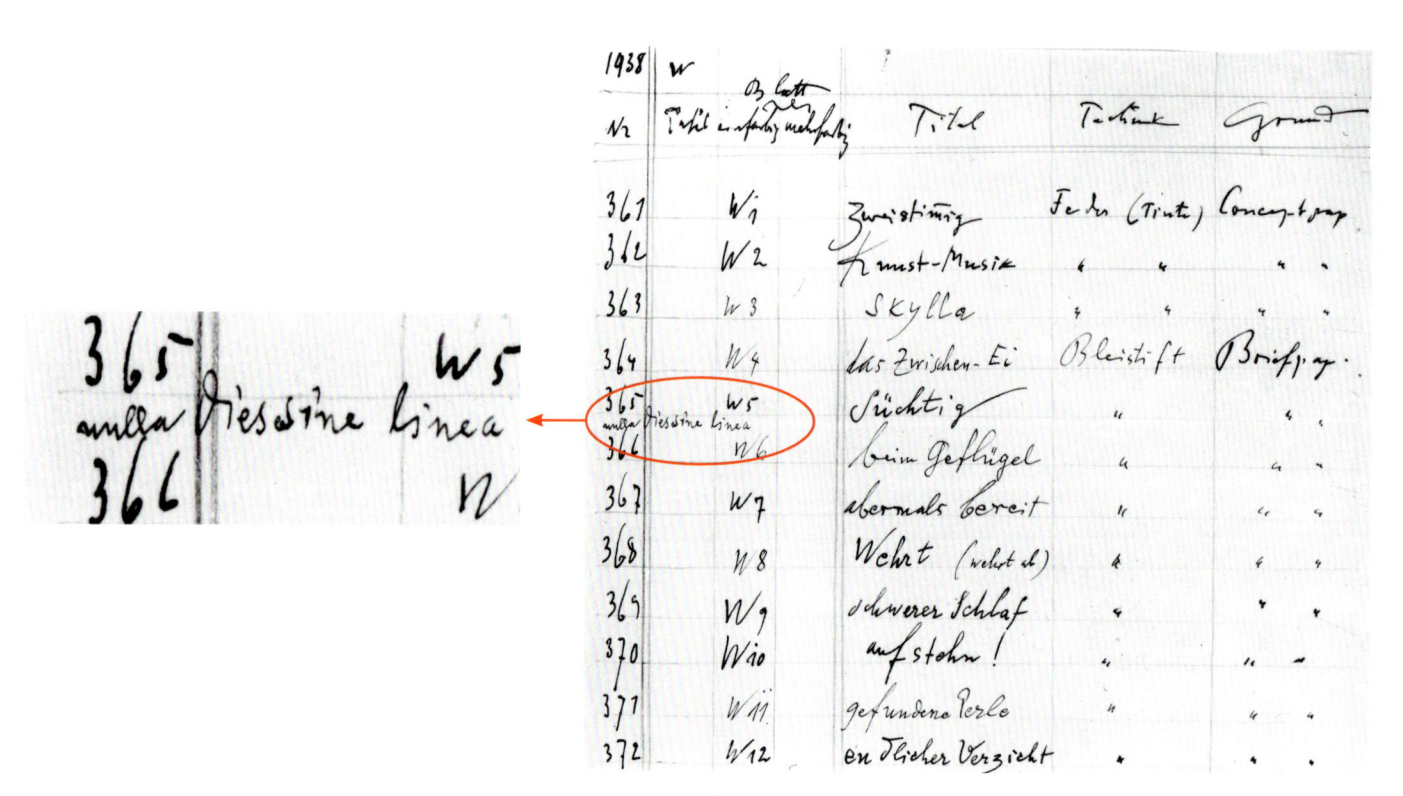

Fig. 173. Page from Paul Klee's catalogue of works for the year 1938 (nos. 361–372) with the comment 'nulla dies sine linea' (no day without a line) below the number 365

he felt very driven to increase his artistic output.[657] Doris Wild writes: 'In the short time that was left to him [van Gogh] between February 1888 and June 1890, he virtually produced his life's work in a creative, euphoric frenzy. He was like one possessed as he created picture after picture, painting in the silence of his humble room, while outside the mistral blew or the sun burned down. At times he even worked right through the night.'[658] Klee felt very affected by van Gogh's fate when he visited two of his exhibitions in Munich in 1908.[659] He wrote in his diary: 'Here a mind is suffering under a blazing star. He escapes into his work. Shortly before his catastrophe.'[660]

In the five years of his illness, Paul Klee produced around 2,500 works. As a proportion of his 9,800 numbered works, this means he completed more than a quarter of his whole oeuvre[661] during the period of his terminal illness.

Illness as Opportunity

'The ancient Greek symbol for crisis is also the sign for opportunity. Crisis and opportunity are so close together,'[662] writes Edgar Heim, continuing: 'Illness is never just a crisis; it is also always an opportunity.'[663] He maintains: 'We also know that illness can activate or deepen creative possibilities. In this way Beethoven's deafness probably stimulated him to produce his monumental work, the 9th Symphony. One of Thomas Mann's most imposing works, "Der Zauberberg" (The Magic Mountain), would not have been conceived without the author's own experiences in a sanatorium, and the paintings which van Gogh produced during his – still not totally explained – periods of sickness are particularly powerful.'[664]

Will Grohmann writes about Paul Klee's passing: 'He has come to the end, but his physical decline has mysteriously freed up superhuman powers of creativity, as if the extinguishing of one light enables a new one to be lit.'[665] The artist was marked both externally and internally by his severe illness. It is admirable how he faced up to illness and adversity with a trenchant 'so what?', and how he mastered his

---

[657] Gerson 1982, pp. 113–116: 'Van Gogh was at his creative peak during his time in Arles between February 1888 and May 1889, although this was also a time when he suffered from unproductive periods of depression. [...] Vincent worked feverishly. [...] On May 3, 1889 he sought help at Dr. Peyron's mental hospital in St.-Rémy. Here too he alternated between periods of depression and periods of health. His work consoled him: "I am working like one possessed, more than ever in a mute frenzy of work. And I think that this will help cure me." (Letter 604).'

[658] Wild 1950, p. 54.

[659] Cf. Grohmann 1965, p. 49.

[660] Klee Diaries, no. 816, also quoted in Grohmann 1965, p. 49, but incorrectly noted as 'Tgb. 822'.

[661] Cf. Helfenstein 1998, p. 12

[662] Heim/ML 1980, p. 233.

[663] Ibid., p. 187.

[664] Ibid.

[665] Grohmann 2003, p. 42.

serious physical illness through mental and spiritual strength and concentrated creative work. Paul Klee really used his illness as an opportunity and thus gained a 'greater health behind the sickness', to quote Friedrich Nietzsche.[666] The Geneva philosopher Jeanne Hersch interprets this 'greater health' as follows: 'Man is a being who is bound to uphold the meaning of life and the meaning of his own life through the way he bears illness and approaching death. This meaning is not health; health is at the service of this meaning. From it, health creates its own meaning and power.'[667]

At this point I would like to draw another interesting parallel, alongside the one already noted with Vincent van Gogh. As a child, the philosopher Karl Jaspers suffered from a severe chronic illness known as bronchiectasis (distortion of the bronchial airways). Symptoms included a chronic cough with emissions of sputum and blood, along with fever and fatigue.[668] Jasper's heart was also weakened by the disease. In a medical paper, the renowned doctor, Prof. Rudolf Virchow, thought it unlikely that the young Karl Jaspers would live beyond thirty.[669] But Jaspers responded to his illness by creating for himself a very well-regulated lifestyle where he avoided all stresses and strains. As a result he lived to the ripe old age of 86! He writes: 'But it was a bitter contest between the hope of overcoming and the melancholy of believing everything would soon be at an end.'[670] Like Klee, Jaspers also managed to achieve greatness despite his crippling ill-health.

It seems to be a personality trait of gifted and hard-working people that they can view sickness as a challenge and even treat it as a stimulus for their work. This is particularly true of artists: when they have real belief in their own ability and impact, nothing will keep them from their work. In this way they accomplish unexpected, almost 'superhuman' feats.

Karl Jaspers' words on greatness and the 'greats' apply to both himself and Paul Klee: 'They [the greats] are of their time but also above their time. Each of them, even the greatest, has his historical place and wears his historical clothes. But the mark of greatness is that it does not seem to be bound by time, rather it is supra-historical. Many of their con-

[666] Quoted in Nager/ML 1998, p. 1591: 'I have time and again met formidable people who were healthy in the deepest sense of the word, despite physical sickness and emotional suffering, infirmities of age and even terminal illness. They have reached the "great health". The thinker and man of sorrows, Friedrich Nietzsche, speaks movingly of this "greater health behind the sickness".'
[667] Quoted in Heim/ML 1980, p. 187.
[668] Cf. Pschyrembel/ML 1998, p. 233.
[669] Cf. Gottschalk 1966, p. 13.
[670] Quoted in ibid.

temporaries may also have appropriated it because of its tangibility, but in the greats it is transformed in a timeless sense. The great is not one whose mind captures his time, but one who uses it to move eternity. So transcendence in work and life allows the great man to become a phenomenon who can speak to every person and every time. […] Like everyone else, a true philosopher is original if he is real and essential. But the great philosopher is original in his originality. This means he brings a new communicability into the world which was not there before. The originality lies in work, in creativeness, which cannot be replicated but which can guide those who come later towards their own originality.'[671]

---

[671] Jaspers 1957, p. 39, quoted in Hersch 1980, p. 126 f.

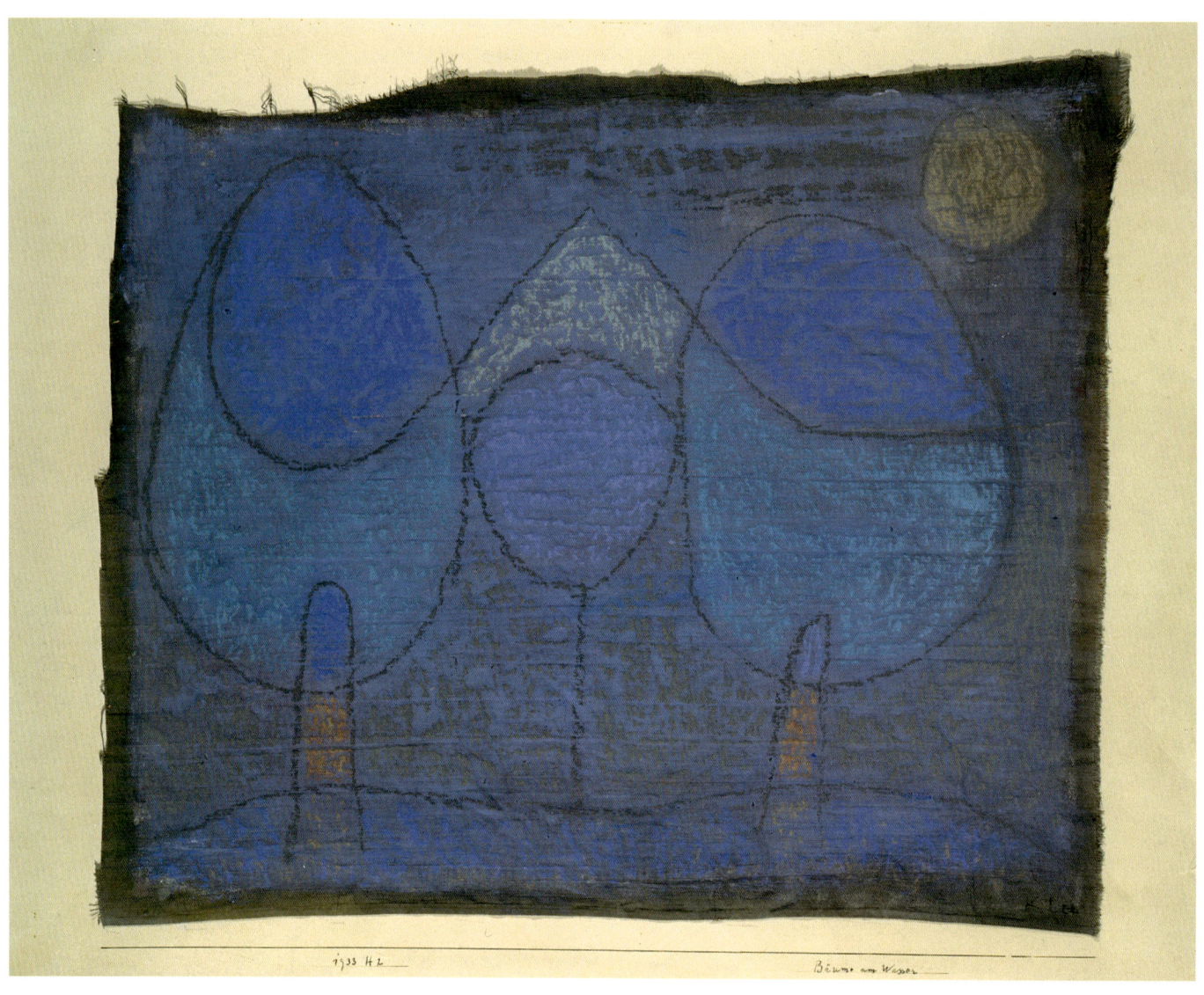

Fig. 174. Trees by the water, 1933, 442

The richly-colored pastel drawing 'Trees by the water' originated in 1933, the year in which Paul Klee had to deal with so much distress and hardship at the hands of the National Socialists. The way he handled his fate and illness is highly admirable and speaks of a rare human greatness. For him, flowers even bloom in the night (fig. 175).

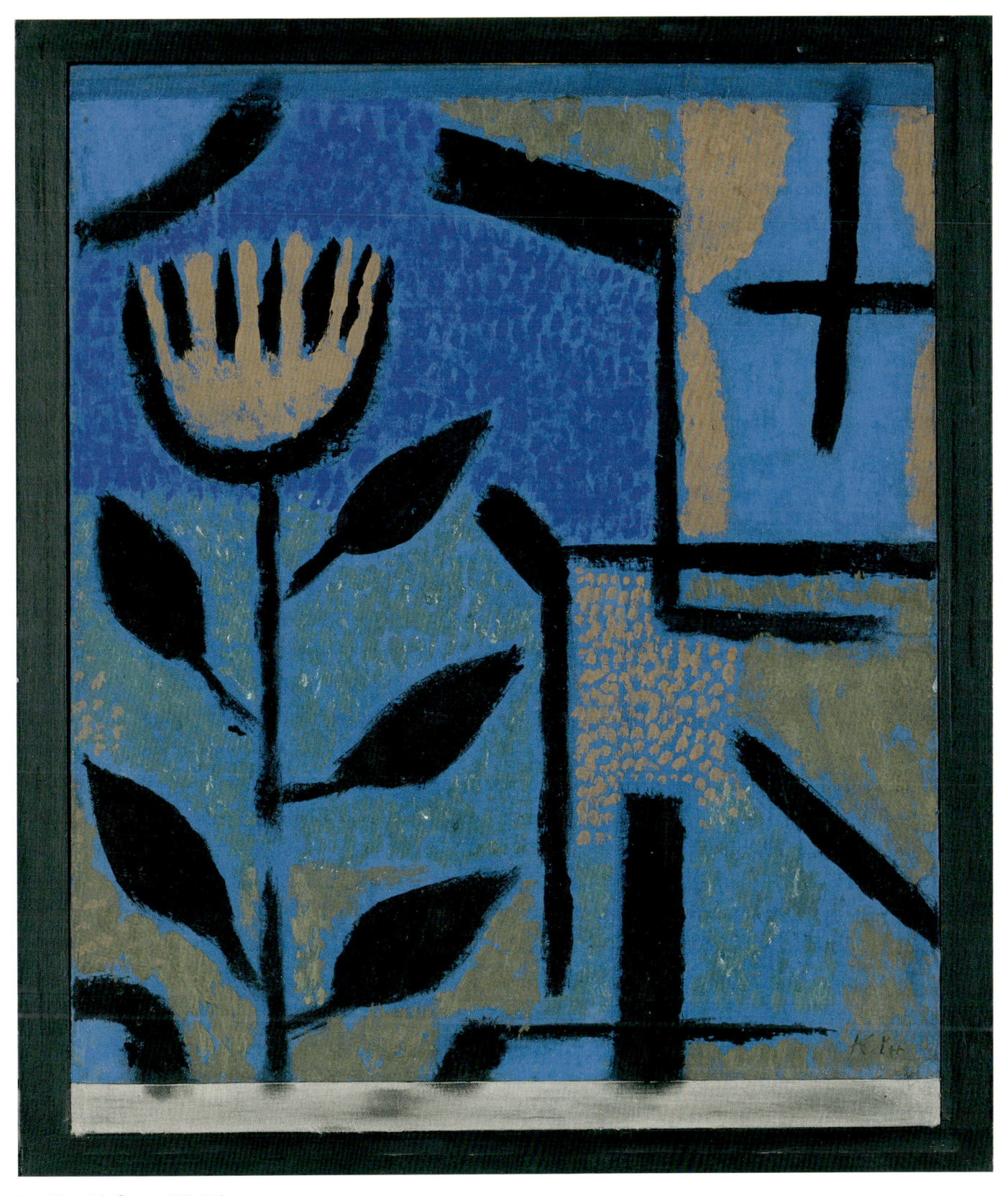

Fig. 175. Night flower, 1938, 118

Fig. 176. Underwater garden, 1939, 746

The painting opposite is another example of how, even while he was ill, Paul Klee was able to produce vital, colorful pictures which had no connection to his physical illness. He often revisited earlier themes such as fish, water and gardens.

Michael Baumgartner writes: 'During his time as a teacher at the Bauhaus, Paul Klee was very interested in the question of movement within different types of environments, whether static, gravity-bound or dynamic. He was particularly interested in the movement of birds and fish, as well as their own particular elements of air and water. He saw water as a kind of intermediate realm where the laws of gravity do not apply and where free movement is possible. "Fish" appears as a theme in more than 60 of Klee's works, and the concept of "water" is equally well used.'[672]

So we see static water in standing bodies of water and dynamic water in streams and rivers. In 'Underwater garden' we get an impression of standing water in an aquarium containing luxuriant and colorful sea plants. The eye is drawn to a red fish, similar to a goldfish, which is suspended in the middle of the picture.

Flowing water reminds us of the axiom attributed to the Greek philosopher Heraclitus[673] 'panta rhei': everything flows; the whole universe is in a state of constant flux, nothing is permanent.[674]

---

[672] Michael Baumgartner in: Zentrum Paul Klee 2005/2, p. 80.
[673] Heraclitus, around 540–480 BC.
[674] Duden, Fremdwörterbuch, 3rd ed., vol. 5, Bibliographisches Institut, Dudenverlag, Mannheim/Wien/Zürich 1974, p. 528, and Zürich 1945–1948, vol. 3, p. 1585.

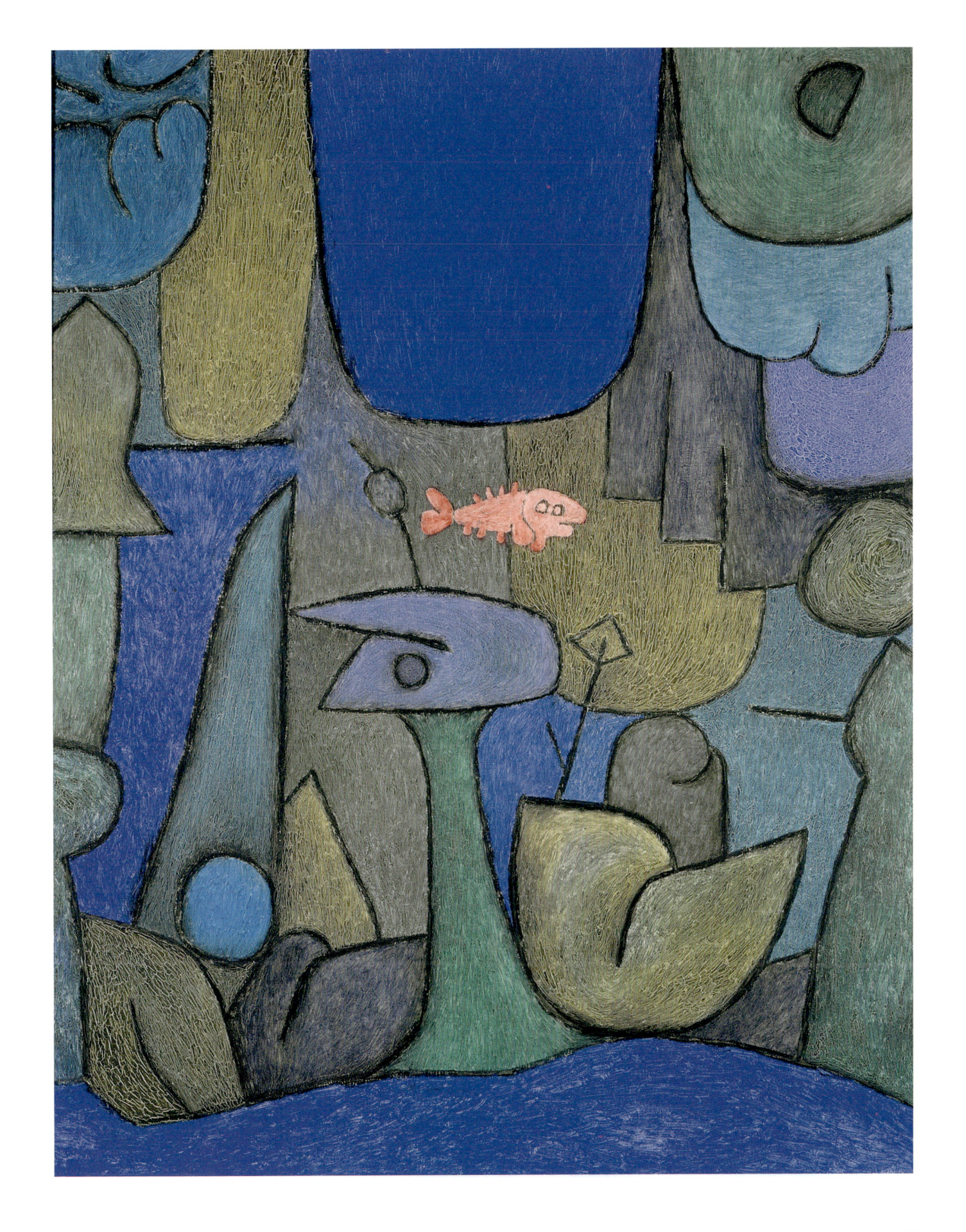

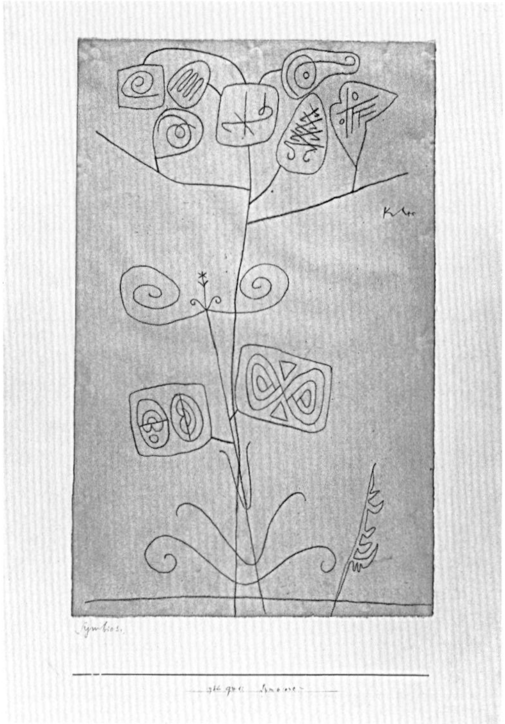

Fig. 177. Symbiosis, 1934, 131

Fig. 178. Flora on the rocks, 1940, 343 ▷

[675] Cf. Ernst-Gerhard Güse in foreword to: Güse 1992, p. 7. Also: Klee, Felix, in: du 2000, p. 63: 'His [Paul Klee's] great knowledge of natural history often appears in the themes of his pictures. He studied botany by pressing plants and he observed animal life.' And: Grohmann 1965, p. 67: 'All around [in Paul Klee's large Bauhaus studio in Weimar] the furniture and shelves were covered with a hundred things which he [Klee] had collected or made over the years, butterflies, shells, roots, pressed plants, masks, ships, homemade models, painted sculptures.'

The last panel painting recorded in Paul Klee's catalogue of works, at the end of April 1940, 'Flora on the rocks', shows a plant structure against bright red and orange surfaces that reminds us of lichen on a tree or rock. The title suggests it is indeed this very common type of rock flora. Lichen is made up of fungi and algae which together create a symbiosis. They are interdependent – the fungi store water and minerals for the algae and the algae provide the fungi with organic nutrients. This symbiosis makes lichen incredibly prolific and robust. Every good partnership can be compared to a symbiosis. Paul and Lily Klee had a harmonious and symbiotic marriage during a difficult time for them both in Bern. Lily did everything she could to make her husband's life easier during his illness. It is interesting to note that in 1934 he gave the title 'Symbiosis' to a drawing of a stylized flower (fig. 177).

Plants were of great importance to the artist. He collected, dried and pressed them and kept them in glass cases. He knew a great deal about botany.[675] Gardens and parks are important motifs in his creative work. Observing the different stages of nature was intrinsic to him, watching the unfolding, growth and decay made him feel at one with nature and creation. This dialogue with nature not only provided a stimulus for his creativity but also gave him strength during his illness. He hints at this in his now famous statement: 'In the here and now I cannot be understood, for I live as well with the dead as with the unborn. Somewhat nearer the heart of creation than normal – and yet not nearly close enough' (see page 186, note 571). Paul Klee finished this painting only a few months before he died. With its freshness and strong colors it conveys to us a last message from the artist: Paul Klee is saying 'yes' to life as well as to dying and to death. He is ready to say goodbye – in the knowledge that in his short life he has made the best use of his abundant talents and has used his creativity to overcome misfortune and illness. This last recorded work can be seen as a tribute to Lily and also as a kind of epilogue.

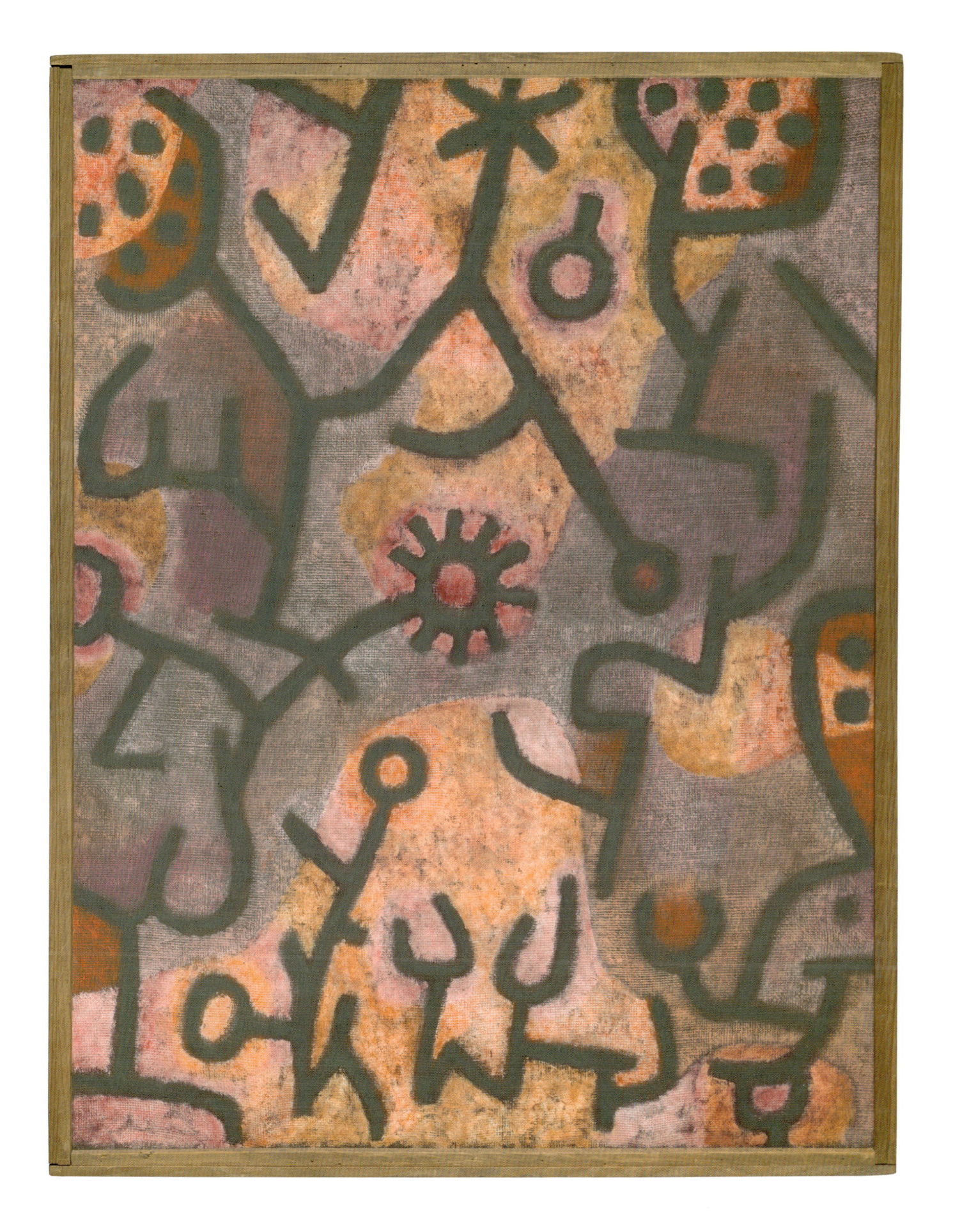

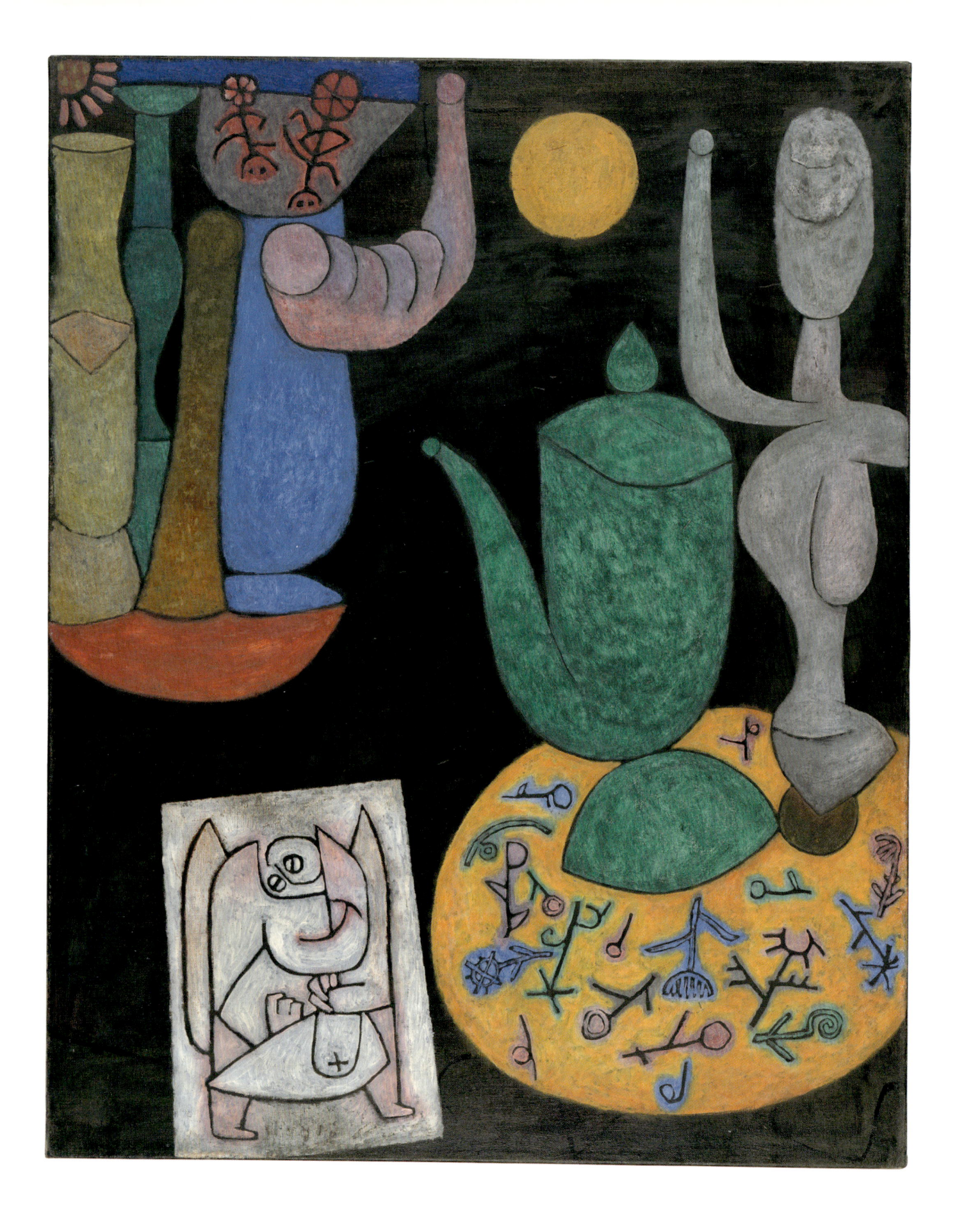

The large oil painting opposite, completed by Paul Klee himself but unsigned, untitled and probably deliberately not recorded in his catalogue of works, was left by the artist on the easel in his studio when he left for his last journey (to Locarno). It is to some extent a retrospective of the last part of his life which was beset by adversity and illness.

It is night. Painted against a black background, the colors are muted, apart from the red and the orange. The painting is full of symbolism. On a table covered in dying, withered flowers there stands a jug and a sculpture of a human form. To the left we can make out other objects, a red bowl and vases. Containers are major symbolic objects in Klee's life: on the one hand he kept his mind open, like a bowl or a vase, while on the other hand he filled his 'pot' with his life's work. The human sculpture alludes to this, with its proudly raised right arm. The cobalt blue vase contains two vermillion-colored flowers. They are unusual flowers. They could also be two people who have fallen into the vase, thrashing around in the water before drowning. They are desperately trying to get a foothold on the edge of the vase. It is reminiscent of the drawing 'Fleeing on wheels' (fig. 114, page 144) from 1939 – the two flowers are almost a copy of these figures 'Fleeing on wheels', albeit upside down, and with the wheels (intentionally or accidentally?) turned into flowers. But it is not possible to flee from fate and illness: fate captures them and brings them back. And yet on the left, next to the drowning flowers, a marguerite daisy appears from the ocher-grey vase like a 'star or wonder flower'. Although it is standing discreetly in the background, it creates a feeling of optimism.

To the right of the vases there is a strange object that brings to mind the lower esophagus and the stomach. The narrowing of the esophagus brought on by his illness was the most painful symptom of all. '[…] my father must have suffered unspeakably (with it)' writes his

◁ Fig. 179. Untitled (Last still life), 1940

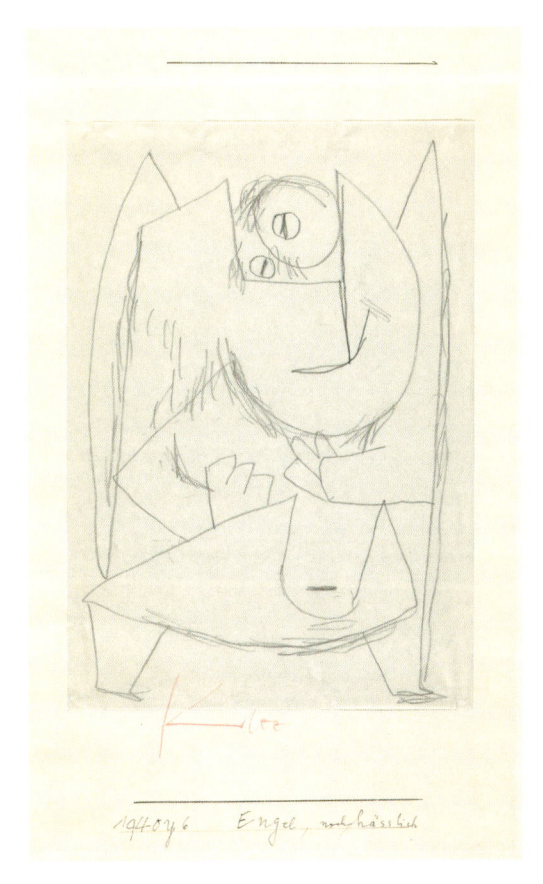

Fig. 180. Angel, still ugly, 1940, 26

son Felix.[676] He also had a stomach ulcer and gastric bleeding. So this 'anatomical' image could be seen as a symbol of Klee's suffering.

At the bottom of the picture the artist has painted a copy of the drawing 'Angel, still ugly' (fig. 180, page 233), which he had completed in the same year. There is, however, a small but very significant difference: in the drawing there is a small horizontal line on the pocket of the angel's robe – is this a minus sign? In the painting, Klee has changed this negative sign into a plus sign (positive sign), as if he wants to say: my suffering is over, my life's work is complete and I see that it is good. The angel has an expression of satisfaction and bliss. He is smiling to himself. Soon he will no longer be 'ugly' in the earthly sense. This inclusion of the angel is also reminiscent of the way artists in the Middle Ages used to depict themselves in the corner of a painting.

Up above, the full moon shines into the black night. It pours its soft, comforting light over the 'still life', imbuing it with that mystical, magical intensity which is so typical of Klee's work. This mysterious painting exudes serenity and tranquility, splendor and peacefulness. It is both retrospective and explicit.[677]

Christine Hopfengart also believes that 'with this classic still life full of color, in which only the fallen, faded petals and the angel are an allusion to death, [Klee] wanted to say goodbye, not as an invalid and sufferer, but as an artist.'[678]

---

[676] Klee 1960/1, p. 110; see also p. 63, note 203.

[677] 'Explicit' signifies (according to Duden, Fremdwörterbuch, 3rd ed., vol. 5, Bibliographisches Institut, Dudenverlag, Mannheim/Wien/Zürich 1974, p. 228) the final words of a medieval manuscript or early printing. The Latin word means 'It is complete, it is finished'.

[678] Verbal communication, Christine Hopfengart to the author, Bern, October 23, 2002 (see also note 680).

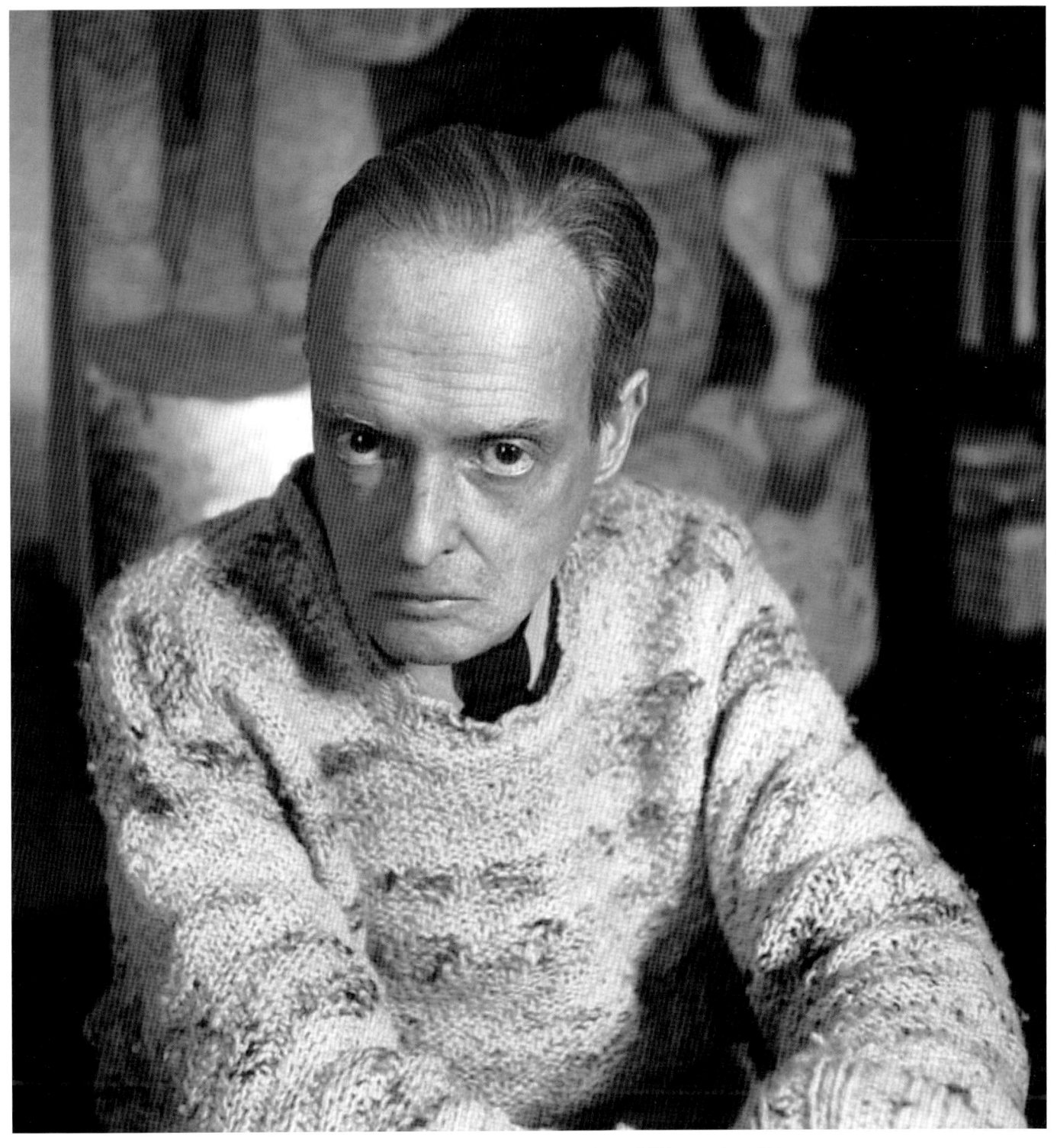

Fig. 181. Paul Klee in his living room in Kistlerweg 6, Bern, in front of the untitled picture (Last still life), December 1939

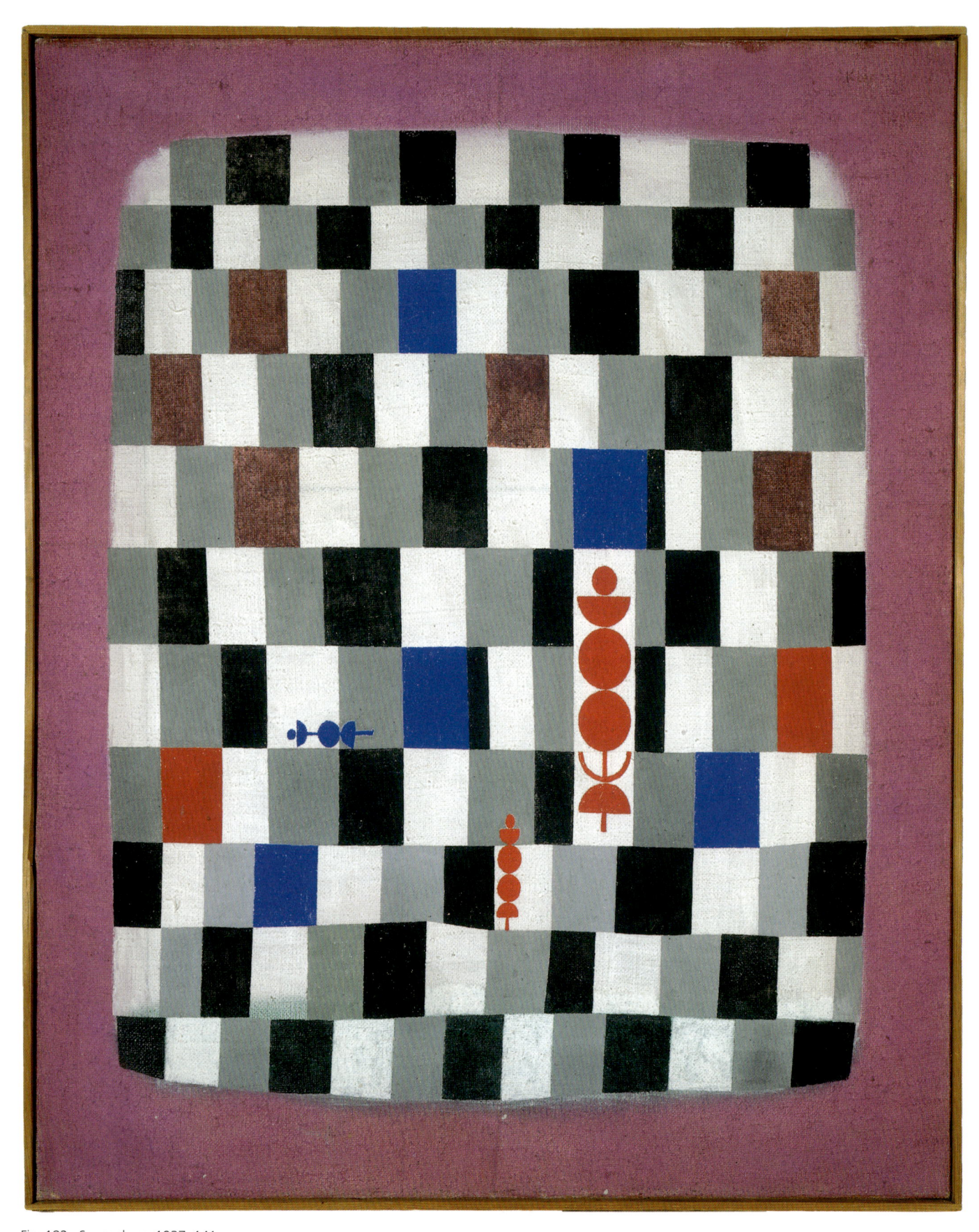

Fig. 182. Super-chess, 1937, 141

6. Summary and Conclusion

In 1933, when Paul Klee was 54 years old, his professional life was suddenly shattered as the National Socialists came to power in Germany. They branded him a 'cultural Bolshevist' and dismissed him from his professorial post at the Düsseldorf Academy of Fine Arts. This led him to emigrate to his 'real home' of Bern in December 1933. In 1935 he became seriously ill with a mysterious disease, which led to his death only five years later. During the last seven years of his life, Paul Klee had to suffer a string of misfortunes and disappointments: defamation by the National Socialists and dismissal from his post as professor at the Düsseldorf Academy of Fine Arts, ridicule of his pictures in the travelling exhibition 'Degenerate Art'[679] which began in Munich in 1937, increasing isolation in Bern due to his illness and the events of the time, a worsening of his personal financial situation as a result of fewer sales at exhibitions, and the sluggish handling of his application for Swiss citizenship. It is certainly conceivable that such an unfortunate chain of events could have triggered Paul Klee's illness and had an influence on its course.

Today it is clear that none of the doctors' medical records relating to Paul Klee are still in existence, so the final diagnosis of his illness must remain hypothetical. However, my comprehensive research, as detailed in this book, confirms that the previous tentative diagnosis of 'scleroderma' was very probably accurate. The research actually allows us to be more precise in the diagnosis: Paul Klee very probably suffered from the rarest and most serious form of the autoimmune connective tissue disease known as 'diffuse systemic sclerosis'. The main evidence for this comes from the letters written by the artist and his wife (as quoted), from important

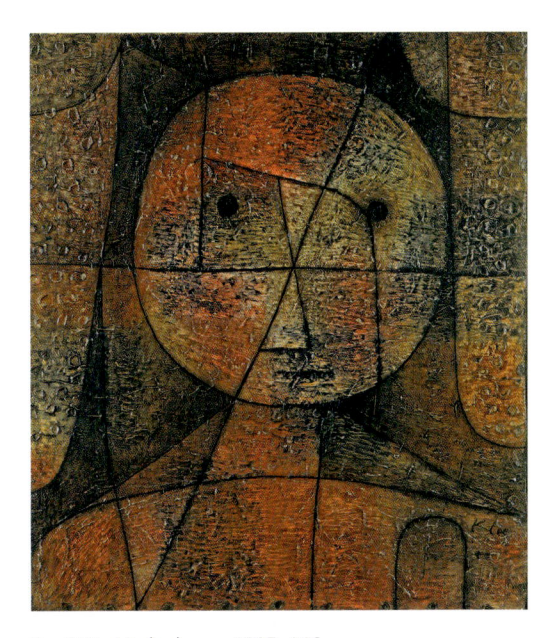

Fig. 183. Marked man, 1935, 146

[679] Klee's pictures were pilloried by the National Socialists in three so-called 'Schandausstellungen' (shame exhibitions) in Mannheim, Chemnitz and Dresden in 1933 (from Josef Helfenstein in: Klee 1998–2004, vol. 6, 2002, p. 10). 17 of Paul Klee's works were also included in the 'Entartete Kunst' (Degenerate Art) exhibition organized by the National Socialists in Munich from July 19 to November 30, 1937. This defamatory show subsequently became a travelling exhibition until 1941, visiting another eight German cities and Salzburg. In 1937, 102 of Klee's works were removed from German museums (quoted in Frey: Bern 1990, p. 114).

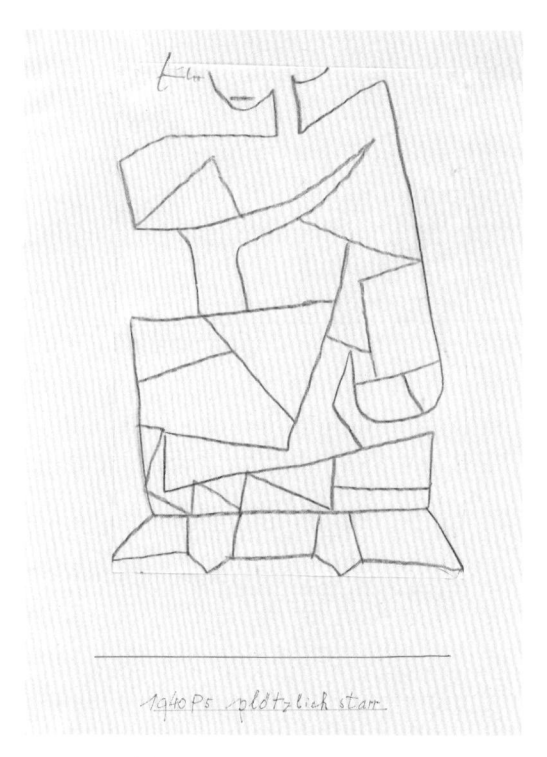

Fig. 184. Suddenly rigid, 1940, 205

information told to me by their only son, Felix Klee, who died in 1990, and from verbal or written comments made by various people who were friends of Klee's or who otherwise knew him personally.

A typical characteristic of this disease is a thickening and hardening of the skin. At the same time, the sufferer starts to form a kind of 'armor' around his body, as if to protect himself from the outside world. The disease not only thickens and hardens the skin, it also makes a relentless attack on the connective tissue of the inner organs. Klee may have stiffened up physically, but mentally and spiritually he remained unrestricted.

Even today, the diffuse form of systemic sclerosis can lead to death within a few years. However, the more common and – in terms of life expectancy – less serious limited form would have made it difficult or even impossible for the artist to carry on drawing and painting. Fortunately, the fact that his hands were not affected allowed him to continue working unhindered during his illness.

Paul Klee was a highly intelligent and sensitive person. But he hid this sensitivity from the outside world, remaining calm, sanguine and tolerant in his outlook even during the most difficult of times. As a person he was reserved, self-disciplined, modest and kind. He bore his suffering and accepted his fate with quiet fortitude.

Bowed but not broken by suffering and adversity. Despite this severe illness, the artist managed to create a substantial and important body of late work which was different from his earlier oeuvre. In part, his drawings and paintings reflect succinctly and visually the course of his illness and the emotions he was experiencing at the time. His late work is also filled with greater spirituality. In his mind, Paul Klee stood above his physical infirmity and as much as possible he distanced himself from it. He rose above it by pouring his worries and distress into the diary-like drawings, by 'putting them down on paper', which then freed him to create the most wonderful paintings full of vitality, freshness and light.

The majority of his output in his final years is not connected to his physical illness. And from time to time we are still treated to a glint of his innate sense of humor!

The art historian Christine Hopfengart notes that with the last still-life which he left on his easel, Paul Klee is saying his goodbyes not as an invalid and sufferer but as an artist.[680] It is a classic still-life full of color and animation, with just a few fallen, faded petals and an angel suggesting death and dying. It was always very important to him to strive for economy, equilibrium and poise in his life and work. Paul Klee used his extraordinary mental composure to deal with the physical symptoms caused by his disease. He was an exceptional tightrope artiste. Even when balancing on the high wire of his avant-garde art he was always confident and assured. The Greek/Latin word 'harmonia' with its many facets of meaning is a perfect description of the artist and his work, encompassing destiny, accord, harmonious sounds, inner and outer concordance, balance, symmetry and unity.

Paul Klee's oeuvre is unique and complete in itself. The viewer is moved, captured, dazzled by its vibrancy. The richness of his works is like a spring which can never run dry. Like the charismatic artist himself, his poetic art is magical and mystical – and yet ultimately so human.

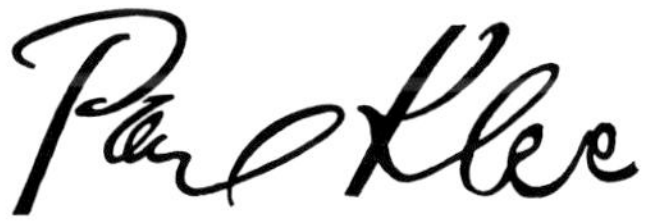

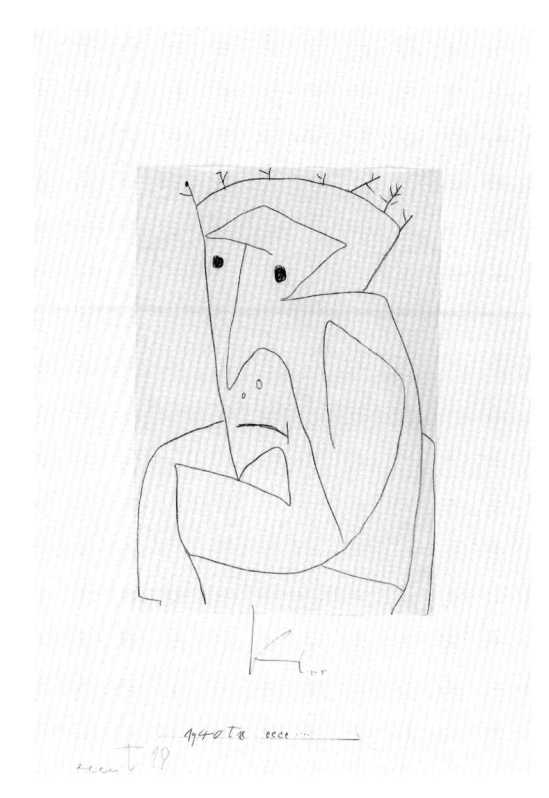

Fig. 185. Ecce ...., 1940, 138

[680] Verbal communication, Christine Hopfengart to the author, Bern, October 23, 2002.

Paul Klee und seine Krankheit

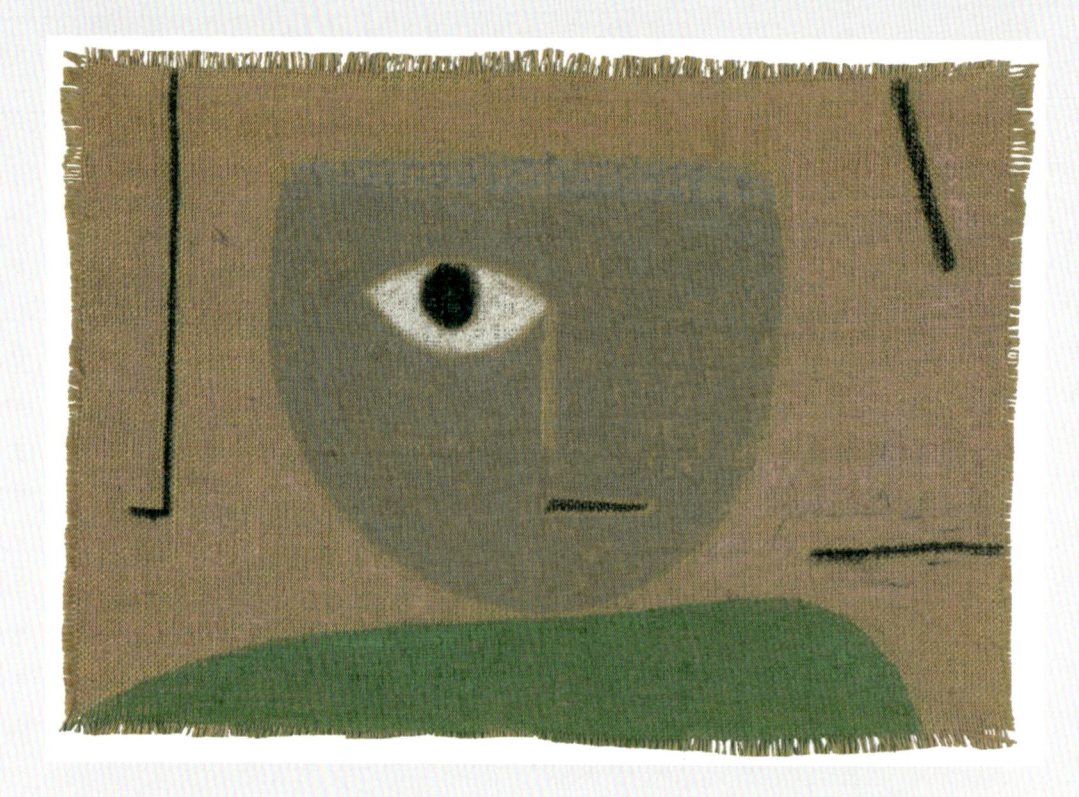

Eine Ausstellung der Medizinischen Fakultät
der Universität Bern
zu ihrem 200-Jahre-Jubiläum

mit Beiträgen des Medizinhistorischen Instituts
der Universität Zürich und des Zentrum Paul Klee

Zentrum Paul Klee, Bern
5. bis 27. November 2005

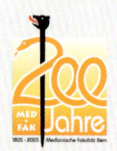

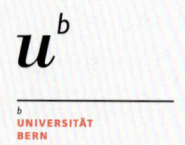

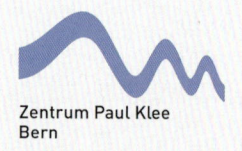

Fig. 186. Poster for the Bern Medical Faculty exhibition in the Zentrum Paul Klee, Bern, November 5–27, 2005

From November 5 to 27, 2005, an exhibition was held at the Zentrum Paul Klee, Bern, entitled 'Paul Klee und seine Krankheit' ('Paul Klee and His Illness'). This exhibition was organized by the Medical Faculty of the University of Bern to mark its 200th anniversary. The Medical History Institute of the University of Zurich contributed exhibits from its 'Paul Klee and Medicine' exhibition which took place at the University of Zurich Medical History Museum from March 31 to October 9, 2005. The Zentrum Paul Klee made available various works by the artist which fit in with the theme of the exhibition. The research contained in this book formed the basis of the Bern exhibition, along with an exposition on the current state of research and knowledge about the disease scleroderma. Patron of the exhibition was the Dean of Bern University Medical Faculty, Professor Martin Täuber.

Contributors:
Dr. Hans Suter, curator.[681]

From the Medical Faculty of the University of Bern: Prof. emerit. Emilio Bossi[682]; Prof. Urs Boschung[683]; Prof. Peter M. Villiger[684], with his colleagues Prof. Michael Seitz[685], Dr. Hans-Rudolf Ziswiler[686], Dr. Stephan Gadola[687], Marlise Bühler[688] and Brigitte Rausch[689]; Prof. Lasse R. Braathen[690] and his colleague Fritz Schweizer[691]; Dr. Peter Frey[692] and his colleague Hans Holzherr[693]; and from the Dean's Office: Marianne Thormann[694] and Petra Bühlmann[695].
From the Medical History Institute and Museum, University of Zurich: Prof. Beat Rüttimann[696]; Prof. Christoph Mörgeli[697], and lic. phil. Walter Fuchs[698].
From the Zentrum Paul Klee: Andreas Marti[699]; Ursina Barandun[700]; Franziska Aebersold[701]; Prof. Tilman Osterwold[702]; Dr. Michael Baumgartner[703]; Osamu Okuda[704]; Mark Isler[705]; Heidi Frautschi[706]; Fabienne Eggelhöfer[707]; Hansruedi Pauli[708]; Murielle Utinger[709]; Martin Blatter[710]; Erwin Schenk[711] and his team, Anita Gasser[712], Myriam Weber[713] and Patrizia Zeppetella[714].
From the Paul Klee's Estate, Bern: Stefan Frey[715].

[681] Specialist in skin diseases, FMH, Fahrni (Bern).
[682] Assistant Dean of the Medical Faculty of the University of Bern and President of the Organizing Committee for the 200th anniversary celebrations of the Bern University Medical Faculty in 2005.
[683] Director of the Institute of Medical History at the University of Bern.
[684] Director and Chief Physician of the University Clinic and Polyclinics of the Department of Rheumatology and Immunology/Allergology, Inselspital, Bern.
[685] Deputy Chief Physician at the above-mentioned University Clinic/Polyclinics, Inselspital, Bern.
[686] Head of Administration at the above-mentioned University Clinic/Polyclinics, Inselspital, Bern.
[687] Senior Academic Physician at the above-mentioned University Clinic/Polyclinics, Inselspital, Bern.
[688] Directors' Assistant at the above-mentioned University Clinic/Polyclinics, Inselspital, Bern.
[689] Occupational Therapist at the above-mentioned University Clinic/Polyclinics, Inselspital, Bern.
[690] Director of the University Clinic and Polyclinic for Dermatology and Venereology, Inselspital, Bern.
[691] Photographer at the Dermatology Clinic, Inselspital, Bern.
[692] Head of the Medical Training Institute and Department of Teaching Media, Inselspital, Bern.
[693] Designer, Department of Teaching Media, Inselspital, Bern.
[694] Executive Secretary, Dean's Office, Medical Faculty, University of Bern.
[695] Secretary, Dean's Office, Medical Faculty, University of Bern.
[696] Director of the Medical History Institute and Museum, University of Zurich.
[697] Curator of the Medical History Museum, University of Zurich.
[698] Curator of the exhibition 'Paul Klee and Medicine' at the Medical History Museum, University of Zurich.
[699] Director of the Zentrum Paul Klee (ZPK), Bern.
[700] Deputy Director, ZPK, Bern.
[701] Events Director, ZPK, Bern.
[702] Art Director, ZPK, Bern.
[703] Curator and Deputy Art Director, ZPK, Bern.
[704] Research Assistant, ZPK, Bern.
[705] Marketing and Sponsoring Director, ZPK, Bern.
[706] Administrator, Photoarchives/Copyright, ZPK, Bern.
[707] Administrator, Photoarchives/Copyright, ZPK, Bern.
[708] Museum technician, ZPK, Bern.
[709] Museum technology staff member, ZPK, Bern.
[710] Buildings technician, ZPK, Bern.
[711] Events and Multimedia Director, ZPK, Bern.
[712] Bookbinder, ZPK, Bern.
[713] Restorer, ZPK, Bern.
[714] Restorer, ZPK, Bern.
[715] Freelance art historian, secretary of the Klee family collection and Paul Klee's Estate, Bern.

Special Medical Terms

Autoimmune disease — Disease caused by the production of antibodies which work against the body's own cells, organs or tissues. Cause unknown in many cases. May possibly be triggered by a combination of factors that weaken the immune system. Today it is possible to identify such a disease using immunofluorescence microscopy to detect 'autoantibodies' in the blood.

Collagen — Connective tissue.

Collagenoses (synonym: connective tissue diseases) — Chronic inflammatory autoimmune diseases of the connective tissue (collagen) of the skin, mucous membranes, blood vessels and internal organs. Classified under rheumatic diseases. Main protagonists: systemic sclerosis, Lupus erythematosus, dermatomyositis/polymyositis.

Connective tissue — Encases and divides organs, holds them in position and connects blood vessels and nerves. Made up of connective tissue cells (fibroblasts, fibrocytes) and matrix and intercellular substances made from them, including intercellular cement (mucopolysaccharides), embedded collagen and elastic fibers. Connects outer and inner cell layers (for instance in blood vessels, and as the dermis between the epidermis and the subcutaneous tissue). (From: Pschyrembel 1998, p. 197.)

Dermatomyositis — An autoimmune connective tissue disease (collagenosis) affecting the skin and muscles: purple lesions on the skin and swelling on the eyelids, cheeks and bridge of the nose, on the upper body, elbows, knees, and backs of the fingers; giant nail-fold capillaries; lachrymose expression. Painful inflammation of the muscles, muscle weakness, muscle wasting, Raynaud's syndrome and arthritis.

Drug-induced exanthema — Undesirable reaction to drugs on the skin or mucous membranes as a result of oversensitivity (allergy) or intolerance. Patches form on the skin with red spots (as in scarlet fever, rubella or measles), or with papules, blisters, bubbles or wheals (such as with urticaria). Often occurs over the whole body. Symptoms improve when the relevant drug is discontinued but may reappear if the same drug or a chemically-related drug is used at a later date.

Esophageal stenosis — Narrowing of the esophagus with painful swallowing. Can be caused by deformity, compression by a tumor or by thickening and hardening of the connective tissue of the lower third of the esophagus due to systemic sclerosis. Accompanied by acid reflux and esophageal inflammation with heartburn or burning pain behind the breastbone.

Fibrosis — Development of excess connective tissue with thickening and hardening of the skin and mucous membranes, in blood vessels, in the esophagus and in internal organs such as the lungs, heart and kidneys.

Lupus erythematosus — Chronic autoimmune disease with inflammation of the connective tissue (collagenosis). Two main types: one type only affects the skin and is cosmetic in nature (chronic discoid Lupus erythematosus with typical discoloring of the face, known as 'butterfly rash', Lupus erythematosus disseminatus which also affects the skin on other parts of the body), and one type which also affects the internal organs, often with serious consequences (systemic Lupus erythematosus).

Malabsorption — Abnormality in absorption of food nutrients across the gastrointestinal tract into the blood and lymphatic vessels. Can result in: diarrhea, weight loss, fatigue, anemia. Can also present with changes to skin and mucosal membranes, for example in the various forms of systemic sclerosis.

Mask face — Typical symptom of systemic sclerosis: stiff, taut facial skin, pointed nose, radial wrinkles around the mouth (tobacco pouch mouth), limited opening and constriction of the mouth, loss of facial expression.

Mixed collagenosis (Mixed Connective Tissue Disease, MCTD; formerly known as Sharp's syndrome) — Combination of symptoms of systemic sclerosis and systemic Lupus erythematosus and/or dermatomyositis/polymyositis. Often also accompanied by Raynaud's syndrome, sclerodactyly and arthritis. Can often develop into classic collagenosis over time.

Morphea (synonym: circumscribed or localized scleroderma) — Collagenosis that normally only affects the connective tissue of the skin, with circumscribed, permanent blotching of the skin, cosmetic in nature. Starts with a red blotch with thickening/hardening of the dermis, then gradual whitening of the center with a 'lilac ring' at the edge, and finally only a whitish hardened patch with thinning of the epidermis.

Inflammation of the heart muscle associated with rheumatic diseases or after an infection. Symptoms: cardiac arrhythmia, cardiac insufficiency with shortness of breath and fatigue.	**Myocarditis**
Concurrent existence of two or more defined collagenoses, for instance systemic sclerosis and systemic Lupus erythematosus.	**Overlap syndrome**
Autoimmune disease affecting the muscles: muscle weakness, muscle pain, mostly around the shoulders and the pelvis as well as the upper arms and the thighs. If it affects the skin, it is known as dermatomyositis.	**Polymyositis**
Another name for systemic sclerosis.	**Progressive systemic scleroderma**
Disease with similarities to the limited form of systemic sclerosis, triggered by the long-term inhalation of organic solvents such as benzol or benzine, of vinyl chloride produced during the manufacture of polyvinyl chloride (PVC), of the industrial solvent trichloroethylene or of quartz dust during mining. Symptoms include: scleroderma-type thickening of the skin, Raynaud's syndrome, finger pad defects with calcium excretion, bone cysts, osteoporosis, reduction of blood platelets and liver damage.	**Pseudoscleroderma**
In systemic sclerosis the arterial wall thickens due to an accumulation of connective tissue in the small arteries (arterioles) of the lungs. This leads to a significant constriction of the blood vessels and – as a consequence – to high blood pressure in the arteries of the lungs. This problem occurs typically in the limited form of systemic sclerosis but it can also be found in the diffuse form. In the latter, it is a consequence of general fibrosis of the lung tissue, in the former the fibrosis is restricted to the wall of the blood vessels. Nowadays, pulmonary arterial hypertension can be detected by an echocardiograph of the heart. It has to be confirmed by a cardiac catheter examination which shows a mean pressure in the pulmonary artery of more than 25 mm Hg at rest and of more than 30 mm Hg during physical exertion. Pulmonary arterial hypertension is a severe complication of systemic sclerosis. Despite new treatment modalities it can be fatal.	**Pulmonary arterial hypertension**
Blood circulation disorder of the fingers with characteristic symptoms, caused by a temporary cramp-like narrowing of the arteries in the fingers due to cold or emotional stress: at first white fingers ('dead finger'), then blue-purple coloring caused by carbonic acid flowing through the blood vessels. As the cramping reduces, oxygen-rich blood flows into the now dilated arteries, resulting in a painful reddening of the fingers. In cold weather the pain can even start during the whitening stage. Can also occur without being linked to an underlying disease, especially in young women, as well as in conjunction with certain diseases such as systemic sclerosis and pseudoscleroderma.	**Raynaud's syndrome**
Hardening of the skin with thick, stiff fingers, especially in the limited form of systemic sclerosis. Tapering of the finger ends ('Madonna fingers'). In serious cases there is bend contracture with limited finger mobility.	**Sclerodactyly**
The name of this disease comes from the Greek 'scleros' meaning hard and 'derma' meaning skin. A chronic, but very rare autoimmune disease with thickening and hardening of the connective tissue of the skin, mucous membranes, blood vessels and internal organs. It is a form of collagenosis. There are various forms: those that only affect the skin (morphea) or those that affect the skin and the mucous membranes, with or without involvement of the internal organs. If the latter are involved, it is these days referred to as 'systemic sclerosis'. Joints and muscles can also undergo changes.	**Scleroderma**
See under 'Lupus erythematosus'.	**Systemic Lupus erythematosus**
See also under 'Scleroderma'. There are two major forms: 'limited' and 'diffuse'. The limited form represents 95% of cases and in addition to the facial skin symptoms ('mask face'), most cases involve the skin on the hands ('sclerodactyly') and forearms. Mucous membranes can also often be affected. Raynaud's syndrome can precede the disease for a long period. Internal organs are rarely affected, usually later on. In the remaining 5% of cases classified as 'diffuse' the skin on the face is affected ('mask face') as well as on the neck and trunk and possibly the whole body. Mucous membranes can be affected. However, sclerodactyly and Raynaud's syndrome are rare. Due to internal organs being affected early the prognosis is poor. Can lead to death within five to ten years.	**Systemic sclerosis**

Index of Terms

Afterlife/hereafter: pages 132, 186, 194, 196, 197, 200, 203, 209, 219
Anemia: 69, 79, 80, 82, 102, 103, 105, 106, 242
Angels: 179, 194, 196–200, 209, 233, 234, 239
Attempt to gain Swiss citizenship: 157, 265, 266
Autoimmune disease: 50, 61, 80, 90, 91, 106, 107, 237, 242, 243, 252
Balance: 56, 94, 127, 135, 139, 141, 211, 239
Bar lines/Broad bars/Black lines: 56, 139, 211, 213
Bauhaus: 20, 36, 58, 117, 119–121, 141, 154, 157, 210, 228, 230
Bronchitis: 39, 61, 79, 80, 105
Catalogue of works: 13, 102, 177–179, 182, 196, 200, 220–222, 230, 233, 237
Clinica Sant' Agnese: 12, 14, 37, 73, 74, 76, 91, 111, 155
Collagenoses: 48, 51, 98, 103, 104, 106, 242, 243
Concentration: 89, 91, 140, 220
Convalescence/holidays: 45, 67, 70, 73, 163, 220
Cosmic: 92, 116, 194, 197, 201, 202, 212
Creation: 17, 21, 116, 163, 186–188, 196, 197, 201, 202, 211, 216, 230
Creative (creativity): 15, 16, 21, 29, 36, 67, 95, 97, 101, 115, 119, 120, 133, 156, 172, 186, 194, 201, 203, 212, 222–225, 230
CREST syndrome: 104, 106
Crisis: 14, 127, 128, 154, 156, 223
Dance: 135, 139, 181, 204
Death: 7, 11, 12, 14, 20, 21, 37, 41, 45, 52, 53, 63, 70, 73–76, 80, 84–86, 91, 104, 106, 114, 117, 132, 139, 150, 151, 154–156, 164, 165, 168, 170, 175–178, 182, 185–192, 196, 197, 200, 203, 204, 208, 210, 216, 224, 234, 237–239, 243
Defamation: 21, 124, 128, 135, 153, 237
Depression: 129, 136, 223
Dermatomyositis: 48, 98, 103, 104, 106, 242, 243
Detailed Passion: 182, 188
Diary: 13, 20, 29, 90, 96, 98, 107, 121, 132, 133, 136, 153, 186, 210, 211, 216, 221, 223, 238
Diary-like drawings/recordings: 136, 210, 211, 216, 238
Diet: 63–65, 68, 83, 105, 118
Diffuse form of systemic sclerosis: 52–54, 60, 73, 79, 106, 238
Drug-induced exanthema/Drug reaction: 41, 42, 54, 103, 242
Eidola: 188, 208, 209
Esophageal stenosis: 62, 242
Exhibition: 14, 21, 28–30, 67, 91, 98, 141, 142, 176, 194, 202, 223, 237, 241
Fate/destiny/misfortune/adversity: 3, 11, 20, 21, 51, 127, 129, 133, 144, 153, 155, 156, 170, 173, 182, 187, 216, 223, 226, 230, 233, 237–239
Fear: 31, 127–132, 157, 185, 187, 188, 203
Fortitude: 57, 85, 154, 238
Friendship: 96, 109, 128, 154, 176
Gastric acid (production/lack of): 64, 79, 105
Gastric bleeding: 65, 69, 79, 105, 234
Gastric ulcer/stomach ulcer: 65, 79, 83, 105, 234
Goodbye: 65, 147, 163, 175, 190, 230, 234, 239
Hope: 11, 12, 15, 44, 45, 48, 74, 76, 84, 94, 97, 129, 132, 133, 136, 139, 143, 156, 170, 178, 190, 197, 203, 224

Humor: 97, 116, 139, 197, 199, 203, 208, 216
Intensity: 130, 185, 201, 210, 212, 220, 234
Intermediate world/realm: 194, 196, 197, 228
Intuition: 156, 163, 164, 172, 186
Isolation: 8, 21, 24, 28, 91, 96, 107, 128, 185, 186, 193, 210, 213, 237
Late work/later works: 15, 30, 91, 128, 133, 170, 185, 186, 194, 206, 210, 211, 213, 216, 217, 238, 239
Leap year: 182, 220, 221
Limited form of systemic sclerosis: 51–54, 58, 60, 78, 80, 104, 106, 238, 243
Malabsorption: 69, 85, 242
Mask face: 52, 53, 57, 103, 105, 106, 242, 243
Masks: 83, 203, 204, 206, 230
Metamorphosis: 178, 187, 197, 209
Metaphysical: 193, 210, 212
Mixed collagenosis/Mixed connective tissue disease: 48, 98–100, 104, 106, 242
Morphea: 50–53, 242, 243
Myocardial fibrosis: 72, 76, 79
Myocarditis: 72, 74, 76, 106, 243
Mystical/mystic: 195, 201, 202, 217, 234, 239
Narrowing of the esophagus: 62–64, 66, 79, 233
National Socialists/Nazis: 21, 24, 86, 124, 130, 135, 153, 157, 158, 160–162, 170, 237, 268
Nature: 143, 187, 194, 201, 202, 230
Nulla dies sine linea: 220–222
Opportunity: 14, 16, 101, 155, 193, 223, 224
Organic solvents: 88–90, 107, 243
Overlap syndrome: 48, 104, 106, 243
Pneumonia: 39, 40, 43, 45, 47, 61, 70, 71, 79, 100, 105
Polymyositis: 48, 98, 103, 104, 106, 242, 243
Production/output: 16, 136, 172, 177, 178, 182, 204, 212, 220, 222, 223, 239
Pseudoscleroderma: 86, 89, 90, 106, 143
Psyche: 15, 93, 115, 127, 129, 133, 206
Pulmonary arterial hypertension: 70, 72, 85, 243
Pulmonary fibrosis: 70–72, 78, 91, 243
Raynaud's syndrome: 60–62, 85, 86, 89, 92, 98–100, 102, 104–106, 242, 243
Renal fibrosis: 73, 80
Sanatorium: 12, 14, 46, 54, 63, 65, 73, 74, 84, 111, 113, 221, 223
Sclerodactyly: 53, 54, 58, 59, 62, 78, 99, 100, 102, 104, 106, 242, 243
Scleroderma: 11, 12, 15, 48, 50–53, 56, 58, 60, 61, 81–83, 86, 87, 89–92, 97, 98, 103, 106, 129, 133, 170, 181, 183, 237, 241–243
Sicca syndrome: 59, 105
Spirituality: 193, 194, 196, 238
Stafne sign: 59
Swallowing difficulties: 63, 84, 98, 100, 103, 106
Systemic Lupus erythematodes: 48, 62, 90, 98–100, 102–104, 106, 242, 243
Systemic sclerosis/Progressive scleroderma: 51–54, 58–64, 67, 69, 70–73, 76, 78–80, 85, 86, 90, 97, 98, 103, 104, 106, 237, 238, 242, 243
The Blue Four (Die Blaue Vier): 20
The Blue Rider (Der Blaue Reiter): 20, 29, 119
The Bridge (Die Brücke): 29
Tightrope walker/artiste: 135, 139–141, 239
Transcendence: 179, 193, 194, 210, 225
Treatment: 12, 42, 53, 61, 65, 74, 81–83, 85, 109, 111, 118
Vasomotor trophic neurosis: 60, 78, 106

Index of Names

Note:
– The names below refer to people mentioned in the text and to people referred to in the notes
– Names printed in italics denote people for whom biographical information is provided (pp. 246–252)

Aebi Christoph: pages 40, 270
Aichinger-Grosch Ju (Juliane Paula): 41, 63, 76, 84, 93, 117, 154–157, 246, 254, 268
Arp Jean: 30, 247, 266, 267
Bachmann Virginia: 12, 13, 264, 270
Barr Alfred: 212, 254
Bätschmann Oskar: 201, 202, 246, 254, 256, 258
Baumgartner Michael: 13, 64, 120, 228, 241, 246, 254, 258, 270
Beer F.-J.: 86, 153, 253, 264
Beethoven Ludwig, van: 223
Benos J.: 129, 253
Bergmann Gustav, von: 119, 246
Hans Bietenhard: 220, 270
Bloesch Hans: 28, 29, 74, 76, 117, 246, 255, 258
Bodmer Diana: 12, 111, 265, 270
Bodmer Heinrich: 221, 255
Bodmer Hermann: 12, 74–76, 108, 111, 113, 246, 259, 264, 265
Boschung Urs: 51, 109, 112, 113, 241, 246, 270
Bossi Emilio: 241
Braathen Lasse R.: 112, 241, 270
Bruderer Hans-Jürgen: 172, 255
Brunner Erika: 270
Bürgi-Bigler Hanni: 28, 154, 176, 246, 255
Bürgi Rolf: 28, 71, 176, 246, 255
Bywaters E.G.L.: 97, 133, 253
Cabane Jean: 246, 269, 270
Campendonk Heinrich: 20, 29, 249
Castenholz Gabriele: 12, 50, 51, 60, 61, 78, 81, 83, 86, 89, 90, 98–100, 102, 153, 246, 253, 268, 270
Charlet Jean: 53, 54, 59, 78, 88, 246, 265
Chiquet Simone: 270
Curzio Carlo: 50
Danuser Brigitta: 78, 86, 88–90, 246, 247, 253, 270
Dula Karl: 267, 270
Dürer Albrecht: 220, 221, 255, 259
Dürring Jacqueline: 270
Edschmid Kasimir: 201, 255, 256
Eggelhöfer Fabienne: 241, 270
Erne Emil: 270
Feininger Lyonel: 20, 119, 120, 247, 251, 255
Feitknecht Thomas: 270
Franciscono Marcel: 177, 178, 188, 255
Frank Herbert: 188, 189, 221, 255
Frautschi Heidi: 241, 270
Frehner Matthias: 270
Frey-Surbek Marguerite: 28, 87, 247, 255, 265
Frey Peter: 241, 270
Frey Stefan: 13, 30, 42, 53, 54, 59, 60, 69, 73, 74, 76, 86, 101, 118, 119, 154, 157, 160, 176, 177, 186, 194, 237, 241, 247, 255, 257, 258, 262, 268–270
Frick-Riedtmann Anna C. R.: 92, 93, 259
Friedli Bendicht: 87, 170, 204, 247, 270
Friedli Susanne: 270
Früh-von Arx Franziska: 267, 270
Fuchs Walter J.: 11, 30, 241, 247, 250, 270

Fueter Max: 28
Gadola Stephan: 48, 51, 52, 58, 60, 61, 69, 70, 72, 73, 80, 85, 103, 104, 241, 253, 270
Geelhaar Christian: 30, 120, 196, 255, 257
Geiser Bernhard: 28, 212, 214, 215, 247, 255
Gerber Urs: 270
Giedion-Welcker Carola: 13, 63, 120, 121, 155, 170, 176, 206, 217, 247, 255, 256, 266
Gintrac Elie: 50
Glaesemer Jürgen: 13, 15, 28, 45, 95, 101, 129–133, 139, 155–157, 160–162, 170, 178, 185, 186, 192, 194, 196, 197, 203, 208–211, 220, 221, 247, 255, 256, 259, 268, 269, 270
Gogh Vincent, van: 188, 189, 221, 223, 224, 247, 250, 255
Gottwald W.: 129, 253
Götz-Gee Eugen: 270
Grandini Sergio: 14, 264
Grohmann Gertrud: 11, 13, 14, 39, 45, 84, 93, 94, 100, 154, 157, 176, 247, 249, 259, 268
Grohmann Will: 11, 13, 14, 16, 20, 21, 39–42, 45, 46, 54, 61, 65, 67, 69, 71–74, 76, 82–84, 92, 95, 96, 107, 116–120, 122, 127, 132, 154, 156, 157, 178, 179, 187, 197, 203, 204, 209, 211, 212, 220, 223, 230, 247, 249, 256, 258, 259, 262, 268–270
Gropius Walter: 120, 247
Grosch Karla: 154
Grote Gertrud: 39, 60, 67, 81, 84, 157, 248
Grote Ludwig: 13, 16, 76, 84, 246, 248, 254–258
Haemmerli Theodor: 74, 108, 113, 248, 259
Haftmann Werner: 194, 197, 217, 256
Haller Hermann: 19, 246, 248
Hartmann Sabine: 270
Heim Edgar: 14, 127, 128–130, 132, 154, 223, 224, 248, 253, 270
Helfenstein Josef: 13, 29, 157, 160, 177, 185, 186, 194, 204, 220, 223, 237, 248, 254–256, 258, 270
Heraclitus: 228, 248
Hersch Jeanne: 224, 225, 248, 256
Hippocrates: 50
Hitler Adolf: 24, 130, 157, 158, 268
Hodler Ferdinand: 29
Hopfengart Christine: 13, 121, 141, 234, 239, 248, 256, 270
Huber Othmar: 122, 256
Huggler Max: 12–14, 28, 29, 31, 53, 58, 78, 102, 163, 177, 194, 211, 248, 256, 259, 264, 266, 270
Hulton Edward and Nika: 194, 258
Hunziker Thomas: 270
Iseli Karl Friedrich: 248, 265
Jackowski Jochen: 253, 267, 270
Jaspers Karl: 193, 224, 225, 248, 256
Jawlensky Alexej, von: 20, 251
Jesus: 183
Jung Ernst G.: 50, 51, 248, 249, 253, 254, 269, 270
Kahnweiler Daniel-Henry: 11, 39, 45, 153, 214, 251, 256
Kállai Ernst: 121, 259
Kandinsky Nina: 39, 40, 45, 46, 48, 63, 67, 71, 80, 81, 83, 84, 94, 101, 117, 118, 249, 251, 256, 267
Kandinsky Wassily: 20, 28, 40, 46, 48, 63, 67, 71, 83, 87, 94, 96, 101, 117, 118, 216, 247, 249–251, 256, 257, 259, 262, 266, 267
Kant Immanuel: 193, 249, 256

Kaposi Moritz: 50, 51
Karger Thomas: 270
Kayser Hans: 28
Kehrli Jakob Otto: 265, 266
Kersten Wolfgang: 139, 249, 255–258
Klee-Coll Aljoscha (Alexander): 7, 249, 259, 269, 270, 271
Klee-Coll Anne-Marie: 263
Klee Euphrosine: 157, 170, 220, 249
Klee Felix: 8, 11–13, 20, 28, 40, 47, 52, 53, 58–60, 63, 76, 78, 87, 89, 93, 95–97, 99–103, 115, 127, 129, 154, 157, 160, 166, 172, 173, 203, 209, 211, 220, 230, 234, 238, 246, 249, 256–259, 263, 264, 268, 270
Klee Hans: 19, 20, 154, 203, 248, 249, 256, 259, 265
Klee-Frick Ida: 19, 21, 249, 259
Klee Lily: 11–13, 19, 21, 24, 27, 28, 36, 39–43, 45–47, 48, 53, 54, 60, 61, 63–65, 67–74, 76, 77, 80–84, 92–96, 100–103, 106, 109, 115, 117, 118, 122, 153, 154, 156, 157, 161, 176, 209, 212, 214, 220, 230, 246–249, 251, 258, 259, 263, 264, 267–269
Klee Mathilde: 19, 20, 28, 93, 119
Kocher Theodor: 110
Kollwitz Käthe: 130, 249
Kort Pamela: 162, 257
Krebs Alfred: 6, 12, 13, 41, 42, 58, 63, 73, 211, 249, 254, 264–266, 269, 270
Kröll Christina: 64, 257
Künzi Theodor: 86, 270
Lautenschlager Deborah: 270
Le Corbusier (Jeanneret Charles-Edouard): 30
LeRoy E. Carwile: 78, 97, 253
Lotmar Fritz: 12, 28, 39, 48, 108, 109, 113, 249, 259, 264
Lotmar Gerold: 109, 264, 270
Lütken Ilona: 270
Macke August: 20, 29, 249, 250
Maier Olivier: 270
Mandach Conrad, von: 31, 266
Marc Franz: 20, 29, 196, 249
McKay Gill: 3, 250, 270
McKay Neil: 3, 250, 270
Meyer-Benteli Hans und Erika: 28, 246
Mittag Hannelore: 183, 254
Moilliet Louis: 20, 28, 249, 250
Moosberger Daniel: 270
Mörgeli Christoph: 241, 270
Morscher Christoph: 92, 93, 96, 254
Mozart Wolfgang Amadeus: 76, 217
Munch Edvard: 130, 132, 250, 255
Münter Gabriele: 20, 119, 250, 257
Naegeli Oscar: 12, 40, 48, 61, 81, 108, 112, 250, 259, 264, 265
Nager Frank: 224, 250, 254
Nebel Hildegard (Hilde): 28, 48, 71
Nebel Otto: 28, 39, 40, 43, 71
Neumann J.B.: 93, 101, 156, 262
Nietzsche Friedrich: 224, 250
Nolde Emil: 29, 212, 250
Novalis Georg Philipp Friedrich: 194, 250
Okuda Osamu: 13, 14, 241, 246, 250, 257, 258, 270
Osterwold Tilman: 241, 250, 251, 257
Pedersen Lisbet Milling: 87, 254
Penrose Roland: 216, 257
Permin Henrik: 87, 254

Petitpierre Petra: 69, 132, 187, 257
Picasso Pablo: 212, 214–216, 247, 251, 255, 257, 259, 263, 266, 268, 269
Pliny the Elder (Gaius Plinius Secundus): 221, 251
Porzig Hartmut: 267, 270
Probst Rudolf: 39, 72, 153, 262
Rabinovitch Gregor: 130, 251
Rausser Fernand: 263, 270
Reiner Michael: 91, 92, 153, 251, 254
Rewald Sabine: 40, 257
Rilke Rainer Maria: 172, 251
Rohrer Heinrich: 255, 270
Roth Peter: 270
Rotzler Willy: 194, 196, 251, 257
Rupf-Wirz Hermann: 28, 41, 45–48, 63, 67, 70, 71, 74, 81, 83, 84, 94, 95, 101, 118, 119, 214, 216, 246, 249, 251, 259–262, 267, 270
Rupf-Wirz Margrit: 28, 41, 44–48, 67, 70, 71, 74, 81, 83, 84, 118, 214, 249, 251, 259–262, 270
Rüttimann Beat: 241, 270
Ryser Markus: 267, 270
Saint Jerome: 220, 221, 259
Sandblom Philip: 86, 88, 254
Schädelin Albert: 76
Schafroth Anna M.: 170, 251, 270
Schatzmann Max: 12, 251, 264
Scheyer Emmy (Galka): 20, 40, 45–47, 61, 72, 102, 154, 157, 251, 259, 262
Schlemmer Oskar: 120, 247, 252
Schmalenbach Werner: 124, 256, 258
Schmid Sebastian: 270
Schmidt Georg: 28, 76, 117, 252, 255, 256, 258
Schmidt-Rottluff Karl: 87
Schmied Wieland: 187, 188, 258
Schorer Gerhard: 12, 13, 39, 40, 42, 43, 46, 48, 49, 60, 71, 72, 78, 81–84, 108–110, 118, 251, 252, 259, 264
Schuppli Madeleine: 122, 252
Schweizer Fritz: 241, 270
Sechehaye Henriette: 252, 264, 258
Seitz Michael: 241, 253, 254, 270
Silver Richard M.: 97, 253
Stämpfli Rudolf: 270
Steiner Juri: 270
Stössel-Schorer Marie-Louise: 110, 264, 270
Streiff Bruno: 58, 270
Surbek-Frey Marguerite: 28, 87, 247, 255, 265
Surbek Victor: 28, 247
Suter Hans: 8, 241, 252, 254, 270, 272
Tavel Hans Christoph, von: 8, 9, 13, 29, 64, 141, 172, 173, 216, 247, 252, 258, 259, 264, 269, 270
Trüssel Fritz: 30, 31, 266
Tyndall Alan: 270, 271
Uehlinger Enrico: 14, 264
Villiger Peter M.: 14, 48, 51 52, 58, 60, 61, 69, 70, 72, 73, 80, 85, 103, 104, 241, 252–254, 270
Virchow Rudolf: 224, 252
Vock Peter: 265, 270
Wada Sadao: 14, 258, 263
Weber Angela: 270
Welti Jakob: 30
Werlen Liobina: 155
Weyden Rogier, van der: 183, 252
Wild Doris: 211, 216, 223, 247, 250, 258
Zollinger-Streiff Kathi: 58, 270
Zschokke Alexander: 161, 252, 258
Zürcher Kaspar: 42, 249

Biographical Details of People Referred to in the Text

Aichinger-Grosch Ju (Juliane Paula)
German actress. Friend of Paul and Lily Klee's since Klee's time as a teacher at the Bauhaus in Weimar. Lived near the Bauhaus. Her husband Franz (Bobby) Aichinger was a student at the Bauhaus under Mies van der Rohe and became an architect. (From: Grote 1959, pp. 48–49.)

Bätschmann Oskar (born 1943)
Professor, PhD, studied Art History in Florence and Zurich; 1978–1984 Curator of the Zurich Museum of Applied Arts; 1979–1983 Lecturer in Art History at the University of Zurich; 1984–1988 Professor of Art History at the University of Freiburg (D); 1988–1991 Professor of Art History at the University of Giessen (D); from 1991 Professor of Contemporary and Modern Art History and Director of the Institute of Art History at the University of Bern. Areas of research: Leon Battista Alberti, Hans Holbein Jr., Nicolas Poussin, history of modern artists, methodological problems in Art History.

Baumgartner Michael (born 1952)
PhD, Bern art historian. 1996–2004 research associate at the Paul Klee Stiftung, Bern Museum of Fine Arts. 2005–2006 Curator and Deputy Artistic Director of the Zentrum Paul Klee in Bern. Since 2007 Artistic Curator at the Zentrum Paul Klee in Bern.

Bergmann Gustav, von (1878–1955)
Professor of Medicine. 1927–1945 Professor of Internal Medicine at the 2nd Charité Medical University Clinic in Berlin; 1945–1953 Professor at the 2nd Medical University Clinic in Munich. At the time one of the most renowned internists in Germany. (From: Lexikon der hervorragenden Ärzte der letzten fünfzig Jahre, Munich-Berlin, 1962, p. 101 f, and Nachtragsband III, Hildesheim-Zurich-New York, 2002, p. 109. Details supplied to the author by Prof. Urs Boschung, Director of the Institute of Medical History at the University of Bern.)

Bloesch Hans Jörg (1878–1945)
PhD, writer and historian from Bern. Formerly Chief Librarian of the Bern State and University Library. 1911 joint editor of Jeremias Gotthelf's extensive collected works. He was a childhood friend of Paul Klee's. (From: Grote 1959, p. 117, and Sorg/Okuda 2005, p. 11.)

Bodmer Hermann Oskar (1876–1948)
Doctor of Medicine, specialist in internal medicine, CH–6600 Locarno (see p. 111).

Boschung Urs (born 1946)
Professor of Medicine. Studied medicine in Freiburg (CH) and Bern. 1973–1974 research associate at the Bern Public Library; 1974–1976 Assistant Professor at the Institute of Medical History, University of Zurich; 1976–1977 Assistant Professor at the Institute of Medical History, University of Bonn; 1978–1985 Curator of the Medical History Collection, University of Zurich, and permanent research associate at the Institute of Medical History, University of Zurich; since 1985 Professor of Medical History and Director of the Institute of Medical History, University of Bern. Main areas of research: Albrecht von Haller, medicine of the 18th to the 20th century.

Bürgi-Bigler Hanni (1880–1936)
Friend of Paul and Lily Klee's and patron to Paul Klee in the final years of his life. (From: Bern/Hamburg 2000, p. 8.)

Bürgi Rolf (1906–1967)
Bern Lawyer. Son of Hanni and Alfred Bürgi-Bigler. Purchased his first work by Paul Klee whilst still at school, later continued his parents' practice of collecting Paul Klee's works. Arranged the exit visas for Paul and Lily Klee to leave Germany in 1933. After 1933 he acted as friend and advisor to the couple in all material matters. After Paul Klee's death he was mandated by Klee's widow and their son Felix Klee to administer the estate. In 1946, shortly before Lily Klee's death, he arranged for the sale of the entire artistic estate to the dedicated collectors Hermann Rupf and Hans Meyer-Benteli of Bern, in order to avoid the liquidation of these artistic assets in favor of the Allies under the terms of the Washington Agreement. In 1947 Rolf Bürgi, the two buyers and the Bern architect Werner Allenbach founded the Paul Klee Stiftung, which from 1952 was housed in the Bern Museum of Fine Arts, moving in 2005 to the Zentrum Paul Klee in Bern. (From: Bern/Hamburg 2000, pp. 8–9.)

Cabane Jean (born 1949)
From 1988 Professor of Medicine at the University Pierre & Marie Curie, Paris 6. Specialist in internal medicine and Chief Physician of the Division of Internal Medicine at the Hôpital Saint Antoine, a hospital of the 'Assistance Publique – Hôpitaux de Paris'. For over 20 years he has specialized in scleroderma research. 1996 founder and from 2005 President of the 'Groupe Français de Recherche sur la Sclérodermie'. Close ties to the French Scleroderma Patients Association. 2007 initiated the French translation of Dr. Hans Suters' book with the title 'Paul Klee et sa maladie'.

Castenholz-von Elsner Gabriele (born 1973)
Doctor of Medicine. Studied medicine in Marburg, Berlin and Frankfurt. Wrote dissertation in 2000 in Marburg on 'Die progressive systemische Sklerose. Analyse und Geschichte unter besonderer Berücksichtigung der Krankheit des Malers Paul Klee (1879–1940)'.

Doctor of Dental Medicine. The last dentist to treat Paul Klee in Bern.	**Charlet Jean (1906–1990)**
Professor of Medicine. Studied medicine in Zurich, further studies to become a specialist in occupational medicine, preventative medicine and public health at the Institute of Hygiene and Occupational Physiology, Zurich Federal Technical College, and at the National Heart and Lung Institute, Brompton Hospital, London. 1996–2003 Assistant Professor at the Institute of Hygiene and Occupational Physiology, Zurich Federal Technical College. 2003 Professor of Occupational Medicine at the French-speaking Institute for Occupational Health at the University of Lausanne. Since 2005, Director of the Institute. Since 2006, President of the Swiss Association for Occupational Medicine, medical expert in her field on national and international committees. Main areas of research: environmental hygiene, lung function, bioaerosols, organic particles, passive smoking, stress prevention.	**Danuser-Nideröst Brigitta (born 1955)**
German-American painter. Came to Germany in 1887, where he studied painting in Hamburg and Berlin, continued his studies in Paris, 1919–1933 teacher at the Bauhaus, member with Paul Klee of 'Der Blaue Reiter' ('The Blue Rider') and 'Die Blaue Vier' ('The Blue Four') artists' groups. 1936 returned to USA (New York). (From: Darmstaedter 1979, p. 223.)	**Feininger Lyonel (1871–1956)**
Painter, drawer and graphic artist in Bern. Wife of the painter Victor Surbek. From 1904 to 1906 she was a private student of Paul Klee's.	**Frey-Surbek Marguerite (1886–1981)**
Bern art historian. From 1981 to 1986 and from 1988 to 1996 freelance research associate at the Paul Klee Stiftung, Bern Museum of Fine Arts; since 1996 doing freelance work and Curator/Secretary of the Klee family collection and the Paul Klee's Estate. Good biographical knowledge of Paul Klee.	**Frey Stefan (born 1957)**
Doctor of Medicine. Studied medicine in Bern. General practitioner in CH–3800 Unterseen (Bern) from 1959–1988. Since then freelance drawer and painter in Unterseen.	**Friedli Bendicht (born 1930)**
MA, Bern art historian. Research associate at the Institute and Museum of Medical History, University of Zurich; Curator of the exhibition 'Paul Klee und die Medizin' in the Museum of Medical History, University of Zurich, March 31 to October 9, 2005; exhibits from this exhibition also used in the exhibition 'Paul Klee und seine Krankheit' at the Zentrum Paul Klee, Bern, November 5–27, 2005.	**Fuchs Walther Johann (born 1963)**
PhD, Bern art historian. Knew Pablo Picasso personally, published 'Picasso, peintre-graveur: Catalogue illustré de l'oeuvre gravé et lithographié, 1889–1931', Bern 1933.	**Geiser Bernhard (1895–1967)**
German art historian. Close contact with contemporary visual artists and poets, such as Paul Klee, László Moholy-Nagy, Hans Arp and James Joyce. Intellectual partnership with her husband, the Swiss art historian Siegfried Giedion. Author of 17 books and over 280 journal articles on modern painting, sculpture and poetry. (From: Giedion-Welcker 2000, p. 173.)	**Giedion-Welcker Carola (1983–1979)**
PhD. From 1971 responsible for the works of Klee at the Bern Museum of Fine Arts, 1972 Curator of the Paul Klee Stiftung, 1977–1988 Curator of the graphic art collection at the Bern Museum of Fine Arts. (From: Nachruf von Hans Christoph von Tavel, in: Kunstmuseum Bern, 1988, pp. 10–11.) Worked extensively on the works of Paul Klee at the Paul Klee Stiftung, documented and published in: Glaesemer 1973, 1976, 1979, 1984.	**Glaesemer Jürgen (1939–1988)**
Dutch painter with a moving story. Suffered mentally with bouts of madness and possibly also epilepsy. Very close to his brother Theo, who was devoted to his wellbeing. Came into contact with the Impressionists in Paris. 1888 moved to Arles in Provence. In the short time remaining to him – from February 1888 to June 1889 – he virtually produced his life's work in a creative frenzy. Painted interiors, locals from the town, himself, irises and sunflowers and the landscape of Provence. 1888 lived in the asylum in St. Rémy. 1890 moved to Auvers-sur-Oise near Paris, where he was cared for by Dr. Gachet who helped him, but could not prevent him dying from an attempted suicide in 1889. (From: Wild 1950, pp. 53–56.)	**Gogh Vincent, van (1853–1890)**
Professor, PhD, German art historian and critic in Dresden and Berlin. Was linked with many artists such as Paul Klee, Wassily Kandinsky and Ernst Ludwig Kirchner. He and his wife Gertrud were close friends of Paul and Lily Klee's. Great patron of modern art. Author of many books about contemporary art. Wrote the first comprehensive monograph about Paul Klee, which appeared in 1954 (Editions des Trois Collines, Geneva, and Kohlhammer, Stuttgart 1954).	**Grohmann Will (1887–1968)**
German-American architect. Founder and first director of the 'Bauhaus school' in Weimar in 1919, and from 1926 to 1928 in Dessau. The idea behind the Bauhaus lay in the combining of fine and applied arts. Gropius asked famous artists such as Paul Klee, Wassily Kandinsky,	**Gropius Walter (1883–1969)**

	Lyonel Feininger, Oskar Schlemmer and Johannes Itten (from Switzerland) to become teachers there. 1934 moved to England, 1937 to the USA, where he worked as a progressive architect. (From: Darmstaedter 1979, p. 291, and Di San Lazzaro 1958, p. 113.)
Grote Ludwig (1893–1974)	PhD. Published 'Erinnerungen an Paul Klee', Prestel Verlag, Munich 1959. He and his wife Gertrud Grote were friendly with Paul and Lily Klee.
Haemmerli-Schindler Theodor (1883–1944)	Doctor of Medicine, specialist in internal medicine, especially cardiology, Zurich (see p. 113).
Haller Hermann (1880–1950)	Honorary doctor, Swiss sculptor. 1899 studied painting with Paul Klee at Heinrich Knirr's private school in Munich, 1901 again with Klee at the Munich Academy of Fine Arts under Franz von Stuck, 1902 masters student of Leopold von Kalckreuth at the Stuttgart Academy of Fine Arts. 1904 with Paul Klee in Rome, where he switched to sculpture. 1909–1914 in Paris, from 1914 in Zurich. 1933 awarded honorary doctorate by the University of Zurich. (From: NZZ 1998, pp. 458–459.)
Heim Edgar (born 1930)	Professor of Medicine. Studied medicine in Bern, Vienna and Paris, 1957–1963 further studies to become a specialist in psychiatry and psychotherapy in Bern; 1963–1965 research and lecturing in psychiatry at the University of Boston (USA); 1966–1968 Assistant Medical Director at the Psychiatric Polyclinic, University of Bern; 1968–1977 Director of the Schlössli Psychiatric Clinic, CH–8618 Oetwil a.S. (Zurich); 1977–1994 Professor of Psychiatry and Psychotherapy and Director of the Psychiatric Polyclinic, University of Bern. Areas of research: psychosomatic medicine, psychotherapy, social psychiatry. Author and editor of numerous books, including 'Krankheit als Krise und Chance', vol. 7 of 'Stufen des Lebens', Kreuz Verlag, Stuttgart/Berlin 1980.
Helfenstein Josef (born 1957)	Professor, PhD, Bern art historian. 1988–2000 Curator of the Paul Klee Stiftung and the graphic art collection at the Bern Museum of Fine Arts; 2000–2003 Director of the Krannert Art Museum and Kinkhead Pavilion, Urbana-Champaign, and professor at the University of Illinois, USA; from 2004 Director of the Menil Collection, 1511 Branard, Houston, Texas 77006, USA.
Heraclitus (ca. 549–480 BC)	Greek philosopher. Taught that the entire universe was in a state of constant flux: 'panta rhei', everything flows. (From: Zürich 1945–1948, vol. 3, p. 1585.)
Hersch Jeanne (1910–2000)	Professor, PhD, Swiss philosopher. Pupil of Karl Jasper's. Studied literature and philosophy in Geneva, Heidelberg and Freiburg (D), 1956–1958; 1960 and 1962–1977 Professor of Philosophy at the University of Geneva; 1959 visiting professor at the Pennsylvania State University, USA, and 1961 at the New York State University. 1966–1968 Director of the Philosophy Department at UNESCO, later represented Switzerland as a member of the Executive Council of the same organization. (From: Luzern 1991–1993, vol. 3, p. 404.)
Hopfengart Christine (born 1955)	PhD, German art historian. 1974–1987 studied art history, German language and literature and classical archeology in Munich, Heidelberg, Berlin and Cologne. 1988–1991 intern at the Berlin National Gallery, 1989 dissertation: 'Klee – vom Sonderfall zum Publikumsliebling'. 1991–1995 research associate and Assistant Director at the Nuremberg Kunsthalle; 1995–2001 Curator at the Bremen Kunsthalle; 2001–2004 Curator of the Paul Klee Stiftung, Bern Museum of Fine Arts; since 2005 Head of Research and Archives at the Zentrum Paul Klee in Bern.
Huggler Max (1903–1994)	Professor, PhD, Bern art historian. 1931–1946 Director of Bern Kunsthalle, 1944–1965 Director of the Bern Museum of Fine Arts. Knew Paul and Lily Klee well, in 1935 organized a welcoming exhibition of 273 of Paul Klee's works in the Bern Kunsthalle (see p. 29 and notes 55 and 56). Publications include 'Paul Klee, Die Malerei als Blick in den Kosmos', Verlag Huber and Co, AG, Frauenfeld/Stuttgart 1969.
Iseli Karl Friedrich (1907–1991)	Teacher and politician in CH–3612 Steffisburg (Bern). Was a student of Hans Klee's at the cantonal teachers' college in Hofwil, Bern.
Jaspers Karl (1883–1969)	Professor of Medicine, honorary doctor and philosopher of German extraction. From 1967 a citizen of Basel. Originally studied law, then switched to the study of medicine in Berlin, Göttingen and Heidelberg; 1916 Professor of Psychology in Heidelberg; 1921 Professor of Philosophy in Heidelberg; 1937 forced into retirement by the National Socialists; 1948 appointment to the University of Basel as Professor of Philosophy. 1958 awarded the Peace Prize of the German Book Trade. Had a natural leaning towards existential philosophy. Main work: 'Von der Wahrheit' (1947). (From: Luzern 1991–1993, vol. 3, p. 646.)
Jung Ernst G. (born 1932)	Professor of Medicine. Born in Winterthur (Zurich). Studied medicine in Lausanne, Kiel and Zurich. Further studies to become a consultant in dermatology and venereology in Zurich. 1965–1975 chief consultant at the Dermatology Clinic of the University of Heidelberg; 1975–

2000 Professor of Dermatology at the Faculty of Clinical Medicine Mannheim, University of Heidelberg, and Director of the Heidelberg Dermatology Clinic. Dean and Dean of Studies of the Medical Faculty of Heidelberg. 1975–1997 Vice Rector of the University of Heidelberg. Main areas of scientific interest: photobiology/dermatology, genetics and dermato-oncology. Editor of a popular textbook on dermatology and of 'Kleine Kulturgeschichte der Haut' (A Short Cultural History of the Skin) containing many of his own original contributions (see p. 253).

Professor. Born in Moscow. Studied law and macroeconomics, 1893 lectureship at the law faculty in Moscow, 1896 resigned, moved to Munich, pupil of Franz von Stuck at the Munich Academy of Fine Arts; 1910 produced first abstract picture; 1911 co-founder of the artists' group 'Der Blaue Reiter' ('The Blue Rider') with Franz Marc, August Macke, Paul Klee, Heinrich Campendonk; 1915–1921 in Moscow; 1922–1933 teacher at the Bauhaus (in Weimar, from 1926 in Dessau, from 1932 in Berlin). 1933 closure of the Bauhaus by the National Socialists, moved to Neuilly-sur-Seine near Paris; 1939 became French citizen. Wassily and his wife Nina were close friends of Paul and Lily Klee's. (From: Kandinsky 1972, p. 81 f.)

Kandinsky Wassily (1866–1944)

Professor, German philosopher. Professor of Logic and Metaphysics in Königsberg. Main work: 'Kritik der reinen Vernunft'. In the 'categorical imperative' he proposes a principle for the moral (ethical) rationale of all actions: 'Live your life as though you would like your rules of conduct to become universal laws!' (From: Luzern 1991–1993, vol. 3, pp. 739 f and 780.)

Kant Immanuel (1724–1804)

Lecturer, PhD, German art historian. 1985–1990 academic research in museums and teaching post at the Institute of Art History, University of Bern; from 1991 lecturer at the Institute of Art History, University of Zurich. Publications include several about Paul Klee. (From Kersten 1990, cover text.)

Kersten Wolfgang (born 1954)

Felix and Euphrosine Klee's only son, Paul and Lily Klee's grandson. As an artist uses the pseudonym Aljoscha Ségard. Painter, drawer, graphic artist, object artist, pictures using wax technique. (From: NZZ 1998, p. 962.)

**Klee Aljoscha
(Alexander, born October 6, 1940, in Sofia)**

Honorary doctor. Paul and Lily Klee's only son, educated at the Bauhaus School in Weimar. Then studied history of music and art. Until 1944 opera director in Germany. From 1948, following military service and time as a prisoner of war, director at Swiss Radio in Bern. Also worked as an actor. 1960 became Swiss citizen. Published his father's diaries and letters. First President of the Paul Klee Stiftung in Bern. 1987 awarded honorary doctorate by the University of Bern. (From: Luzern 1991–1993, vol. 4, p. 5.)

**Klee Felix
(Munich, November 30, 1907 to August 13, 1990, Bern)**

Paul Klee's father. Originally from Thüringen (D). Wanted to be a singer but due to external circumstances decided to become a teacher. Taught for over 50 years as music teacher at the cantonal teachers' college in Hofwil, Bern. (From: Grohmann, 1965, p. 26.) With his open, cheerful personality and sense of humor he became a very popular teacher. Also produced some literary works: 'Hans Klee, Jugend Verse, Lyrisches, Lenz und Liebe' (self-published, undated).

Klee Hans (1849–1940)

Paul Klee's mother. Native of Basel with family links to the South of France and possibly even to North Africa. Musically trained, inspired Paul Klee's love of music and encouraged him to play the violin. (From: Grohmann 1965, p. 26.)

Klee-Frick Ida Maria (1855–1921)

Paul Klee's wife. Daughter of the Munich physician Dr. Ludwig Karl August Stumpf. Pianist and piano teacher. Got to know Paul Klee in Munich in 1889 and married him on September 15, 1906. Lively exchange of letters with friends such as Will and Gertrud Grohmann, Wassily and Nina Kandinsky, Hermann and Margrit Rupf.

**Klee-Stumpf Lily Karoline Sophie Elisabeth
(Munich, October 10, 1876 to September 22, 1946, Bern)**

Professor, German painter and graphic artist. 1919 appointed professor while living in Berlin. Had a preference for social motifs in her work, with an intrinsically expressive style. (From: Darmstaedter 1979, p. 376.)

Kollwitz Käthe (1867–1945)

Professor of Medicine, specialist in dermatology, venereology and internal medicine. Studied medicine in Bern. 1970–1989 Director of the University of Bern Dermatology Clinic. Main areas of research: drug eruptions, psoriasis. Author of a handbook on the side effects of internal drugs on the skin (together with Dr. Kaspar Zürcher).

Krebs Alfred (born 1923)

PD, specialist in psychiatry and neurology in Bern (see p. 109).

Lotmar Fritz (1878–1964)

German painter, member of the artists' group 'Der Blaue Reiter' ('The Blue Rider'). Studied at the Düsseldorf Academy of Fine Arts; 1907 studied under Lovis Corinth in Berlin; 1907–1908 in Paris, where he came into contact with the Impressionists, the Fauves and the Cubists; from

Macke August (1887–1914)

	1909 in Bonn, Munich and Bavaria; 1912 traveled with Franz Marc to Paris; 1914 traveled with Paul Klee and Louis Moilliet to Kairouan in Tunisia. 1914 killed in the War, aged 27. (From: Darmstaedter 1979, p. 433.)
McKay Gill (born 1960)	BA (Hons), native of England. 1978–1981 studied Modern Languages and Literature at the University of Bristol; 1981–1993 worked in banking, retail and manufacturing sectors in the UK; 1994–2002 yoga teacher and nutrition clinic administrator; 2002–2006 Business English language trainer and business skills trainer in Germany; 2006–2007 business skills trainer and internal communications manager in retail sector, Kuwait City; from 2007 freelance language consultant, translator and proof-reader based in Stuttgart.
McKay Neil (born 1958)	BA (Hons), Dip ION, native of England. 1978–1981 studied Modern Languages and Literature at the University of Bristol; 1981–1993 worked in banking and retail sectors in the UK; 1994–1996 studied Nutritional Medicine at the Institute for Optimum Nutrition in London; 1996–2002 Nutrition Consultant in private practice in Kendal; 2002–2006 Business English language trainer and business skills trainer in Germany; 2006–2007 Strategy Management and HR Director in retail sector, Kuwait City; from 2007 freelance language consultant, translator and proof-reader based in Stuttgart.
Moilliet Louis (1880–1962)	Bern painter. Met Paul Klee at grammar school in Bern. 1900 went to technical college in Bern; 1901 studied under Fritz Mackensen at the Artists' Colony Worpswede; 1902 studied at the Düsseldorf Academy of Fine Arts, then at the Weimar Academy of Fine Arts; 1903 in Berlin again; 1904 back in Worpswede, masters student of Leopold von Kalckreuth at the Stuttgart Academy of Fine Arts; 1905 studied under Adolf Hölzel in Stuttgart; 1909 in Bern again and with August Macke in Paris; 1913 at Lake Thun; 1914 traveled with Paul Klee and August Macke to Tunisia; 1920 with Hermann Hesse in Tessin; 1936 in the Black Forest; 1938 in Lugano; 1939 in Corsier-sur-Vevey. Known especially for his finely wrought watercolors and stained-glass windows. (From: NZZ 1998, p. 733 f.)
Munch Edvard (1863–1944)	Most important Norwegian artist of modern times. Knew van Gogh and Gaugin in Paris. His work is similar to that of the Fauves. Became father of the German Expressionist movement. Suffered from nervous disorders. Lived in Oslofjord and the area around Oslo. Powerful, expressive works, portraits and landscapes. Themes include: birth, love, jealousy, emotional need, death. (From: Wild 1950, pp. 77–90.)
Münter Gabriele (1877–1962)	German painter. Strongly influenced by the early work of her long-time companion Wassily Kandinsky, member of the artist group 'Der Blaue Reiter' ('The Blue Rider'). (From: Darmstaedter 1979, p. 498, and Luzern 1991–1993, vol. 4, p. 689.)
Naegeli Oscar Emanuel Viktor (1885–1959)	Professor of Medicine, specialist in dermatology and venereology (see p. 112).
Nager Frank (born 1929)	Professor of Medicine, specialist in internal medicine, especially cardiology, CH–6402 Merlischachen (Luzern). 1971–1994 Chief Physician of the Medical Clinic at Luzern Cantonal Hospital. 1976 Professor at the University of Zurich. Numerous medical and sociomedical papers, including: 'Der heilkundige Dichter – Goethe und die Medizin', 'Das Herz als Symbol', 'Gesundheit, Krankheit, Heilung, Tod – Betrachtungen eines Arztes'. (From: Heusser 2000, p. 523.)
Nietzsche Friedrich (1844–1900)	Professor, PhD, German philosopher. Studied theology and classical philology. 1870 Professor of Classical Philology in Basel; 1879 resigned on health grounds, moved to Sils-Maria in the Engadine (Grisons). Also spent periods living in Northern Italy and on the Riviera. 1889 mental breakdown followed by symptoms of insanity. 1900 died in Weimar. Nietzsche was primarily recognized as the spokesman for Nihilism. Main work 'Also sprach Zarathustra'. His writings had a lasting influence on philosophy of existence and life as well as on psychoanalysis. (From: Luzern 1991–1993, vol. 3, pp. 812 f.)
Nolde Emil (actually Hansen Emil) (1867–1956)	German painter and graphic artist. One of the main exponents of German Expressionism. (From: Darmstaedter 1979, p. 516.)
Novalis Georg Philipp Friedrich (1772–1801)	German poet. One of the most important lyric and prose poets of Early Romanticism. (From: Luzern 1991–1993, vol. 4, p. 834 f.)
Okuda Osamu (born 1951)	Japanese art historian. From 1983 in Bern, studied art history at the University of Bern. 1996–2004 research assistant at the Paul Klee Stiftung, Bern Museum of Fine Arts; since 2005 research associate at the Zentrum Paul Klee in Bern. Surveyed the last home of Paul Klee, Kistlerweg 6, in Bern, reconstructed Klee's last studio together with Walther Fuchs, and in 2005 organized with Walther Fuchs the exhibition 'Paul Klee und die Medizin' at the Medical History Museum, University of Zurich. (March 31 to October 9). (From: Sorg/Okuda 2005, p. 284.)

Professor, PhD. Studied art history, archeology, philosophy and psychology in Innsbruck and Hamburg; 1971–1973 Curator and Deputy Director of the Wilhem-Lehmbruck-Museum in Duisburg; 1973–1993 Director of the Württembergischer Kunstverein in Stuttgart; 1993 Honorary Professor at the University of Stuttgart; 1995–1997 Artistic Director of the Kunsthalle Museum Fridericianum, Kassel; 2003–2004 Artistic Curator-in-waiting at the Zentrum Paul Klee in Bern. 2005–2006 Artistic Curator at the Zentrum Paul Klee in Bern. Numerous exhibitions and publications relating to Paul Klee and contemporary art. Since 2007 freelance art historian.	**Osterwold Tilman (born 1943)**
Spanish painter, graphic artist and sculptor. From 1904 in France. Co-creator of Cubism, from 1901 'blue period', from 1905 'rose period', around 1909 'analytical Cubism', around 1917 classical style with delicate line drawings, from the 1920s increased emotional intensity with distortions and garish colors. Extensive, multifaceted, influential and very important works. (From: Darmstaedter 1979, p. 552.)	**Picasso Pablo (1881–1973)**
Roman writer and historian. Died during the eruption of Mt. Vesuvius in 79 AD. Only preserved work the extensive 37-volume 'Naturalis historia'. (From: Luzern 1991–1993, vol. 5, p. 190.)	**Pliny the Elder (Gaius Plinius Secundus) (23–79 AD)**
Doctor of Law. Son of Jewish parents, born and raised in Russia; trained to be an artist in Munich and to be an architect in St. Petersburg; studied law in Moscow; 1905 took part in the Russian Revolution; 1914 in Paris and Austria; 1915 in Zurich; 1916 in Geneva; from 1917 settled in Zurich. Worked with Max Gubler, Otto Morach and Karl Geiser. 1929 became Swiss national. Favored social themes, expressionist style, virtuoso fine etchings, including depictions of the horrors of war. (From: NZZ 1998, p. 844.)	**Rabinovitch Gregor (1884–1958)**
Doctor of Medicine. Studied medicine in Lausanne and Basel, further studies to become a specialist in internal medicine, specializing in endocrinology and diabetology, in Lausanne, Bern and Geneva. 1967–1968 Senior Physician at the Geneva Medical Polyclinic; 1968–1970 endocrinology research residency at the Hammersmith Hospital, London; 1970–1974 Senior Physician at the Medical University Clinic, Inselspital, Bern; 1974–1999 Chief Physician at the Regional Hospital CH–6850 Mendrisio (Tessin); from 2000 working in private practice as consultant in endocrinology and bone densitometry. In 1990 organised the exhibition 'Paul Klee. Ultimo decennio – Letztes Jahrhundert 1930–1940' at the Mendrisio Museum of Art, April 7 to July 8, 1940.	**Reiner Michael (born 1934)**
Austrian poet. Influential German-speaking lyric poet of the first half of the 20th century. Came to Switzerland in 1919. (From: Luzern 1933, vol. 5, p. 371.) Rilke met Paul Klee in Munich in 1921 (according to Pfeiffer-Belli 1978, p. 385).	**Rilke Rainer Maria (1875–1926)**
PhD, Basel art historian. 1948–1961 Curator of the Zurich Museum of Applied Arts; 1962–1968 editor of the Swiss art and culture journal 'du'; 1969 arts writer and lecturer at the University of Zurich; 1982–1983 at the Graduate School, City University, New York. (From: Luzern 1991–1993, vol. 5, p. 427.)	**Rotzler Willy (1917–1994)**
Honorary doctor, Bern businessman. Attended business school in Bern; 1901 bank clerk in Frankfurt; 1903/1904 further studies in Paris; 1905 returned to Bern, partner in haberdashery business with his brother-in-law Rudolf Hossman; 1907 first customer of the art dealer Daniel-Henry Kahnweiler at the opening of the his gallery in Paris; 1908 visited by Pablo Picasso and Daniel-Henry Kahnweiler; 1909–1932 art critic at the 'Berner Tagwacht'; 1909 marriage to Margrit Wirz (1877–1961). Built an important art collection together with his wife. 1913 first meeting with Paul Klee. 1954 creation of the Hermann und Margrit Rupf-Stiftung, which is housed in the Bern Museum of Fine Arts. Hermann Rupf was also a patron of music in the City of Bern. 1957 awarded honorary doctorate by the University of Bern. The couple were friends with Paul and Lily Klee, Wassily and Nina Kandinsky and Daniel-Henry Kahnweiler. (From: Kunstmuseum Bern 1998, p. 22.)	**Rupf Hermann (1880–1962)**
MA, Bern art historian. Studied art history in Bern. Regular speaker on the subject of Paul Klee at home and abroad and publisher of research papers, alongside her work as Exhibition Curator at the Bern Museum of Fine Arts, the Coninx Museum in Zurich and the Oskar Reinhart Museum am Stadtgarten in Winterthur. 2005–2006 working at the Zentrum Paul Klee, Bern. Publications include papers on Paul Klee, Werner Neuhaus, Albert Schnyder, Emil Zbinden and Louis Moilliet.	**Schafroth Anna Magdalena (born 1961)**
Doctor of Medicine, specialist in internal medicine in Bern. Locum to Dr. Gerhard Schorer. There is no evidence that he also treated Paul Klee.	**Schatzmann Max (1886–1953)**
German-American art dealer and collector. In 1924 founded the artists' group 'Die Blaue Vier' ('The Blue Four') in Weimar with Lyonel Feininger, Alexej Jawlensky, Wassily Kandinsky and Paul	**Scheyer Emmy Esther (Galka) (1889–1945)**

	Klee. In the same year emigrated to Hollywood, USA, publicized the four artists in the USA, actively championed them for 20 years and paved the way for them in the USA. (From: Bern/Düsseldorf 1997, pp. 8–12.)
Schlemmer Oscar (1888–1943)	Professor, German painter and sculptor. 1920–1928 teacher at the Bauhaus in Weimar/Dessau; 1929–1932 Professor at the Breslau Academy of Fine Arts, 1933 at the Berlin Academy of Fine Arts. 1933 lost job due to the National Socialists. (From: Darmstaedter 1979, p. 638.)
Schmidt Georg (1896–1965)	Professor, PhD, honorary doctor, Basel art historian. 1939–1961 Director of the Basel Public Art Collection and Museum of Fine Arts, judiciously built an important collection at the Basel Museum of Fine Arts. 1958 Professor of History of Art at the Munich Museum of Fine Arts. 1946 awarded honorary doctorate by the Federal Technical College in Zurich. (From: Luzern 1991–1993, vol. 5, p. 593, and from: Schmidt 1966, p. 328.)
Schorer Gerhard (1878–1959)	Doctor of Medicine, specialist in internal medicine In Bern (see p. 110).
Schuppli Madeleine (born 1965)	Zurich art historian. Studied art history in Geneva, Hamburg and Zurich. Research work in various museums, 1996–1999 Curator at the Basel Kunsthalle; 2000–2007 Director of the Thun Museum of Fine Arts, from 2007 Director of the Aarau Museum of Fine Arts. Board member of the Swiss Visual Arts Association and member of the board of trustees of the Swiss cultural foundation Pro Helvetia.
Sechehaye Henriette (1907–1999)	Painter. Paul Klee's last student in Bern. Friend of the Klee family. (Vatter-Jensen 2005.)
Suter Hans (born 1930)	Doctor of Medicine and honorary doctor. Specialist in dermatology and venereology. Studied medicine in Geneva, Bern and Vienna. Further studies to become consultant in dermatology and venereology in Bern, Thun and Zurich; 1965–2004 dermatology practice in Thun; from 1972–2005 involved in student education at the Dermatology Clinic, University of Bern, where he was employed as an external senior physician (1975–1990), as a lecturer (from 1998) and as an examiner for state exams (1978–2002). Involved for many years in art associations, sometimes as president; coauthor and copublisher of books on art. With his wife Marlis Suter, built an extensive collection of 20th century Swiss art which, since 2004, the couple have opened to the public in various exhibitions at the Wichterheer Museum in CH–3653 Oberhofen am Thunersee. Patron of regional art. 2003 the couple were awarded the City of Thun Culture Prize. 2006 awarded honorary doctorate by the University of Bern. 2006 published 'Paul Klee und seine Krankheit', Stämpfli Verlag AG, Bern. 2007 translation of the book into French 'Paul Klee et sa maladie', 2010 translation into English 'Paul Klee and His Illness', S. Karger AG, Basel.
Tavel Hans Christoph, von (born 1935)	PhD, Bern art historian. Studied in Bern and Munich, 1961–1965 coeditor of the 'Künstler-Lexikon der Schweiz XX. Jahrhundert' (Verlag Huber & Co. AG, Frauenfeld 1958–1967), 1965–1968 Curator of the Bern Museum of Fine Arts; 1968–1980 Editor and Head of Library at the Swiss Institute for Art History in Zurich; 1972–1974 teaching position at the University of Zurich; 1980–1995 Director of the Bern Museum of Fine Arts; 1996–2000 in Rome; 2004–2005 Director of the Istituto Svizzero di Roma.
Villiger Peter Matthias (born 1955)	Professor of Medicine. Studied medicine in Bern, further studies in Switzerland and the USA; from 1999 Director and Chief Physician of the Clinic and the Polyclinics of the Department of Rheumatology and Immunology/Allergology, Inselspital, Bern, Professor of Rheumatology and Clinical Immunology at the University of Bern; 2006 President of the Swiss Association of Rheumatology; Vice Dean of postgraduate education at the Medical Faculty of Bern. Main area of research: pathogenic mechanisms in systemic autoimmune diseases.
Virchow Rudolf (1821–1902)	Professor of Medicine, German physician and politician. From 1856 professor at the medical faculty, University of Berlin. Seminal studies into pathological anatomy, founder of cellular pathology, campaigner for better hygiene (disinfection, etc.). (From: Luzern 1991–1993, vol. 6, p. 486.)
Weyden Rogier, van der (around 1400–1464)	Dutch painter. Master of the Old Dutch School of painters. (From: Darmstaedter 1979, p. 762.)
Zschokke Alexander (1894–1981)	Professor, Basel sculptor. 1913 began architecture studies in Munich; trained to be a painter in Basel; switched to sculpture in Berlin in 1919; linked with 'Die Brücke' ('The Bridge') artists' group; 1931–1937 Professor at the Düsseldorf Academy of Fine Arts and therefore colleague of Paul Klee from 1931 to 1933; returned to Basel in 1937. (From: NZZ 1998, pp. 1168–1169.)

Bibliography

Note: In the notes the bibliographical references are shown in an abridged form with the relevant page numbers. Abridged medical references are indicated by the letters 'ML'.

Medical Literature (ML)

Beer/ML 1980
Beer, F.-J., Le centenaire de Paul Klee, in: Médecine et Hygiène, vol. 38, no. 1362, 23.1.1980, pp. 247 f.

Bernoulli/ML 1955
Bernoulli, E., and Lehmann, H., Übersicht der gebräuchlichen und neueren Arzneimittel, 8th ed., Benno Schwabe & Co.-Verlag, Basel 1955.

Bovenzi/ML 1995
Bovenzi, M., et al., Scleroderma and occupational exposure, Scand. J. Work Environ Health 1995, 21, pp. 289–292.

Brasington and Thorpe-Swenson/ML 1991
Brasington, R.D., and Thorpe-Swenson, A.J., Systemic sclerosis associated with cutaneous exposure to solvent: case report and review of the literature, in: Arthritis and Rheumatism, vol. 34, no. 5, May 1991, pp. 631–633.

Braun-Falco, Plewig, Wolff/ML 1996
Braun-Falco, O., Plewig, G., Wolff, H.H., Dermatologie und Venerologie, ch. 18: Erkrankungen des Bindegewebes, Springer-Verlag, Berlin/Heidelberg/New York, pp. 697–765.

Büchi/ML 2000
Büchi, S., Villiger, P.M., Kauer, Y., Klaghofer, R., Sensky, T., Stoll, T., PRISM (Pictorial Representation of Illness and Self Measure) – a novel visual method to assess the global burden of illness in patients with systemic Lupus erythematosus, Lupus 2000, 9, pp. 368–373.

Burckhardt/ML 1961/1
Burckhardt, W., Die beruflichen Hautkrankheiten, in: Handbuch der Haut- und Geschlechtskrankheiten, J. Jadassohn, supp. series, ed. by A. Marchionini, vol. 2, part 1, Springer-Verlag, Berlin/Göttingen/Heidelberg 1961, pp. 269–474.

Burckhardt/ML 1961/2
Burckhardt, W., Arzneimittelexantheme, in: Handbuch der Haut- und Geschlechtskrankheiten, J. Jadassohn, supp. series, ed. by A. Marchionini, vol. 2, part 1, Springer-Verlag, Berlin/Göttingen/Heidelberg 1961, pp. 545–596.

Bywaters/ML 1987
Bywaters, E.G L., Paul Klee: The effect of scleroderma on his painting, in: Appelbloom, T. (ed.), Art, History and Antiquity of Rheumatic Diseases, Brussels 1987, pp. 49 f.

Castenholz/ML 2000
Castenholz, G., Die progressive systemische Sklerose. Analyse und Geschichte unter besonderer Berücksichtigung der Krankheit des Malers Paul Klee (1879–1940), Dissertation, Marburg 2000.

Conrad/ML 1994
Conrad, K., et al., Nichtorganspezifische Autoantikörper in Seren von Uranerzbergarbeitern mit und ohne Sklerodermie, in: Stuttgart 1994, pp. 18–23.

Cronin/ML 1980
Cronin, E., Contact Dermatitis, Churchill Livingstone, Edinburgh/London/New York 1980.

Danuser/ML 2000
Danuser, B., Von den Gefahren des Künstlerberufs: Paul Klee und die Sklerodermie, Arbeitsmedizinische Betrachtungen, in: Newsletter, Institut für Hygiene und Arbeitsphysiologie ETH Zurich, November 2000, pp. 17–20.

Degens and Baur/ML 1994
Degens, P., Baur, X., Zur Epidemiologie und Statistik der Sklerodermie als mögliche Berufskrankheit, in: Stuttgart 1994, pp. 27–33.

Dirschka/ML 1994
Dirschka, Th., et al., Systemische Sklerodermie im Uranerzbergbau. Klinisch-dermatologische Befunde, in: Stuttgart 1994, pp. 12 f.

Gadola and Villiger/ML 2006
Gadola, S.D., and Villiger, P.M., Konnektivitiden ('Kollagenosen'), in: Villiger and Seitz/ML 2006, pp. 74–94.

Gottwald and Benos/ML 1974
Gottwald, W., und Benos, J., Die neurologischen und pyschiatrischen Syndrome der Sklerodermie, in: Fortschritte der Neurologie, Psychiatrie, vol. 42, no. 5, Stuttgart 1974, pp. 225–263.

Haustein/ML 1990
Haustein, U.-F., et al., Silicea-induced scleroderma, J. Am. Acad. Dermatol. 1990, 22.

Haustein/ML 1996
Haustein, U.-F., Raynaud-Phänomen und Sklerodermie, in: 'Der Hautarzt', Berlin/Heidelberg/New York, no. 47, 1996, pp. 336–340.

Heim/ML 1980
Heim, E., Krankheit als Krise und Chance, Stufen des Lebens, vol. 7, ed. by Hans Jürgen Schultz, Kreuz-Verlag, Stuttgart/Berlin 1980.

Hinton/ML 1963
Hinton, J.M., The physical and mental distress of the dying, in Quart. J. Med., Neue Folge 32, no. 125, 1963, pp. 1–20.

Jackowski/ML 2002
Jackowski, J., Summary of clinical and radiological symptoms of systemic scleroderma in the mouth, jaw and facial areas for a lecture on March 22, 2002 at the annual conference of the Schweiz. Gesellschaft für dento-maxillofaziale Radiologie in Lausanne, entitled 'Die radiologischen Zeichen der systemischen Sklerodermie im Mund-, Kiefer- und Gesichtsbereich'.

Jadassohn/ML
Jadassohn, J., Handbuch der Haut- und Geschlechtskrankheiten, suppl. series, ed. by A. Marchionini, vol. 2, part 1, Springer-Verlag, Berlin/Göttingen/Heidelberg 1961.

Jung/ML 1991
Autoimmunkrankheiten, in: Jung, E.G. (ed.), Dermatologie, 2nd ed., Hippokrates Verlag, Stuttgart, 1991, pp. 84–101.

Jung/ML 2005
Jung, E.G., Sklerodermien in Sage und Gegenwart. Aktuelle Dematologie 2005, 31, Georg Thieme Verlag KG, Stuttgart 2005, pp. 573–575.

Jung/ML 2007
Jung, E.G. (dir.), Kleine Kulturgeschichte der Haut, Steinkopf Verlag, Darmstadt 2007.

Krieg/ML 1996
Krieg, T., Erkrankungen des Bindegewebes, in: Braun-Falco, Plewig, Wolff/ML 1996, pp. 697–735.

Kumer/ML 1944
Kumer, L., Sclerodermia (Darrsucht), in: Bindegewebshypertrophien (Bindegewebswucherungen), in: idem, Dermatologie, 6–10th ed., Verlag Wilhelm Maudrich, Vienna 1944, pp. 313–315.

LeRoy/Silver/ML 1996
LeRoy, E.C., and Silver, R.M., Paul Klee and Scleroderma, in: Bulletin on Rheumatic Diseases, vol. 45, no. 6, 1996, pp. 4–6.

Lesser/ML 1900
Lesser, E., Scleroderma, ch. 4, in: Lehrbuch der Haut und Geschlechtskrankheiten, 10th ed., Verlag von F.C.W. Vogel, Berlin 1900, pp. 105–111.

Maddison/ML 2000
Maddison, P.J., Mixed connective tissue disease: overlap syndromes, Baillière's Clinical Rheumatology; 14 (1), pp. 111–124.

Masi/ML 1980
Masi, A.T., Rodnan, G.P., Medsger, T.A. Jr., et al., Subcommittee for Scleroderma Criteria of the American Rheumatism Association Diagnostic and Therapeutic Criteria Committee: Preliminary criteria for the classification of systemic sclerosis (scleroderma), Arthritis and Rheumatism 1980; 23, pp. 581–590.

Maurer and Mühlemann/ML 1999
Maurer, A.-M., and Mühlemann, K., Masernausbruch in Rekrutenschulen, in: Bulletin des Schweizerischen Bundesamtes für Gesundheit, Abt. Epidemiologie und Infektionskrankheiten, no. 4, 25.1.1999, Bern 1999.

Mayr/ML 1935
Mayr, J.K., Sklerodermie, in: idem, Kurzgefasstes Lehrbuch der Haut- und Geschlechtskrankheiten, 3rd ed., Verlag von Rudolph Müller & Steinicke, Munich 1935, pp. 72–74.

Melhorn/ML 1994
Melhorn, J., 'Quarzinduzierte' Progressive Systemische Sklerodermie, in: Stuttgart 1994, pp. 8–11.

Meurer/ML 1996
Meurer, M., Lupus erythematodes, Dermatomyositis, Mixed Connective Tissue Disease (MCTD, Sharp-Syndrom), in: Braun-Falco, Plewig, Wolff/ML 1996, pp. 736–756.

Mittag and Haustein / ML 1998
Mittag, M., and Haustein, U.-F., Die progressive systemische Sklerodermie – prognosebestimmender Befall innerer Organsysteme, in: 'Der Hautarzt', Springer-Verlag, Berlin/Heidelberg/New York, no. 49, 1998, pp. 454–551.

Mittag / ML 2001
Die Haut im medizinischen und kulturgeschichtlichen Kontext, ed. by Hannelore Mittag, 2nd ed., text no. 103 of the University Library, Marburg, Marburg 2001.

Moll / ML 1991 / 1
Moll, I., Progressive systemische Sklerodermie (PSS), in: Dermatologie, ed. by E.G. Jung, 2nd ed., Hippokrates Verlag, Stuttgart 1991, pp. 92–98.

Moll / ML 1991 / 2
Moll, I., Dermatomyositis, ed. by E.G. Jung, 2nd ed., Hippokrates Verlag, Stuttgart 1991, pp. 99–101.

Morscher / ML 1994
Morscher, C., Paul Klee und die Hypothese der morphischen Resonanz, Pychotherapie, Psychosomatik, Medizinische Psychologie, Georg Thieme Verlag, Stuttgart/New York 1994, pp. 200–206.

Nager / ML 1998
Nager, F., Das Geheimnis Gesundheit, in: Schweiz. Ärztezeitung, Schweiz. Ärzteverlag AG, Basel 1998; 79: 34, p. 1591.

Oestensen and Villiger / ML 2001
Oestensen, M., Villiger, P.M., Nonsteroid anti-inflammatory drugs in systemic Lupus erythematosus, Lupus 2001 10 (3), pp. 135–139, Review.

Pedersen and Permin / ML 1988
Pedersen, Milling, L., and Permin, H., Rheumatic Disease, Heavy-Metal Pigments, and the Great Masters, in: The Lancet, 4.6.1988, pp. 1267–1269.

Peter / ML 1996
Peter, H.-H., Overlap-Syndrom, in: Klinische Immunologie, ed. by Peter, H.-H., and Pichler, W.J., 2nd ed., Verlag Urban & Schwarzenberg, Munich/Vienna/Baltimore 1996, pp. 373–380.

Pongratz / ML 1996
Pongratz, D., Overlap-Syndrom, in: Klinische Immunologie, ed. by Peter, H.-H., and Pichler, W.J., 2nd ed., Verlag Urban & Schwarzenberg, Munich/Vienna/Baltimore 1996, pp. 393–396.

Pschyrembel / ML 1998
Pschyrembel, Klinisches Wörterbuch, Verlag Walter de Gruyter, Berlin/New York 1998.

Reiner / ML 1990
Reiner, M., Dämmerblüten. Versuch einer Pathographie Paul Klees, in: Mendrisio 1990, n. pag. [pp. 35–38].

Rihs / ML 1994
Rihs, H.-P., et al., Unterschiedliche HLA-D-Phänotypfrequenzen bei anti-Scl-70- und ACA-positiven Patienten mit progressiver systemischer Sklerodermie mit und ohne Tätigkeit im Uranerzbergbau, in: Stuttgart 1994, pp. 23–25.

Röther and Peter / ML 1996
Röther, E., and Peter, H.-H., Progressive Systemsklerose, in: Klinische Immunologie, ed. by Peter, H.-H., and Pichler, W.J., 2nd ed., Verlag Urban & Schwarzenberg, Munich/Vienna/Baltimore 1996, pp. 381–390.

Ruzicka / ML 1996
Ruzicka, T., Calcinosis dsytrophica/Thibierge-Weissenbach-Syndrom/CREST-Syndrom, in: Braun-Falco, Plewig, Wolff/ML 1996, pp 1200 f.

Sandblom / ML 1990
Sandblom, P., Kreativität und Krankheit, Springer-Verlag, Berlin/Heidelberg 1990, pp 155–158.

Seemann and Hillenbach / ML 1994
Seemann, U., Hillenbach, C., Auswertung von Autopsiefällen aus dem Uranerzbergbau, in: Stuttgart 1994, p. 14.

Sharp / ML 1972
Sharp, G.C., Irving, W., Tan, E., Gould, R.G., Holman, H.R., Mixed connective tissue disease: an apparently distinct rheumatic disease syndrome associated with a specific antibody to an extractable nuclear antigen (ENA), American Journal of Medicine 1972; 52, pp. 148–159.

Stoll / ML 2001
Stoll, T., Kauer, Y., Büchi, S., Klaghofer, R., Sensky, T., Villiger, P.M., Prediction of depression in systemic Lupus erythematosus patients using SF-36 Mental Health scores, Rheumatology (Oxford), 2001 June; 40 (6), pp. 695–698.

Suter / ML 1998
Suter, H., Vom Leiden gezeichnet – und dennoch! Zur Krankheit von Paul Klee, Med. Report, Organ für ärztliche Fortbildungskongresse, vol. 22, no. 31, Blackwell Wissenschafts-Verlag GmbH, Berlin 1998, pp. 20 f.

Suter / ML 2003
Suter, H., Die Hände waren nicht befallen. Zur Krankheit von Paul Klee, Der Bund, Dec. 20, 2003, Verlag Der Bund, Bern 2003, p.16.

Stuttgart / ML 1994
Arbeitsmedizin, Sozialmedizin, Umweltmedizin, special ed. 22, Gentner Verlag, Stuttgart 1994.

Tan / ML 1982
Tan, E.M., Cohen, A.S., Fries, J.F., et al., The 1982 revised criteria for the classification of systemic Lupus erythematodes, Arthritis and Rheumatism 1982; 25, pp. 1271–1277.

Villiger and Stucki / ML 1996
Villiger, P.M., Stucki, G., Therapy of rheumatoid arthritis (chronic polyarthritis), Schweiz. Rundschau Med. Praxis, Sept. 10, 1996; 85 (37), pp. 1102–1107.

Villiger / ML 1997
Villiger, P. M., Rheumatoid arthritis: one disease – two view points, Schweiz. Med. Wochenschrift, Dec. 22, 1997; 127 (51–52), pp. 2117–2118.

Villiger and Seitz / ML 2006
Villiger, P.M., Seitz, M., Rheumatologie in Kürze, 2nd ed., Thieme, Stuttgart/New York 2006.

Wais / ML 2003
Wais, T., Fierz, W., Stoll, T., Villiger, P.M., Subclinical disease activity in systemic Lupus erythematosus: immunoinflammatory markers do not normalize in clinical remission, J. Rheumatol. 2003 Oct.; 30 (10), pp. 2133–2139.

Welcker / ML 2001
Welcker, M., Klinisches Bild des systemischen Lupus erythematodes, in: Elias. Journal der Pharmacia Diagnostics GmbH & Co, Freiburg, no. 2, Aug. 2001, pp. 3 f.

Wiebe / Ml 1994
Wiebe, V., Systemische Sklerodermie im Uranerzbergbau. Radiologische Lungenbefunde, in: Stuttgart 1994, pp. 15–17.

Zürcher and Krebs / ML 1992
Zürcher, K., and Krebs, A., Cutaneous Drug Reactions, 2nd ed., Verlag S. Karger AG, Basel/Freiburg/Paris/London/New York/New Dehli/Bangkok/Singapore/Tokyo/Sydney 1992. 1st ed. 1980: Hautnebenwirkungen interner Arzneimittel/Cutaneous Side effects of Systemic Drugs.

Art History / Philosophy Literature / Lexica

Aichinger-Grosch
Aichinger-Grosch, Ju, in: Grote 1959, pp. 48–55.

Bätschmann 2000
Bätschmann, Oskar, Grammatik der Bewegung. Paul Klees Lehre am Bauhaus, in: Bätschmann/Helfenstein 2000, pp. 107–124.

Bätschmann / Helfenstein 2000
Paul Klee. Kunst und Karriere. Beiträge des Internationalen Symposiums in Bern, ed. by Oskar Bätschmann and Josef Helfenstein (Schriften und Forschungen zu Paul Klee, vol. 1, pub. by the Paul Klee Stiftung, Bern Museum of Fine Arts, Stämpfli Verlag AG, Bern 2000).

Barr 1941
Barr, Jr., Alfred H., Introduction, in: Paul Klee, catalogue of the travelling exhibition organised by the Museum of Modern Art, New York 1941, pp. 4–6.

Baumgartner 1984
Baumgartner, Marcel, L'Art pour L' Aare, Bernische Kunst im 20. Jahrhundert, Kantonalbank von Bern, Bern 1984.

Baumgartner 1999
Baumgartner, Michael, Josef Albers and Paul Klee – zwei Lehrpersönlichkeiten am Bauhaus, in: Josef and Anni Albers, Europa und Amerika, Bern Museum of Fine Arts, Bern, Nov. 6, 1998 to Jan. 31, 1999, DuMont Buchverlag, Cologne 1998, pp. 165–186.

Basel 1965
Paul Klee, Spätwerke, Galerie Beyeler, Basel 1965.

Basel / Hannover 2003 / 2004
Paul Klee, Die Erfüllung im Spätwerk, exhibition catalogue. Fondation Beyeler, Riehen/Basel Aug. 10 to Nov. 9, 2003, Sprengel Museum Hannover Nov. 22, 2003 to Feb. 15, 2004, Benteli Verlags AG, CH–3084 Wabern/Bern.

Berggruen 1999
Berggruen, Heinz, Hauptweg und Nebenwege, Erinnerungen eines Kunstsammlers, Nicolaische Verlagsbuchhandlung Beuermann GmbH, Berlin 1999.

Berlin 1998
Klee aus New York, Hauptwerke der Sammlung Berggruen, Nicolaische Verlagsbuchhandlung Beuermann GmbH, Berlin, and Staatliche Museen zu Berlin, Berlin 1998.

Bern 1990
Paul Klee. Das Schaffen im Todesjahr, Bern Museum of Fine Arts, Bern, Aug. 17 to Nov. 4, 1990.

Bern / Düsseldorf 1997
Die Blaue Vier, catalogue for the exhibition of the same name in the Bern Museum of Fine Arts, Bern, and in the Kunstsammlung Nordrhein-Westfalen, Düsseldorf, 1997/1998, DuMont Buchverlag, Cologne 1997.

Bern / Hamburg 2000
Paul Klee. Die Sammlung Bürgi, exhibition catalogue. Bern Museum of Fine Arts, Bern, Feb. 4 to April 16, 2000; Hamburger Kunsthalle, Hamburg, May 5 to July 23, 2000.

Bern 2001 / 2002
Picasso und die Schweiz, ed. by Marc Fehlmann and Toni Stooss, Bern Museum of Fine Arts, Bern, Oct. 5, 2001 to Jan 6, 2002, Stämpfli-Verlag AG, Bern 2001.

Bhattacharya-Stettler 2001
Bhattacharya-Stettler, Therese, '…C'est comme un Corot!' – Picasso und Bern, in: Picasso und die Schweiz, exhibition catalogue. Bern Museum of Fine Arts, Bern, Oct. 5, 2001 to Jan. 6, 2002, pp. 75–89.

Bloesch / Schmidt 1950
Paul Klee, 1879–1940, Reden zu seinem Todestag am 29. Juni 1940 von Dr. Hans Bloesch und Dr. Georg Schmidt, Verlag Benteli AG, Bern 1950, also printed in: Mendrisio 1990, n. pag. [pp. 174–179].

Bodmer 1944
Bodmer, Heinrich, Dürer, Wilhelm Goldmann Verlag, Leipzig 1944.

Brockhaus 1894–1897
Brockhaus' Konversations-Lexikon in 17 volumes, F.B. Brockhaus, Leipzig/Berlin/Vienna 1894–1897.

Bruderer 1990
Bruderer, Hans-Jürgen, Konstruktion – Intuition, in: Paul Klee, Konstruktion – Intuition, exhibition catalogue, Städtische Kunsthalle, Mannheim, Dec. 9, 1990 to March 3, 1991, Verlag Gerd Hatje, Stuttgart 1990, pp. 9–24.

Bürgi 1948
Bürgi, Rolf, 1922–1933–1939, in: Du 1948, pp. 25 f.

Bürgi 2002
Paul Klee, Das 'Skizzenbuch Bürgi', 1924/25, with a commentary on the facsimile by Wolfgang Kersten, ed. by Stefan Frey, Wolfgang Kersten and Alexander Klee, Klee-Studien, vol. 1, ZIP (Zurich InterPublishers), Zurich 2002.

Bütikofer / Frey / Nyffenegger 1992
Bütikofer, Katharina; Frey, Stefan; Nyffenegger, Katharina, 'Zum Beispiel: Paul Klee', Verlag Aare, Solothurn 1992.

Darmstaedter 1979
Darmstaedter, Robert, Reclams Künstlerlexikon, Verlag Philipp Reclam jun., Stuttgart 1979.

Di San Lazzaro 1958
Di San Lazzaro, G., Paul Klee, Leben und Werk, special edition for the Ex Libris Book Club, Droemersche Verlaganstalt Th. Knaur Nachf., Munich-Zurich 1958.

Doschka 2001
Doschka, Roland, Der Lyriker im Paradiesgärtlein und der Dramatiker in Arkadien. Gedanken zum schöpferischen Prozess im Werk von Paul Klee und Pablo Picasso, in: Paul Klee. Jahre der Meisterschaft 1917–1933, exhibition catalogue, Stadthalle, Balingen, Munich, July 28 to Sept. 30, 2001, pp. 15–20.

Du 1948
Du, Schweizerische Monatsschrift, Zurich, vol. 8, no. 10, Oct. 1948, Verlag Conzett & Huber, Zurich 1948.

du 1961
du, Kulturelle Monatsschrift, vol. 21, no. 248, Oct. 1961, Verlag Conzett & Huber, Zurich 1961.

du 1986
du, Die Zeitschrift für Kunst und Kultur 12/1986, Dec. 1986, Verlag Conzett & Huber, Zurich 1986.

du 2000
du, Die Zeitschrift der Kultur, no. 703, Feb. 2000, Verlag TA-Media AG, Zurich 2000.

Düsseldorf 1964
Paul Klee, Kunstsammlung Nordrhein-Westfalen, 2nd ed., pub. by the Kunstsammlung Nordrhein-Westfalen, Düsseldorf 1964.

Edschmid 1920
Edschmid , Kasimir (ed.), Tribüne der Kunst und Zeit, Erich Reiss Verlag, Berlin 1920.

Eggum 1998
Eggum, Arne, in: Edvard Munch, exhibition catalogue for the Museo d'Arte Moderna, Città di Lugano, Sept. 19 to Dec. 13, 1998, ed. by Rudy Chiappini, Skira Verlag, Geneva-Milan 1998.

Feininger 1959
Feininger, Lyonel, in: Grote 1959, pp. 71–75.

Franciscono 1990
Franciscono, Marcel, Klees Krankheit und seine Bilder des Todes, in: Bern 1990, pp. 13–25.

Frank 1999
Van Gogh, Vincent, mit Selbstzeugnissen und Bilddokumenten, presented by Herbert Frank, Rowohlt Taschenbuch Verlag GmbH, Reinbek near Hamburg, 1976, 13th ed. 1999.

Frauenfeld 1958–1967
Künstlerlexikon der Schweiz. XX. Jahrhundert in two volumes, Verlag Huber & Co. AG, Frauenfeld 1958–1967.

Frey-Surbek 1976
Frey-Surbek, Marguerite, Im Hause Klee. Bern 1904, in: Literarische Skizzen von Marguerite Frey-Surbek, ed. by Heinrich Rohrer, Director of the Bern Public Library, private publication, Bern 1976, pp. 13–15.

Frey 1990
Frey, Stefan, Paul Klee. Chronologische Biographie (1933–1941), in: Bern 1990, pp. 111–132.

Frey 2003
Frey, Stefan, and Hüneke, Andreas, Paul Klee, Kunst und Politik in Deutschland 1933. Eine Chronologie, in: Paul Klee 1933, exhibition catalogue, Städtisches Museum im Lenbachhaus, Munich, Feb. 8 to May 4, 2003/ext. until May 18, 2003; Bern Museum of Fine Arts, Bern, June 4 to Aug. 17, 2003; Schirn Kunsthalle, Frankfurt a.M., Sept. 18 to Nov. 30, 2003; Hamburger Kunsthalle, Hamburg, Dec. 11, 2003 to July 3, 2004, pp. 268–306.

Frey Zitate
Frey, Stefan, Zitate zur Krankengeschichte, 35 pp., Zentrum Paul Klee, Bern, Paul Klee's Estate, Bern.

Frey / Helfenstein 1991
Paul Klee. Verzeichnis der Werke des Jahres 1940, pub. by the Paul Klee Stiftung, Bern Museum of Fine Arts, Bern, compiled by Stefan Frey and Josef Helfenstein, assisted by Irene Rehmann, Stuttgart 1991.

Geelhaar 1979
Geelhaar, Christian, 'Diesseitig gar nicht fassbar? Zur Wirkungsgeschichte Paul Klees', Basler Magazin, no. 50, Basel, Dec. 15, 1979.

Geiser 1961
Geiser, Bernhard, Picasso besucht Paul Klee in Bern 1937, in: du 1961, pp. 53, 88 and 90.

Geiser 1987
Geiser, Bernhard, Besuch bei Paul Klee in Bern, in: Das Genie lässt bitten, Erinnerungen an Picasso, Verlag Philipp Reclam jun., Leipzig 1987, pp. 76–82.

Gerson 1982
Gerson, Horst, Gogh Vincent Willem van, in: Kindlers Malerei Lexikon, vol. 5, Deutscher Taschenbuch Verlag GmbH & Co. KG, Munich 1982, pp. 106–117.

Giedion-Welcker 2000
Paul Klee. In Selbstzeugnissen und Bilddokumenten, presented by Carola Giedion-Welcker, 19th ed., Rowohlt Taschenbuch Verlag GmbH, Reinbek near Hamburg 2000 (Rowohlts Monographien 52).

Glaesemer 1973
Glaesemer Jürgen, Paul Klee, Handzeichnungen I. Kindheit bis 1920, Bern Museum of Fine Arts, Bern 1973.

Glaesemer 1976
Glaesemer, Jürgen, Paul Klee. Die farbigen Werke im Kunstmuseum Bern. Gemälde, farbige Blättter, Hinterglasbilder und Plastiken, Bern Museum of Fine Arts, Bern, pub. by the Schweiz. Mobilar Versicherungsgesellschaft in association with Verlag Kornfeld u. Cie, Bern, Bern 1976.

Glaesemer 1979
Glaesemer, Jürgen, Paul Klee. Handzeichnungen III. 1937–1940, Bern Museum of Fine Arts, Bern 1979.

Glaesemer 1984
Glaesemer, Jürgen, Paul Klee. Handzeichnungen II. 1921–1936, Bern Museum of Fine Arts, Bern 1984.

Glarus 1995
Othmar Huber collection, Glarner Kunstverein, Glarus 1995.

Gottschalk 1966
Gottschalk, Herbert, Karl Jaspers, Colloquium Verlag Otto H. Hess, Berlin 1966 (Köpfe des XX. Jahrhunderts, vol. 43).

Grohmann 1965
Grohmann, Will, Paul Klee, Editions des Trois Collines, Geneva, and Kohlhammer, Stuttgart 1954, 4th ed. 1965, special edition by the Büchergilde Gutenberg, Zurich 1965.

Grohmann 1966
Grohmann, Will, Der Maler Paul Klee, Verlag M. DuMont Schauberg, Cologne 1966.

Grohmann 2003
Grohmann, Will, Der Maler Paul Klee, revised, Verlag M. DuMont Schauberg, Cologne 2003.

Grote 1959
Erinnerungen an Paul Klee, ed. by Ludwig Grote, Prestel Verlag, Munich 1959.

Güse 1992
Paul Klee, Wachstum regt sich. Klees Zwiesprache mit der Natur, ed. by Ernst-Gerhard Güse, 2nd ed., Prestel Verlag, Munich 1992.

Gutbrod 1968
Lieber Freund. Künstler schreiben an Will Grohmann, ed. by Karl Gutbrod, Verlag M. DuMont Schauberg, Cologne 1968.

Haftmann et al. 1957
Haftmann, Werner, Giedion-Welcker, Carola, Grohmann, Will, Schmalenbach, Werner, Schmidt, Georg, Im Zwischenreich. Aquarelle und Zeichnungen von Paul Klee, Verlag M. DuMont Schauberg, Cologne 1957, 2nd ed. 1959.

Haftmann 1961
Haftmann, Werner, Paul Klee. Wege bildnerischen Denkens, Prestel Verlag, Munich 1950, published by the Fischer Bücherei KG, Frankfurt am Main and Hamburg 1961.

Haldi/Schindler 1920
Berner Album, ed. by Chr. Haldi and Peter Schindler, Büchler-Verlag, Bern 1920.

Hamburg 1967
Jahrbuch der Hamburger Kunstsammlungen, vol. 12, Hamburg 1967.

Helfenstein 1990
Helfenstein, Josef, Das Spätwerk als 'Vermächtnis'. Klees Schaffen im Todesjahr, exhibition catalogue, Bern Museum of Fine Arts, Bern, Aug. 17 to Nov. 4, 1990, pp. 59–75.

Helfenstein 1998
Helfenstein, Josef, Foreword, in: Catalogue of works Paul Klee, vol. 1: 1883–1912, pub. by the Paul Klee Stiftung, Bern Museum of Fine Arts, Bern, Benteli Verlags AG, Bern 1998, pp. 11–17.

Helfenstein 2000
Helfenstein, Josef, 'Ein kleines Publikum aus feinen Köpfen'. Klees Bildertausch mit befreundeten Künstlern, in: Bätschmann/Helfenstein 2000, pp. 125–145.

Hersch 1980
Hersch, Jeanne, Karl Jaspers, R. Piper & Co. Verlag, Munich 1980.

Hertel 1959
Hertel, Christof, in: Grote 1959, pp. 97–100.

Heusser 2000
Heusser, Peter (ed.), Goethes Beitrag zur Erneuerung der Naturwissenschaften, Verlag Paul Haupt, Bern/Stuttgart/Vienna 2000.

Hopfengart 1989
Hopfengart, Christine, Klee. Vom Sonderfall zum Publikumsliebling. Stationen seiner öffentlichen Resonanz in Deutschland 1905–1960, Verlag Philipp von Zabern, Mainz 1989.

Huggler 1969
Huggler, Max, Paul Klee. Die Malerei als Blick in den Kosmos, Verlag Huber & Co. AG, Frauenfeld/Stuttgart 1969.

Insel 294
Paul Klee, Handzeichnungen, Insel Bücherei no. 294, Insel-Verlag, Frankfurt am Main, Wiesbaden branch (without date).

Insel 800
Paul Klee, Traumlandschaft mit Mond, Insel Bücherei no. 800, Insel-Verlag, Frankfurt am Main 1964.

Jaspers 1957
Jaspers, Karl, Drei Gründer des Philosophierens: Plato, Augustin, Kant, R. Piper & Co. Verlag, Munich 1957, licensed edition by the Deutscher Bücherbund, Stuttgart-Hamburg, without year [1957], unabridged special edition of the section 'Die fortzeugenden Gründer des Philosophierens: Plato, Augustin, Kant' from: 'Die grossen Philosophen', vol. 1.

Jaspers 1973
Jaspers, Karl, Philosophie, vol. 1 (of 3), Berlin 1932, 4th ed. Berlin/Heidelberg/New York 1973 (quoted by Hersch, Jeanne, in: Karl Jaspers, Eine Einführung in sein Werk, R. Piper & Co. Verlag, Munich 1980).

Kahnweiler 1950
Klee, Collection: Palettes, Texte de Daniel-Henry Kahnweiler, Les Editions Braun & Cie, Rue Louis Le Grand, Paris 1950.

Kandinsky 1972
Kandinsky, Aquarelle und Zeichnungen, Galerie Beyeler, Basel 1972.

Kandinsky 1976
Kandinsky, Nina, Kandinsky und ich, Kindler Verlag GmbH, Munich 1976.

Kerkovius 1959
Kerkovius, Ida, in: Grote 1959, pp. 56 f.

Kersten 1990
Kersten, Wolfgang, Paul Klee, Übermut, Fischer Taschenbuch Verlag GmbH, Frankfurt am Main 1990.

Kindler 1982
Kindlers Malerei Lexikon, vol. 5, Deutscher Taschenbuch Verlag GmbH & Co. KG, Munich 1982, licensed edition authorized by the Kindler Verlag AG, Zurich 1982.

Klee Hans
Klee, Hans, Jugend Verse, pub. at the suggestion of former pupils of the author's in his capacity as music teacher at the cantonal teachers' college, Bern, private publication, undated.

Klee 1920
Klee, Paul, article, in: Schöpferische Konfession, Erich Reiss Verlag, Berlin 1920 (=Tribüne der Kunst und Zeit. A collection of writings, ed. by Kasimir Edschmid, XIII), pp. 28–40, re-printed in Klee 1976, pp. 118–122.

Klee 1923
Klee, Paul, Wege des Naturstudiums, in: Staatliches Bauhaus in Weimar, 1919–1923, Bauhaus-Verlag, Weimar-Munich 1923, pp. 24–25.

Klee 1924
Klee, Paul, Vortrag Jena [facsimile und transcription], in: Paul Klee in Jena 1924. Der Vortrag, Jena 1999 (=Minerva. Jenaer Schriften zur Kunstgeschichte, vol. 10), pp. 11–69, first published under the title 'Paul Klee, über die moderne Kunst', Benteli Verlag, Bern 1945 (2nd ed. 1979). 'On modern art', translated by Douglas Cooper, Benteli, Bern 1945.

Klee 1927/2002
Paul Klee, Das Jahr 1927/Das Jahr 2002, Galenica AG, CH–3027 Bern 2002.

Klee 1948
Klee, Felix, Erinnerungen an meinen Vater, in: Du 1948, p. 14; re-printed in: du 2000, pp. 62 f.

Klee 1956
Klee, Paul, Das bildnerische Denken, ed. and compiled by Jürg Spiller, Benno Schwabe & Co. Verlag, Basel-Stuttgart 1956.

Klee 1957/1
Paul Klee, Engel bringt das Gewünschte, 2nd ed., Woldemar Klein Verlag, Baden-Baden 1957.

Klee 1957/2
'Im Zwischenreich', Aquarelle und Zeichnungen von Paul Klee, Verlag M. DuMont Schauberg, Cologne 1957.

Klee 1960/1
Klee, Felix, Paul Klee, Leben und Werk in Dokumenten, selected from posthumous documents and unpublished letters, Diogenes Verlag, Zurich 1960.

Klee 1960/2
Klee, Paul, Gedichte, ed. by Felix Klee, Peter Schifferli Verlags AG, 'Die Arche' Zurich, Zurich 1960.

Klee 1965
Paul Klee, Pädagogisches Skizzenbuch, ed. by Hans M. Wingler, Florian Kupferberg Verlag, Mainz/Berlin 1965.

Klee 1976
Klee, Paul, Schriften, Rezensionen und Aufsätze, ed. by Christian Geelhaar, Verlag M. DuMont Schauberg, Cologne 1976.

Klee 1979
Klee, Paul, Briefe an die Familie 1893–1940. Vol. 2: 1907–1940, ed. by Felix Klee, Verlag M. DuMont Schauberg, Cologne 1979.

Klee 1987
Paul Klee, Leben und Werk, pub. by the Paul Klee Stiftung, Bern Museum of Fine Arts, and the Museum of Modern Art, New York, 1987.

Klee 1989
Klee, Felix, in: Rewald, Sabine, Paul Klee. Die Sammlung Berggruen im Metropolitan Museum of Art, New York, und im Musée National d'Art Moderne, Paris, Verlag Gerd Hatje, Stuttgart 1989, pp. 19–48.

Klee 1990/1
Klee, Felix, Das späte Werk von Paul Klee (1930–1940), in: Mendrisio 1990, n. pag. [pp. 20–30].

Klee 1990/2
Paul Klee, Das Schaffen im Todesjahr, Bern Museum of Fine Arts, Bern 1990, Verlag Gerd Hatje, Stuttgart 1990.

Klee 1996
Paul Klee, Die Zeit der Reife, ed. by Manfred Fath, Prestel-Verlag, Munich-New York 1996.

Klee 1998–2004
Paul Klee, Catalogue of works in 9 volumes, pub. by the Paul Klee Stiftung, Bern Museum of Fine Arts, Benteli Verlags AG, Bern 1998–2004.

Klee Tgb.
Paul Klee, Tagebücher (Diaries) 1898–1918. New edition with commentary, pub. by the Paul Klee Stiftung, Bern Museum of Fine Arts, Bern, compiled by Wolfgang Kersten, Stuttgart/Teufen 1988.

Kornfeld 1962
Kornfeld, Eberhard W., Bern und Umgebung, Aquarelle und Zeichnungen von Paul Klee, 1897–1915, Verlag Stämpfli & Cie AG, Bern 1962.

Kornfeld 1973
Kornfeld, Eberhard W., Paul Klee in Bern, Verlag Stämpfli & Cie AG, 2nd ed., Bern 1973 (1st ed. 1962, 3rd ed. 2006).

Kort 2003
Kort, Pamela, Paul Klee und die Zeichnungen zur 'nationalsozialistischen Revolution', in: Munich et al. 2003/2004, Verlag der Buchhandlung Walther König, Cologne 2003, pp. 182–216.

Kröll 1968
Kröll, Christina, Die Bildtitel Paul Klees. Eine Studie zur Beziehung von Bild und Sprache in der Kunst des zwanzigsten Jahrhunderts, Dissertation, Rheinische Friedrich-Willhelms-University, Bonn 1968.

Kuhr 1959
Kuhr, Fritz, in: Grote, 1959, pp. 94–96.

Kunstmuseum Bern 1984
Berner Kunstmitteilungen no. 227, Jan. 1984, Feb. 1984, Bern Museum of Fine Arts, Bern 1984.

Kunstmuseum Bern 1984/1985
Berner Kunstmitteilungen nos. 234–236, Dec. 1984, Jan. 1985, Feb. 1985, Bern Museum of Fine Arts, Bern 1985.

Kunstmuseum Bern 1988
Berner Kunstmitteilungen nos. 262/263, May 1988, June 1988, Bern Museum of Fine Arts, Bern 1988.

Kunstmuseum Bern 1990/1
Berner Kunstmitteilungen no. 276, Sept./Oct. 1990, Bern Museum of Fine Arts, Bern 1990.

Kunstmuseum Bern 1990/2
Berner Kunstmitteilungen no. 277, Nov./Dec. 1990, Bern Museum of Fine Arts, Bern 1990.

Kunstmuseum Bern 1997
Berner Kunstmitteilungen no. 312, Nov. 1997, Dec. 1997, Bern Museum of Fine Arts, Bern 1997.

Kunstmuseum Bern 1998
Berner Kunstmitteilungen no. 316, Sept. 1998, Oct. 1998, Bern Museum of Fine Arts, Bern 1998.

Kunstmuseum Bern 2001
Berner Kunstmitteilungen no. 332, Oct. 2001, Nov. 2001, Dec. 2001, Bern Museum of Fine Arts, Bern 2001.

Kuthy 1984
Kandinsky und Klee: Aus dem Briefwechsel der beiden Künstler und ihrer Frauen 1912–1940, ed. and introduced by Sandor Kuthy, commentary by Stefan Frey, in: Kunstmuseum Bern 1984/1985 pp. 1–24.

Lang 1987
Das Genie lässt bitten, Erinnerungen an Picasso, ed. by Lothar Lang, Verlag Philipp Reclam jun., Leipzig 1987.

Luzern 1991–1993
Schweizer Lexikon in six volumes, Verlag Schweizer Lexikon Mengis + Ziehr, Lucerne 1991–1993.

Mendrisio 1990
Paul Klee. Ultimo decennio – Letztes Jahrzehnt 1930–1940, exhibition catalogue, Museo d'arte, Mendrisio, April 7 to July 8, 1990.

Munich 1970/1971
Paul Klee, exhibition catalogue, Haus der Kunst, Munich, Oct. 10, 1970 to Jan. 3, 1971.

Munich 1979/1980
Paul Klee, Das Frühwerk 1883–1922, exhibition catalogue, Städtische Galerie im Lenbachhaus, Munich 1979/1980.

Munich 1986
Deutsche Kunst im 20. Jahrhundert, Prestel-Verlag, Munich 1986.

Munich et al. 2003/2004
Paul Klee 1933, exhibition catalogue, Städtische Galerie im Lenbachhaus, Munich Feb. 8 to May 4, 2003; Bern Museum of Fine Arts, Bern, June 4 to Aug. 17, 2003; Schirn Kunsthalle, Frankfurt a.M., Sept. 18 to Nov. 30, 2003; Hamburger Kunsthalle, Hamburg, Dec. 11, 2003 to March 7, 2004.

Münter 1959
Münter, Gabriele, in: Grote 1959, pp. 40–42.

Muth 1959
Muth, Hermann, in: Grote 1959, p. 47.

NZZ 1998
Biografisches Lexikon der Schweizer Kunst in two volumes, pub. by the Schweiz. Institut für Kunstwissenschaft, Zurich and Lausanne, Verlag Neue Zürcher Zeitung, Zürich 1998.

Okuda 2000
Okuda, Osamu, 'Exzentrisches Zentrum'. Paul Klee als Lehrer, in: Pfäffikon 2000, pp. 233–257.

Osterwold 1979
Osterwold, Tilman, Paul Klee, Ein Kind träumt sich, Verlag Gerd Hatje, Stuttgart 1979.

Osterwold 1990
Osterwold, Tilman, Paul Klee, Spätwerk, Verlag Gerd Hatje, Stuttgart 1990.

Osterwold 2005
Paul Klee, Kein Tag ohne Linie, pub. by the Zentrum Paul Klee, Bern, with Tilman Osterwold, Verlag Hatje Cantz, Stuttgart 2005.

Penrose 1981
Penrose, Roland, Pablo Picasso. Sein Leben – sein Werk, Munich 1981 (Penrose, Roland, Picasso: His Life and Work, University of California Press 1981; ed. 1958).

Petitpierre 1957
Petitpierre, Petra, Aus der Malklasse von Paul Klee, Benteli Verlag, Bern 1957.

Pfäffikon 2000
Paul Klee. Die Kunst des Sichtbarmachens. Materialen zu Klees Unterricht am Bauhaus, exhibition catalogue, Seedam Kulturzentrum Pfäffikon, CH–8808 Pfäffikon (Schwyz), May 14 to July 30, 2000, Benteli Verlag, Bern 2000.

Pfeiffer-Belli 1978
Pfeiffer-Belli, Erich, Paul Klee, in: Zürich 1978, pp. 384–397.

Ponente 1960
Ponente, Nello, Klee, Biographisch-kritische Studie, Editions d'Art Albert Skira, Geneva 1960.

Rewald 1989
Rewald, Sabine, Paul Klee, Die Sammlung Berggruen im Metropolitan Museum of Art, New York, und im Musée d'Art Moderne, Paris, Tate Gallery Publishing, New York 1989.

Roethel 1971
Roethel, Hans Konrad, Paul Klee in: München, Verlag Stämpfli & Cie AG, Bern 1971.

Rotzler 1986
Rotzler. Willy, Engelbilder bei Paul Klee, in: du 1986, p. 52.

Schawinsky 1959
Schawinsky, Alexander (Xanti), in Grote: 1959, pp. 67–70.

Schmalenbach 1986
Schamalenbach, Werner, Paul Klee. Die Düsseldorfer Sammlung, Prestel-Verlag, Munich 1986.

Schmied 1986
Schmied, Wieland, in: Deutsche Kunst im 20. Jahrhundert, Malerei und Plastik, 1905–1985, ed. by Christos M. Joachimides, Norman Rosenthal, Wieland Schmied, Prestel-Verlag, Munich 1986.

Schmidt 1966
Schmidt, Georg, Umgang mit Kunst, Walter-Verlag AG, CH–4600 Olten 1966.

Sorg / Okuda 2005
Sorg, Reto, Okuda, Osamu, Die satirische Muse. Paul Klee, Hans Bloesch und das Editionsprojekt 'Der Musterbürger', ed. by Stefan Frey, Wolfgang Kersten and Alexander Klee, Klee-Studien, vol. 2, ZIP (Zürich InterPublishers), Zürich 2005.

Spiller 1962
Spiller, Jürg, Paul Klee, Gebrüder Weiss Verlag Lebendiges Wissen, Berlin-Munich 1962.

Stettler 1997
Stettler, Michael, Lehrer und Freunde, Essays, Stämpfli Verlag AG, Bern 1997.

Vatter-Jensen 2005
Vatter-Jensen, Inga, Henriette Sechehaye, Die letzte Schülerin von Paul Klee, ArchivArte Verlag, Bern 2005.

von Tavel 1969
Von Tavel, Hans Christoph, Ein Jahrhundert Schweizer Kunst, Schweizerische Volksbank, Bern, pub. by Editions d'art Albert Skira, Geneva 1969.

von Tavel 1983
Von Tavel, Hans Christoph, Wege zur Kunst im Kunstmuseum Bern, Taschenbücher vol. 3, Verlag Der Bund, Bern 1983.

von Tavel 1988
Von Tavel, Hans Christoph, Der sanfte Trug des Berner Milieus. Berner Künstler 1910–1920, for the exhibition at the Bern Museum of Fine Arts, Bern, Feb. 26 to May 15, 1988, in: Der sanfte Trug des Berner Milieus, Bern Museum of Fine Arts, Bern 1998, pp. 9–23.

von Tavel 1990
Von Tavel, Hans Christoph, Felix Klee zum Gedenken, in: Kunstmuseum Bern 1990/2.

von Tavel 2001
Von Tavel, Hans Christoph, Paul Klee. Vom Leben und Sterben in seinen Stillleben, manuscript for a lecture given in Rome on Feb. 22, 2001, and in Bologna on Feb. 27, 2001 (12 pp.).

Wada 1975
Wada, Sadao, The Last Moments of Paul Klee, in: 'Mizue' (a monthly review of the fine arts), July 7, 1975, no. 844, Tokyo.

Walter-Ris 2003
Walter-Ris, Anja, Kunstleidenschaft im Dienst der Moderne. Die Geschichte der Galerie Nierendorf, Berlin/New York 1920–1995, ed. by Stefan Frey, Wolfgang Kersten and Alexander Klee, Klee-Studien, vol. 3, ZIP (Zürich InterPublishers), Zürich 2003.

Wedekind 2000
Wedekind, Gregor, Kosmische Konfession. Kunst und Religion bei Paul Klee, in: Bätschmann/Helfenstein 2000, pp. 226–238.

Werckmeister 1987
Werckmeister, Otto Karl, Von der Revolution zum Exil, in: Klee 1987, pp. 31–55.

Wiederkehr Sladeczeck 2000
Wiederkehr Sladeczeck, Eva, Der handschriftliche Oeuvre-Katolog von Paul Klee, in: Bätschmann/Helfenstein 2000, pp. 146–158.

Wild 1950
Wild, Doris, Moderne Malerei, Büchergilde Gutenberg, Zürich 1950.

Wingler 2002
Wingler, Hans, Das Bauhaus, Verlag Gebr. Rasch & Co. and M. DuMont Schauberg, 4th ed., Cologne 2002.

Zahn 1920
Zahn, Leopold, Paul Klee. Leben/Werk/Geist, Gustave Kiepenhauer Verlag, Potsdam 1920.

Zentrum Paul Klee 2005 / 1
Publication to commemorate the opening, Zentrum Paul Klee, Bern (pub.), Ursina Barandun, Michael Baumgartner (ed.), Hatje Cantz Verlag, Ostfildern-Ruit 2005.

Zentrum Paul Klee 2005 / 2
Short guide, Zentrum Paul Klee, Bern (pub.), Ursina Barandun, Michael Baumgartner (ed.), Hatje Cantz Verlag, Ostfildern-Ruit 2005.

Zschokke 1948
Zschokke, Alexander, Begegnung mit Paul Klee, in: Du 1948, pp. 27 f, 74, 76.

Zürich 1945–1948
Schweizer Lexikon in seven volumes, Encyclios-Verlag AG, Zürich 1945–1948.

Zürich 1967 / 1968
Sir Edward and Lady Hulton Collection, London, Exhibition from Dec. 3, 1967 to Jan. 7, 1968, Kunsthaus, Zürich.

Zürich 1978
Die Grossen der Weltgeschichte, ed. by Kurt Fassmann, Kindler-Verlag AG, Zürich 1978.

Index of Documents Quoted in Abridged Form

Klee 1935 / 1936
Klee, Lily, Fiebertabelle, (records of Paul Klee's body temperature from Oct. 18, 1935 to April 18, 1936), notebook, 17 pp. (NFKB).

Klee 1940
Klee, Paul, Lebenslauf (biography), Jan. 7, 1940, facsimile in: Grohmann 1965, pp. 11–14.

Klee [from 1942]
Klee, Lily, Lebenserinnerungen (memoirs), from 1942, 186-page manuscript (copy: NFKB).

List of Illustrations

Frontispiece: Paul Klee, July 1939

1	Symbiosis, 1934, 131	Page 6
2	Aljoscha Klee	7
3	Dr. Hans Christoph von Tavel	8
4	This star teaches bending, 1940, 344	10
5	Lily Klee-Stumpf, 1906	12
6	Paul/Lily Klee with Bimbo the cat, 1935	12
7	Dr. h.c. Felix Klee, 1940	13
8	Dr. Will and Gertrud Grohmann, 1935	14
9	Dr. Max Huggler, 1944	14
10	Dr. Jürgen Glaesemer, 1987	15
11	Marked man, 1935, 146	16
12	Ecce …., 1940, 138	17
13	Bern, Federal Parliament Building, Alps	18
14	Paul Klee, 1892	19
15	Hans Klee, 1880	20
16	Poem by Hans Klee about his children	20
17	Ida Klee-Frick, 1879	21
18	Struck from the list, 1933, 424	22
19	Scholar, 1933, 286	23
20	Rigidity, 1933, 187	25
21	Emigrating, 1933, 181	26
22	Paul and Lily Klee, 1930	27
23	Last residence of Paul/Lily Klee in Bern	27
24	Exhibition poster, Kunsthalle Bern, 1935	28
25	Extract from the minutes of the Bern Municipal Council meeting, July 5, 1940	31
26	Klee's biography, January 7, 1940	32–35
27	Swiss landscape, 1919, 46	36
28	Bern old town with the town hall	37
29	A sick man makes plans, 1939, 611	38
30	Measles: 'Koplik's spots'	40
31	Measles: rash with red spots	40
32	Fine flaking of the rash after measles/drug-induced exanthema	41
33	Rash by drug-induced exanthema	41
34	Handbook: Cutaneous Drug Reactions	42
35	Paul Klee's temperature chart from November 1–11, 1935	43
36	Plant according to rules, 1935, 91	44
37	From a letter from L. Klee to E. Scheyer	47
38	P. Klee, F. Klee, H. & M. Rupf-Wirz, 1937	47
39	Letter from G. Schorer to P. Klee, 1936	49
40	Dermatology Clinic of Bern, ca. 1930	49
41	Morphea, inflammation stage	50
42	Morphea, with lilac ring	50
43	Morphea, final stage	51
44	Systemic sclerosis: mask face	53
45	Paul Klee, 1925	54
46	Paul Klee, 1939	55
47	The eye, 1938, 315	56
48	Mask: pain, 1938, 235	57
49	Systemic sclerosis: sclerodactyly	58
50	Systemic sclerosis: limited form with sclerodactyly and finger contracture	58
51	Systemic sclerosis: sclerodactyly with 'rat-bite necrosis' and ulceration	59
52	Systemic sclerosis: dry, cracked tongue	59
53	Raynaud's syndrome: 'dead finger'	61
54	Systemic sclerosis: sclerodactyly with bleeding in the cuticles in the nail-fold	62
55	Nail-fold capillaroscopy	62
56	Systemic sclerosis: blood vessel with thickening of the wall tissue	63
57	X-ray of a normal esophagus	64
58	Systemic sclerosis: rigid esophagus, X-ray	64
59	Postcard from P. Klee to L. Klee, 1940	65
60	Herring, for me?!, 1939, 658	Page 66
61	Never again that dish!, 1939, 659	66
62	Page 2 of a diet plan, presumably prepared by Lily Klee for Paul Klee	68
63	Systemic sclerosis: X-ray of pulmonary fibrosis	71
64	Systemic sclerosis: microscopic section of a kidney filter	73
65	Sanatorium Viktoria, Locarno-Orselina	74
66	Clinica Sant' Agnese, Locarno-Muralto	74
67	Paul Klee's death certificate	75
68	Paul Klee's cremation certificate	75
69	Paul Klee's obituary notice, June 29, 1940	76
70	Paul Klee's last studio in Bern	77
71	Paul/Lily Klee's memorial plate in Bern	77
72	Paul Klee, December 1939	78
73	Paul Klee drawing, 1931	78
74	Paul Klee painting, 1939	79
75	Prescription from G. Schorer for P. Klee	83
76	Vessel for salve, 1940, 169	84
77	Anna C.R. Frick-Riedtmann, 1880	93
78	Lily and Paul Klee, 1930	94
79	Paul Klee and Will Grohmann, 1935	95
80	Wassily Kandinsky and Paul Klee, 1929	96
81	Paul Klee, July 1939	99
82	Paul Klee's hands, July 1939	100
83	Letter from Paul Klee to his son, Felix, November 29, 1938	101
84	Systemic Lupus erythematosus	102
85	Dermatomyositis	103
86	Paul Klee, July 1939	105
87	Paul Klee and Will Grohmann, 1938	107
88	Dr. Fritz Lotmar	109
89	Dr. Gerhard Schorer	110
90	Dr. Hermann Bodmer	111
91	Prof. Oscar Naegeli	112
92	Dr. Theodor Haemmerli	113
93	Hand puppets made by Paul Klee from 1925/1916/1923	114
94	Ernst Kállai, Caricature of Paul Klee	121
95	Mourning, 1934, 8	123
96	Marked man, 1935, 146	125
97	Manhunt, 1933, 115	126
98	Outbreak of fear, 1939, 27	130
99	Outbreak of fear III, 1939, 124	131
100	Poem by Paul Klee from 1914	133
101	Dances caused by fear, 1938, 90	134
102	Rise from the dead!, 1938, 478	136
103	Difficult resurrection, 1939, 221	136
104	Oh! above me!, 1939, 201	137
105	Something better is nigh, 1939, 204	137
106	High spirits, 1939, 1251	138
107	Do I fall, too?, 1940, 119	139
108	Alas, rather downwards, 1939, 846	139
109	The tightrope walker, 1923, 121	140
110	Unstable signpost, 1937, 45,	141
111	Shattered, 1939, 1065	142
112	SOS, the last signal, 1939, 652	143
113	Dialogue between tree and man, 1939, 403	143
114	Fleeing on wheels, 1939, 653	144
115	Flight, 1940, 121	145
116	He can't escape, 1940, 231	145
117	Mon dieu!, 1939, 551	145
118	The grey man and the coast, 1938, 125	146
119	Departure of the adventurer, 1939, 735	147
120	Rower in the narrowness, 1939, 728	148
121	Navigatio mala, 1939, 563	148
122	River gorge near Y, 1939, 734	149
123	Rowing competition, 1940, 172	150
124	Sick man in a boat, 1940, 66	151
125	The unlucky star, 1939, 538	152
126	This star teaches bending, 1940, 344	152
127	Drinking companion, 1931, 280	Page 158
128	Accusation in the street, 1933, 85	159
129	Violence, 1933, 138	159
130	Tribute, 1933, 299	160
131	'He' a dictator too!, 1933, 339	161
132	Supposed celebrities, 1933, 151	162
133	Target recognized, 1933, 350	163
134	Lonely end, 1934, 183	164
135	The soul departs, 1934, 211	165
136	Revolution of the viaduct, 1937, 153	167
137	Symptom, to be diagnosed in good time, 1935, 17	168
138	Black signs, 1938, 114	169
139	Insula dulcamara, 1938, 481	171
140	Early sorrow, 1938, 318	174
141	Taking leave, 1938, 352	175
142	Paul Klee's catalogue of works, 1940, first page	177
143	Paul Klee's catalogue of works, 1940, last page	179
144	Eyes in the landscape, 1940, 41	180
145	Final renunciation, 1938, 372	180
146	Dancing fruits, 1940, 312	181
147	Suddenly rigid, 1940, 205	181
148	Detailed passion: touched to the core, 1940, 180	182
149	Stick it out!, 1940, 337	182
150	Ecce …., 1940, 138	183
151	Whence? where? whither?, 1940, 60	184
152	Death and fire, 1940, 332	191
153	Cemetery, 1939, 693	192
154	Ibid. [turned through 90° to the right]	193
155	Twilight flowers, 1940, 42	195
156	In the antechamber of angelhood, 1939, 845	196
157	Under grand protection, 1939, 1137	197
158	Forgetful angel, 1939, 880	198
159	Bell angel, 1939, 966	199
160	Untitled (Angel of death), ca. 1940	200
161	Chronometric dance, 1940, 133	205
162	Masks at twilight, 1938, 486	207
163	Eidola: erstwhile philosopher, 1940, 101	208
164	Monologue of the kitten, 1938, 426	208
165	Old man counting, 1929, 60	209
166	Catching a dreary scent, 1940, 112	209
167	Animals in captivity, 1940, 263	213
168	Pablo Picasso, 1963	214
169	Paul Klee, 1912	215
170	Villa R, 1919, 153	218
171	Glass façade, 1940, 288	219
172	Albrecht Dürer, 'Saint Jerome in his study', 1514	221
173	Paul Klee's catalogue of works, 1938, nos. 361–372	222
174	Trees by the water, 1933, 442	226
175	Night flower, 1938, 118	227
176	Underwater garden, 1939, 746	229
177	Symbiosis, 1934, 131	230
178	Flora on the rocks, 1940, 343	231
179	Untitled (Last still life), 1940	232
180	Angel, still ugly, 1940, 26	233
181	Paul Klee, December 1939	235
182	Super-chess, 1937, 141	236
183	Marked man, 1935, 146	237
184	Suddenly rigid, 1940, 205	238
185	Ecce …., 1940, 138	239
186	Poster for the Bern Medical Faculty exhibition, November 5–27, 2005	240

Tables

1	The different forms of scleroderma	53
2	Paul Klee's creative output during his illness	222

Alphabetical Index of Illustrations of Works of Paul Klee

Accusation in the street, 1933, 85
Chalk on paper on cardboard
16.9 x 25 cm
Zentrum Paul Klee, Bern   page 159

Alas, rather downwards, 1939, 846
Pencil on paper on cardboard
29.5 x 21 cm
Zentrum Paul Klee, Bern   page 139

Angel, still ugly, 1940, 26
Pencil on paper on cardboard
29.6 x 20.9 cm
Zentrum Paul Klee, Bern   page 233

Animals in captivity, 1940, 263
Coloured paste on paper on cardboard
31.2 x 48.3 cm
Private collection, Switzerland   page 213

A sick man makes plans, 1939, 611
Pencil on paper on cardboard
20.9 x 29.7 cm
Private collection, Switzerland, on extended
loan to the Zentrum Paul Klee, Bern   page 38

Bell angel, 1939, 966
Pencil on paper on cardboard
29.5 x 21 cm
Zentrum Paul Klee, Bern   page 199

Black signs, 1938, 114
Oil on cotton on cardboard
15 x 24 cm
Private collection, Switzerland, on extended
loan to the Zentrum Paul Klee, Bern   page 169

Catching a dreary scent, 1940, 112
Chalk on paper on cardboard
21.7 x 29.5 cm
Zentrum Paul Klee, Bern   page 209

Cemetery, 1939, 693
Coloured paste on paper on cardboard
37.1 x 49.5 cm
Zentrum Paul Klee, Bern   pages 192, 193

Chronometric dance, 1940, 133
Chalk on paper on cardboard
29.7 x 20.2 cm
Zentrum Paul Klee, Bern   page 205

Dances caused by fear, 1938, 90
Watercolour on paper on cardboard
48 x 31 cm
Zentrum Paul Klee, Bern   page 134

Dancing fruits, 1940, 312
Coloured paste on paper on cardboard
29.5 x 41.8 cm
Kunstmuseum Bern, Hermann und
Margrit Rupf-Stiftung   page 181

Death and fire, 1940, 332
Oil and coloured paste on burlap
Original frame
46.7 x 44.6 cm
Zentrum Paul Klee, Bern   page 191

Departure of the adventurer, 1939, 735
Watercolour and pencil on paper
on cardboard
21.5 x 27 cm
Private collection, Germany   page 147

Detailed passion: touched to the core,
1940, 180
Chalk on paper on cardboard
29.5 x 21 cm
Zentrum Paul Klee, Bern   page 182

Dialogue between tree and man, 1939, 403
Pencil on paper on cardboard
20.9 x 29.7 cm
Zentrum Paul Klee, Bern
Livia Klee Donation   page 143

Difficult resurrection, 1939, 221
Pencil on paper on cardboard
21.5 x 27 cm
Zentrum Paul Klee, Bern   page 136

Do I fall, too?, 1940, 119
Pen on paper on cardboard
21.4 x 27 cm
Zentrum Paul Klee, Bern   page 139

Drinking companion, 1931, 280
Chalk on paper on cardboard
32.9 x 20.9 cm
Zentrum Paul Klee, Bern   page 158

Early sorrow, 1938, 318
Oil, watercolour and scratched drawing
on primed burlap on cardboard
34.4 x 45 cm
Zentrum Paul Klee, Bern   page 174

Ecce …., 1940, 138
Chalk on paper on cardboard
29.7 x 21.1 cm
Zentrum Paul Klee, Bern
Livia Klee Donation   pages 17, 183, 239

Eidola: erstwhile philosopher, 1940, 101
Chalk on paper on cardboard
29.7 x 21 cm
Zentrum Paul Klee, Bern   page 208

Emigrating, 1933, 181
Chalk on paper on cardboard
32.9 x 21 cm
Zentrum Paul Klee, Bern   page 26

Eyes in the landscape, 1940, 41
Wax paint on primed burlap
32 x 85 cm
Kunstmuseum Winterthur
Legat Dr. E. und C. Friedrich-Jezler   page 180

Final renunciation, 1938, 372
Pencil on paper on cardboard
29.9 x 20.9 cm
Private collection, Switzerland, on extended
loan to the Zentrum Paul Klee, Bern   page 180

Fleeing on wheels, 1939, 653
Pencil on paper on cardboard
20.9 x 29.7 cm
Zentrum Paul Klee, Bern   page 144

Flight, 1940, 121
Pen on paper on cardboard
21.4 x 27 cm
Zentrum Paul Klee, Bern   page 145

Flora on the rocks, 1940, 343
Oil and tempera on burlap; original frame
90.7 x 70.5 cm
Kunstmuseum Bern   page 231

Forgetful angel, 1939, 880
Pencil on paper on cardboard
29.5 x 21 cm
Zentrum Paul Klee, Bern   page 198

Glass façade, 1940, 288
Wax paint on burlap on canvas
71.3 x 95.7 cm
Zentrum Paul Klee, Bern   page 219

Hand puppets (untitled, from l to r):
Genie of the matchbox, 1925, 27 cm
Mr. Death, 1916, 35 cm
Bandit, 1923, 58 cm
all Zentrum Paul Klee, Bern
Livia Klee Donation   page 114

'He' a dictator too! 1933, 339
Pencil on paper on cardboard
29.5 x 21.8 cm
Zentrum Paul Klee, Bern
Livia Klee Donation   page 161

He can't escape, 1940, 231
Chalk on paper on cardboard
29.6 x 21 cm
Private collection, Switzerland, on extended
loan to the Zentrum Paul Klee, Bern   page 145

Herring, for me?!, 1939, 658
Pencil on paper on cardboard
29.5 x 21 cm
Location unknown   page 66

High spirits, 1939, 1251
Oil and coloured paste on paper on burlap
Original frame
101 x 130 cm
Zentrum Paul Klee, Bern   page 138

In the antechamber of angelhood,
1939, 845
Pencil on paper on cardboard
29.5 x 21 cm
Zentrum Paul Klee, Bern   page 196

Insula dulcamara, 1938, 481
Oil and coloured paste on paper on burlap
Original frame
88 x 176 cm
Zentrum Paul Klee, Bern   page 171

Lonely end, 1934, 183
Pencil on paper on cardboard
20.6/21.2 x 46.8/45.3 cm
Zentrum Paul Klee, Bern   page 164

Manhunt, 1933, 115
Pencil on paper on cardboard
23/23.2 x 32.3 cm
Zentrum Paul Klee, Bern   page 126

Marked man, 1935, 146
Oil and watercolour on primed
gauze on cardboard
32 x 29 cm
Kunstsammlung Nordrhein-
Westfalen, Düsseldorf   pages 16, 125, 237

Mask: pain, 1938, 235
Chalk on paper on cardboard
21 x 27.1 cm
Zentrum Paul Klee, Bern   page 57

Masks at twilight, 1938, 486
Coloured paste on cardboard
48.3 x 34.7 cm
Private collection, Switzerland   page 207

Monologue of the kitten, 1938, 426
Pencil on paper on cardboard
29.9 x 20.9 cm
Zentrum Paul Klee, Bern
Livia Klee Donation   page 208

Mon dieu!, 1939, 551
Pencil on paper on cardboard
29.7 x 20.9 cm
Zentrum Paul Klee, Bern   page 145

Mourning, 1934, 8
Watercolour and gouache
on paper on cardboard
48.7 x 32.1 cm
Zentrum Paul Klee, Bern   page 123

Navigatio mala, 1939, 563
Pencil on paper on cardboard
20.9 x 29.7 cm
Zentrum Paul Klee, Bern   page 148

Never again that dish!, 1939, 659
Pencil on paper on cardboard
36 x 19 cm
Private collection, Switzerland   page 66

Night flower, 1938, 118
Coloured paste on primed canvas
on cardboard
32.4 x 28.5 cm
Sprengel Museum, Hannover   page 227

Oh! above me!, 1939, 201
Pencil on paper on cardboard
29.7 x 20.9 cm
Zentrum Paul Klee, Bern   page 137

Old man counting, 1929, 60
Pen and pencil on paper
on cardboard
Location unknown   page 209

Outbreak of fear, 1939, 27
Pen on paper on cardboard
27 x 21.5 cm
Zentrum Paul Klee, Bern   page 130

Outbreak of fear III, 1939, 124
Watercolour on primed paper
on cardboard
63.5 x 48.1 cm
Zentrum Paul Klee, Bern   page 131

Plant according to rules, 1935, 91
Watercolour on paper
on cardboard
25.8 x 36.9 cm
Kunstmuseum Bern, Hermann und
Margrit Rupf-Stiftung   page 44

Revolution of the viaduct, 1937, 153
Oil on primed cotton
60 x 50 cm
Hamburger Kunsthalle   page 167

Rigidity, 1933, 187
Pencil on paper on cardboard
32.9 x 20.9 cm
Zentrum Paul Klee, Bern   page 25

Rise from the dead!, 1938, 478
Pen on paper on cardboard
29.8 x 20.9 cm
Zentrum Paul Klee, Bern   page 136

River gorge near Y, 1939, 734
Watercolour and pencil
on paper on cardboard
27 x 21.3 cm
Zentrum Paul Klee, Bern
Private loan   page 149

Rower in the narrowness, 1939, 728
Pencil on paper on cardboard
27 x 21.5 cm
Zentrum Paul Klee, Bern   page 148

Rowing competition, 1940, 172
Chalk on paper on cardboard
21 x 29.5 cm
Zentrum Paul Klee, Bern   page 150

Scholar, 1933, 286
Watercolour and brush
on primed
gauze on wooden panel
Original frame
35 x 26.5 cm
Private collection, Switzerland   page 23

Shattered, 1939, 1065
Chalk on paper on cardboard
29.6 x 42 cm
Zentrum Paul Klee, Bern   page 142

Sick man in a boat, 1940, 66
Chalk on paper on cardboard
20.5 x 41.6 cm
Zentrum Paul Klee, Bern   page 151

Something better is nigh, 1939, 204
Pencil on paper on cardboard
29.7 x 20.9 cm
Zentrum Paul Klee, Bern   page 137

SOS, the last signal, 1939, 652
Pencil on paper on cardboard
20.9 x 29.7 cm
Zentrum Paul Klee, Bern   page 143

Stick it out!, 1940, 337
Pastel on paper on cardboard
29.6 x 20.9 cm
Zentrum Paul Klee, Bern   page 182

Struck from the list, 1933, 424
Oil on paper on cardboard
31.5 x 24 cm
Zentrum Paul Klee, Bern
Livia Klee Donation   page 22

Suddenly rigid, 1940, 205
Chalk on paper on cardboard
29.6 x 21 cm
Zentrum Paul Klee, Bern   pages 181, 238

Super-chess, 1937, 141
Oil on burlap; original frame
120 x 110 cm
Kunsthaus Zürich   page 236

Supposed celebrities, 1933, 151
Pencil on paper on cardboard
24.1 x 20.8 cm
Private collection, Switzerland, on extended
loan to the Zentrum Paul Klee, Bern   page 162

Swiss landscape, 1919, 46
Watercolour on primed linen
on paper on cardboard
Location unknown   page 36

Symbiosis, 1934, 131
Pencil on paper on cardboard
48.2 x 32 cm
Location unknown   pages 6, 230

Symptom, to be diagnosed
in good time, 1935, 17
Pencil on paper on cardboard
17.9 x 27.9 cm
Zentrum Paul Klee, Bern   page 168

Taking leave, 1938, 352
Coloured paste on paper
on cardboard
50.7 x 7.3/9.3 cm
Zentrum Paul Klee, Bern   page 175

Target recognized, 1933, 350
Pencil on paper on cardboard
24.4 x 27.5 cm
Zentrum Paul Klee, Bern   page 163

The eye, 1938, 315
Pastel on burlap
45/46 x 64.5/66.5 cm
Private collection, Switzerland, on extended
loan to the Zentrum Paul Klee, Bern   page 56

The grey man and the coast, 1938, 125
Coloured paste on burlap
105 x 71 cm
Zentrum Paul Klee
Livia Klee Donation   page 146

The soul departs, 1934, 211
Watercolour on primed cardboard
Original frame
30.5 x 49.3 cm
Zentrum Paul Klee, Bern   page 165

261

The tightrope walker, 1923, 121
Oil transfer drawing, pencil and
watercolour on paper on cardboard
48.7 x 32.2
Zentrum Paul Klee, Bern page 140

The unlucky star, 1939, 538
Pencil on paper on cardboard
29.7 x 20.9 cm
Zentrum Paul Klee, Bern page 152

This star teaches bending,
1940, 344
Coloured paste on paper
on cardboard
37.8 x 41.3 cm
Zentrum Paul Klee, Bern
Livia Klee Donation pages 10, 152

Trees by the water, 1933, 442
Pastel on primed canvas
on cardboard
45 x 55 cm
Private collection, Italy page 226

Tribute, 1933, 299
Chalk on paper on cardboard
27.3 x 27 cm
Zentrum Paul Klee, Bern page 160

Twilight flowers, 1940, 42
Wax paint on burlap
35 x 80 cm
Kunstmuseum Bern
Livia Klee Donation page 195

Under grand protection,
1939, 1137
Chalk on paper on cardboard
29.5 x 20.8 cm
Zentrum Paul Klee, Bern page 197

Underwater garden, 1939, 746
Oil on canvas
Original frame
100 x 80 cm
Private collection, Switzerland page 229

Unstable signpost, 1937, 45
Watercolour on paper on cardboard
43.8 x 20.9/19.8 cm
Private collection, Switzerland, on extended
loan to the Zentrum Paul Klee, Bern page 141

Untitled (Angel of death), ca. 1940
Oil on canvas
51 x 66.4 cm
Private collection, Switzerland, on extended
loan to the Zentrum Paul Klee, Bern page 200

Untitled (Last still life), 1940
Oil on canvas
100 x 80.5 cm
Zentrum Paul Klee, Bern
Livia Klee Donation page 232

Vessel for salve, 1940, 169
Wax paint on burlap on cardboard
28.2 x 12/13.8 cm
Zentrum Paul Klee
Livia Klee Donation page 84

Villa R, 1919, 153 (Inv. Nr. 1744)
Oil on cardboard
26.5 x 22 cm
Kunstmuseum Basel page 218

Violence, 1933, 138
Chalk on paper on cardboard
17.1 x 20.9 cm
Zentrum Paul Klee, Bern page 159

Whence? where? whither?, 1940, 60
Watercolour, red chalk and chalk
on paper on cardboard
29.7 x 20.8 cm
Private collection, Switzerland page 184

Abbreviations for Document Locations

AWG	Archive Will Grohmann
BK/CGPP	Bibliothèque Kandinsky Centre Georges Pompidou, Paris
HMRS	Hermann und Margrit Rupf-Stiftung (Foundation), Kunstmuseum Bern
MoMAANY/VP	Museum of Modern Art Archives, New York/Valentin Papers
MoMAANY/NP	Museum of Modern Art Archives, New York/Neumann Papers
NFKB	Nachlass-Verwaltung Familie Klee (Paul Klee's Estate, Bern)
NSMP	Norton Simon Museum Pasadena – The Blue Four Galka Scheyer Collection
PBD	Privatbesitz, Deutschland (Private collection, Germany) (Rudolf Probst Estate)
SFB	Stefan Frey, Bern
SLB/SLA	Schweizerische Landesbibliothek (Swiss State Library), Bern/Schweizerisches Literaturarchiv (Swiss Literary Archive), Bern
ZPKB/SFK	Zentrum Paul Klee, Bern/ Schenkung Familie Klee (Klee Family Donation)

Photographic Credits

Frontispiece: Charlotte Weidler, New York, N.Y.

Fig.		Page
2.	Anne-Marie Klee-Coll	7
3.	Peter Friedli, Bern	8
5.	Photographer unknown	12
6.	Fee Meisel	12
7.	Court photographer Blankhorn, Göttingen	13
8.	Felix Klee	14
9.	Emil Vollenweider, Bern	14
10.	Kunstmuseum Bern Photographer unknown	15
11.	Kunstsammlung Nordrhein-Westfalen, Walter Klein, Düsseldorf	16
13.	Fernand Rausser, Bolligen (Bern), from: Liebesbriefe an Bern Verlag Stämpfli + Cie AG Bern, Bern 1995, p. 91	18
14.	M. Vollenweider & Son, Bern	19
15.	M. Vollenweider, Bern	20
17.	M. Vollenweider, Bern	21
22.	Photographer unknown	27
23.	Felix Klee	27
28.	Fernand Rausser, Bolligen (Bern), from: Liebesbriefe an Bern, Verlag Stämpfli + Cie AG Bern, Bern 1995, p. 90	37
30.	Pediatric Clinic of the University of Bern	40
31.	From: Pediatric Dermatology, 3rd edition (Ed. Schachner, Lawrence, A., and Hansen, Ronald, C.), Mosby-Verlag (Elsevier Company) 2003, p. 1060	40
32.	Dermatology Clinic, University of Bern	41
33.	Dermatology Clinic, University of Bern	41
38.	Lily Klee	47
40.	Photographer unknown	49
41.	Dermatology Clinic, University of Bern	50
42.	Dermatology Clinic, University of Bern	50
43.	Dermatology Clinic, University of Bern	51
44.	Dermatology Clinic, University of Bern	53
45.	Felix Klee	54
46.	Walter Henggeler, © Keystone, Zurich	55
49.	Dermatology Clinic, University of Bern	58
50.	Dermatology Clinic, University of Bern	58
51.	Rheumatology Clinic, University of Bern	59
52.	Rheumatology Clinic, University of Bern	59
53.	Rheumatology Clinic, University of Bern	61
54.	Dermatology Clinic, University of Bern	62
55.	Rheumatology Clinic, University of Bern	62
56.	Rheumatology Clinic, University of Bern	63
57.	Rheumatology Clinic, University of Bern	64
58.	Rheumatology Clinic, University of Bern	64
63.	Rheumatology Clinic, University of Bern	71

Fig.		Page
64.	Rheumatology Clinic, University of Bern	73
65.	Photographer unknown	74
66.	Photographer unknown	74
70.	Jürg Spiller	77
71.	Sadao Wada	77
72.	Walter Henggeler, © Keystone Zurich	78
73.	Felix Klee	78
74.	Felix Klee	79
77.	Photographer unknown	93
78.	Photographer unknown	94
79.	Lily Klee	95
80.	Lily Klee	96
81.	Charlotte Weidler, New York, N.Y.	99
82.	Charlotte Weidler, New York, N.Y.	100
84.	Dermatology Clinic, University of Bern	102
85.	Dermatology Clinic, University of Bern	103
86.	Charlotte Weidler, New York, N.Y.	105
87.	Felix Klee	107
88.	Photographer unknown	109
89.	Photographer unknown	110
90.	E. Steinemann, Locarno	111
91.	Dermatology Clinic, University of Bern	112
92.	Photographer unknown	113
94.	Photographer unknown	121
96.	Kunstsammlung Nordrhein-Westfalen, Walter Klein, Düsseldorf	125
136.	Hamburger Kunsthalle, Elke Walford	167
144.	Kunstmuseum Winterthur, Hans Humm, Zurich	180
168.	From: Klaus Gallwitz, Picasso Laureatus, p. 214, no. 375, Verlag C. J. Bucher AG, Luzern 1971, Photographer unknown	214
169.	Postcard 'Der Sturm' (The Storm)	215
170.	Kunstmuseum Basel, Martin P. Bühler	218
175.	Sprengel Museum, Hannover, Michael Herling, Aline Gwose	227
181.	Walter Henggeler, © Keystone, Zurich	235
182.	Kunsthaus Zürich	236
183.	Kunstsammlung Nordrhein-Westfalen, Walter Klein, Düsseldorf	237

Inside back flap: Fernand Rausser, Bolligen (Bern)

Note:
All reproductions of the works of Paul Klee, unless otherwise stated:
Peter Lauri, Bern,
and Department of Image and Media Technology, University of Basel

Appendices

Research into Paul Klee's Illness

8. Conversations between Professor Alfred Krebs, the author and Felix Klee, Bern, November 9, 1979 and July 23, 1981.

9. Telephone conversation between Dr. Dietrich Schorer, Zollikofen (Bern), son of Dr. Gerhard Schorer, and Professor Alfred Krebs, Bern, in 1979: there were no medical records for Paul Klee among his father's papers.

    Telephone conversation between Dr. Dietrich Schorer, Zollikofen (Bern), and the author, September 8, 1998: his father had never talked to the family about Paul Klee's treatment or illness.

    Letter from Dr. Hans Christoph von Tavel, CH–1169 Yens (Waadt) to the author, February 16, 2000: his uncle, Dr. Gerhard Schorer, had left no records relating to Paul Klee's illness.

    Verbal communication between Marie Stössel-Schorer, Bern, and the author: as Dr. Gerhard Schorer's daughter she also had no specific knowledge about Paul Klee's illness.

10. Telephone conversation between Professor Hans Jürg Schatzmann, Bern, son of Dr. Max Schatzmann, and Professor Alfred Krebs in 1979: he had no written records of his father's relating to Paul Klee's treatment.

    Telephone conversation between Professor Hans Jürg Schatzmann, Bern, and the author, April 28, 2001: his father had been friends with Dr. Gerhard Schorer. He could imagine that his father might have seen Paul Klee in his capacity as Dr. Schorer's locum. He remembered his father saying that Dr. Schorer had spoken to him about Paul Klee's illness. His father had, however, never referred to a diagnosis or tentative diagnosis. Author's note: F.-J. Beer mentioned in his article 'Le centenaire de Paul Klee' (Beer/ML 1980, p. 247) that Paul Klee had had two doctors (without quoting a source): Dr. Gerhard Schorer and Dr. Max Schatzmann. Beer possibly got this information from Felix Klee. However, the latter could not confirm to the author on November 9, 1979 whether Dr. Schatzmann had ever treated his father as locum to Dr. Schorer. There is also no evidence of this in Paul and Lily Klee's letters.

11. Telephone conversation between Gerold Lotmar, Zurich, grandson of Dr. Fritz Lotmar, and the author, April 17, 2001: he had no documents of his grandfather's relating to Paul Klee's illness. In addition to his private practice, Dr. Lotmar held a teaching position at the University of Bern. Cf. 'Festschrift der Schweiz. Zeitschrift für Neurologie und Psychiatrie', vol. 18, Zurich 1949: 'Dedicated to Dr. Fritz Lotmar, lecturer, on the occasion of his 70th birthday, October 26, 1948'. This is the first time that Dr. Lotmar's position as a lecturer at the University of Bern is mentioned in writings about Paul Klee.

    Telephone conversation between Paula Lotmar, CH–8802 Kilchberg (Zurich), daughter of Dr. Fritz Lotmar, and the author, May 3, 2001: she confirmed Gerold Lotmar's statement. Her father had never treated Paul Klee, but had spoken to him about his illness on numerous occasions.

12. Professor Oscar Naegeli had no children. It has not been possible to make contact with any of his close relatives.

13. Telephone conversation between Sister Virginia Bachmann (Mother Superior of the Clinica Sant' Agnese in Locarno-Muralto from 1967 to 1983) and Professor Alfred Krebs, Bern, in 1979: there were no medical records for Paul Klee at the clinic. All that was found were the results of a urine test which had been taken during the last days of the artist's life. Sister Virginia subsequently sent these test results to Professor Krebs in Bern. I would like to thank Sister Virginia Bachmann for her endeavors and Sister Andrea Holbein, archivist at the Kloster Ingebohl (Schwyz), for the information she provided about Sister Virginia Bachmann's time as Mother Superior at the Clinica Sant' Agnese, November 24, 2001.

    Telephone conversation between Sister Virginia Bachmann and the author, April 29, 1981: despite a renewed search, no more documents had come to light since 1979 relating to Paul Klee's period of hospitalization at the Clinica Sant' Agnese. In 1940 the clinic was a secondary hospital with no resident chief physician. The attending physicians would have taken the records of their hospital patients back to their practices and stored them there.

14. Conversation in Bern, September 20, 1983. Felix Klee's comments are referred to separately throughout the text.

15. Telephone conversation between Professor Max Huggler, CH–7554 Sent (Grisons), and the author, August 15, 1981. These comments are also referred to separately in the text.

16. Telephone conversation between Maja Allenbach, Bern, and the author, August 15, 1981: she had no knowledge of Paul Klee's illness. At the artist's request they never spoke about it.

    Verbal communication between Henriette Sechehaye, CH–3653 Oberhofen near Thun, and the author in 1981: she had been Paul Klee's last private student (1940). He had made a deep impression on her. She could not say anything about his illness. There is also no information on this subject in an article by Stefan Haenni, Oberhofen am Thunersee, and Heidi Zingg-Messerli, Thun, on the occasion of the painter's 90th birthday in the Thuner Tagblatt of April 3, 1997, or in the monograph which appeared in 2005 in the Bern Archiv-Arte 'Henriette Sechehaye (1907–1999). Paul Klee's last student' by Inga Vatter-Jensen.

    Telephone conversation between Agnes Inderbitzin, CH–6440 Brunnen (Schwyz) and the author, April 29, 1981: in 1940 she had been governess at the Sanatorium Viktoria in Locarno-Orselina. She remembered Paul Klee as a 'friendly, very entertaining patient'. However, she knew nothing about his illness.

    Telephone conversation between Gertrud Wyss-Trachsel, Bern, and the author, July 24, 1981, confirmed in writing, July 31, 1981: her late husband, Paul Wyss-Trachsel, had been an art master at Bern Grammar School. The couple had lived near to Paul and Lily Klee, at Kistlerweg 36. They had met Paul Klee several times, but had not noticed any signs of illness. One of her friends, Elsa Amman, was a seamstress and had been to the Klees' house on several occasions. But, when asked, she was also unable to give any more specific information about the artist's illness, other than that he ate little and often. She had not noticed any changes to his hands.

17. Letter from Elisabetta Uehlinger, widow of Dr. Enrico Uehlinger, Locarno-Minusio, to the author, November 20, 1980: 'Unfortunately, I have to disappoint you. As you can see from the enclosed article [Grandini, Sergio, "Il soggiorno di Paul Klee nel Ticino" in an (unknown) Ticino newspaper, February 9, 1980] there are no more documents held at the Clinica Sant' Agnese.' In this article, Grandini quotes the answer he received from Dr. Enrico Uehlinger, referred to in note 28 (p. 14), after he asked him if he could give him any information about Paul Klee's illness or about his stay at the Clinica Sant' Agnese. In 1978 Dr. Uehlinger was Chief of Internal Medicine at the Clinica Sant' Agnese in Locarno-Muralto. I would like to thank Mrs. Elisabetta Uehlinger for her letter and for Sergio Grandini's article.

    Telephone conversation between Dr. Fritz Speck, CH–6945 Origlio (Ticino), and the author, June 4, 1981: two years after Paul Klee's death he had worked as a doctor at the Clinica Sant' Agnese. He could not say anything about Paul Klee's illness. What he could say, however, was that in 1981 none of the attending physicians who worked at the Clinica Sant' Agnese in 1940 were still alive, and that the attending physicians – including Dr. Hermann Bodmer – did not keep the medical records of their clinic patients at the clinic itself, but at their private practices.

    Telephone conversation between Giovanna Sciaroni, widow of Dr. Roberto Sciaroni, Locarno-Muralto, and the author, July 23, 1981: her husband had been Chief of Surgery at the Clinica Sant' Agnese. She knew nothing specific about Paul Klee's illness.

    Telephone conversation between Dr. Walter Hadorn, Bern, Emeritus Professor at the Medical Clinic, Inselspital, Bern, and the author, August 15, 1981: he had not known Paul Klee personally and could give no particulars about his illness.

Telephone conversation between Hanny Charlet-Zubrügg, Bern, widow of Dr. Jean Charlet (1906–1990), the last dentist to treat Paul Klee in Bern, and the author, September 14, 1998: there were no records of Paul Klee's treatment in her husband's estate.

Telephone conversation between Esther Hirt-Charlet, Lausanne, daughter of Dr. Jean Charlet, and the author, May 3, 2001: she confirmed her mother's statement. Her father had been a close friend of Paul Klee's. He had always given him special treatment, seeing him on Saturdays and sometimes at Klee's home. The artist had been grateful to her father for his attentive treatment. Paul Klee had been a fine man. I would like to thank Hanny Charlet and Esther Hirt for their research and for the information they provided.

Telephone conversations between Sister Paula Maria Rohner, Kloster Ingebohl (Schwyz), and the author, March 24, 2001, and March 28, 2001: in the 1940 annual report of the Clinica Sant' Agnese there was no mention of Paul Klee. Around 1985 the Clinic became a private convalescent home called 'Casa per convalescenza Sant' Agnese'. The former Sanatorium Viktoria in Locarno-Orselina was sold to a group of doctors around 1991, re-named 'Clinica Santa Croce' and run by Menzinger nuns. I would like to thank Sister Paula Maria Rohner for her research and for the information she provided.

[18] Telephone conversation between the director of the Tarasp Sanatorium (Grisons) and Professor Alfred Krebs in 1979: the records from Paul Klee's stay in 1936 no longer existed.

[19] As Chief Physician of the Dermatology Clinic of the University of Bern, Professor Alfred Krebs had access to the Clinic's archives in 1979: there were no medical records or other documents referring to the examination of Paul Klee in 1936 by Professor Oscar Naegeli.

[20] Professor Krebs received this information in 1979 from the Institute for Diagnostic Radiology, Inselspital, Bern.

Letter from Professor Peter Vock, Director of the Institute for Diagnostic Radiology, University of Bern DRNN, Inselspital, Bern, to the author, June 20, 2001: 'Since around 2001 we have been forced to destroy all patient files which have been inactive for more than 20 years, due to lack of space. It was therefore very unlikely that we would find any examination records for Paul Klee. However, we asked our Senior Archivist to look into your request. He has now informed us that he was unable to find any documents relating to the artist. This does not prove one way or the other whether Paul Klee was ever examined at the Institute of Radiology at the Inselspital, as the relevant administrative documents would have been destroyed anyway due to lack of space, as they are more than twenty years old.' I would like to thank Professor Vock and the Senior Archivist of his institute for their efforts. I would also like to thank Dr. Anton J. Seiler, cantonal doctor, Bern, at the Cantonal Archive in Bern, for his clarification of the regulations pertaining to the keeping of medical records in 1940: at that time there was no legal obligation to keep records: cf. letter from Dr. Seiler to the author, February 6, 2002.

[21] Telephone conversation between Monika Giger and Elisabeth Voland of the 'Centre Valaisan de Pneumologie' in Montana (Wallis) and the author, December 13, 2001: the 'Clinique Cécil' no longer existed. In earlier times it had been a 'Dépendance' of the then 'Sanatorium Valaisan de Pneumologie' (now 'Centre Valaisan de Pneumologie'). No patient records from that time still existed.

Telephone conversation between Drs. Gabriel and Gilberte Barras, CH–3963 Montana (Wallis) – Dr. Gabriel Barras was Chief Physician of the above-mentioned sanatorium from 1954 to 1986 – and the author, December 13, 2001: they confirmed what Mrs. Giger and Mrs. Voland had said. The first Chief Physician of the sanatorium had been Dr. Mauderli, who had died about 20 years earlier. Even the sanatorium's administrator from that time, Mr. Duc, was no longer alive. The former 'Clinique Cécil' had been sold 25 years earlier to the Montana municipality, and the local council now had its offices there.

Telephone conversation between Daniel Barras, secrétaire de la commune de Montana (clerk to the municipality) and the author, December 13, 2001: no patient records had been given to the municipality upon purchase of the building 25 years earlier.

Telephone conversations between Hans Robert Ammann, Public Archivist in CH–1950 Sion (Wallis) and the author, December 13 and 19, 2001: the 'Pension Cécil' had originally been a private hotel. It was purchased by the Wallis Canton in 1946. Until 1965 it had however been known as the 'Clinique Cécil' (as mentioned above) and had been a 'Dépendance' of the then 'Sanatorium Valaisan de Pneumologie' for non-infectious tuberculosis patients. The 'Clinique Cécil' had closed in 1965 [Mr. Amman was kind enough to send me photocopies of archive extracts, ref. 5710–2, pp. 12 and 13]. Patient records had been kept at the 'Sanatorium Valaisan de Pneumologie'. In the public archive only the names of the patients who had taken treatment at the 'Clinique Cécil' were recorded. Paul Klee's name is not among them [he was in Montana in 1936 and the 'Clinique Cécil' did not exist as a 'clinic' until 1946]. I would like to thank the people mentioned above for their willingness to help, their research and the information they provided.

[22] Letter from Diana Bodmer, daughter of Dr. Hermann Bodmer, Zurich, to the author, June 8, 2001: she had no medical records of her father's relating to Paul Klee and knew nothing about his illness, as she was still a child in 1940. In her father's obituary, written by Dr. Otto Hug in the Schweiz. Medizin. Wochenschrift 1948; 21: 523, which Diana Bodmer kindly sent to me, there is no mention of Paul Klee.

[23] See note 13. The test results are referred to on p. 73.

Hans Klee's Personality

[34] One of his students at the cantonal teachers' college in Hofwil, Karl Friedrich Iseli, characterized Hans Klee in the following way: humorous, a little sarcastic, an outstanding teacher, an 'original' (personal communication by Karl Friedrich Iseli to the author, CH–3617 Fahrni, July 6, 1988). The artist Marguerite-Frey Surbek, who as a young artist regularly had her works appraised by Paul Klee, had a similar impression: 'Klee's father's irrepressible humor could be at its most waspish if any spirit of excess or vacuousness tried to make inroads into his clear and logical appraisal methods, and he was particularly wary of the hero worship which at that time was starting to cloud people's judgment in artistic circles. […] It is essential for anyone researching Paul Klee's early years to delve deeply into his father's amazing personality, not only through the recollections of his friends, but above all by reviving memories of the 53 years he spent at the college. Bernese writer Simon Gfeller devotes an enjoyable chapter to him entitled "Hans Imbart", which expands on his merciless way of making judgements and his striking sense of humor.' (Frey-Surbek 1976, p. 13 f). See also page 203, note 605.

Paul Klee's Efforts to Gain Swiss Citizenship

[65] Kehrli, Jakob Otto, Why Paul Klee's desire to die as a Swiss citizen could not be fulfilled, in: 'Der Bund' no. 6, Bern, January 5, 1962.

[66] Ibid. Dr. Jakob Kehrli wrote in his newspaper article of January 5, 1962: '[…] On July 11, 1939, Paul Klee was officially interviewed [by the Security and Criminal Investigation Department of the Bern police]. […] The very next day the Security and Criminal Investigation Department wrote a report on his assimilation: "The applicant was born and raised in Bern and completed his schooling there. He then studied in Munich and was appointed to the post of professor at the Bauhaus School in Weimar in 1920. Until his return in 1933 he was a profes-

sor at the Düsseldorf Academy of Fine Arts. He relinquished this position because he was temporarily suspended and would certainly have been subsequently dismissed, as his work was considered to be '"degenerate art"' by the regime in Germany at that time. After a repetition of the reasons which led him to return to Bern, the report continues: Professor Conrad von Mandach, Curator of the Bern Museum of Fine Arts, described him (Klee) as an outstanding artist. He is no longer recognized in Germany because his art is '"beyond all understanding"', and because he is somewhat left-leaning, so his art is branded '"degenerate art"'. The Bern Police Security and Criminal Intelligence Department has no prejudicial information on the above-named [Paul Klee] [...]."'

Letter from Dr. Max Huggler to the cantonal police headquarters in Bern, attn. Mr. Krebs, lawyer, Bern, November 3, 1939 (Swiss Federal Archive): 'Following a phone call from Officer Hofstetter, I have taken the liberty of giving you below my estimation of the artist, Professor Paul Klee.

Klee represents an artistic movement which is clearly recognized and understood by experts to be a feasible and legitimate art form. Along with Kandinsky and Picasso, Klee is one of the few truly productive artists of this movement who are continuing to work even after a somewhat artificial boom in demand has subsided, who are developing in a legitimate way and whose international reputation remains undiminished.

As far as the fears that have been communicated to me are concerned, please allow me to make the following observations. Nobody should seriously think that there will be some kind of damage to local or Swiss art. There is already a general impression both in Switzerland and abroad that Klee is of Swiss nationality. The appreciation of his work is limited to a very small number of friends and collectors who will not allow a change in his nationality or residence to affect their art purchases or their interest in him. This and other similar artistic movements will not gain strength at the moment, and probably not even in the foreseeable future, as true understanding and support for them will remain limited to a small number of die-hard enthusiasts.

Klee has directly and indirectly stimulated and challenged artists from totally different fields through his paintings, his outstanding personality and his remarkable knowledge of all things artistic.

Klee has already earned himself a clearly defined place in the art history of the last decade, and his significant contribution to the development of art deserves to be recognized.

If you require any further information, please do not hesitate to contact me.

Yours respectfully, Dr. Huggler, Director of the Bern Kunsthalle.'

[67] One of the policemen involved in the Paul Klee naturalization case wrote in a report to the Federal Justice and Police Department, October 31, 1939: 'Des peintres bien connus de chez nous estiment que cette "Neue Richtung" fantaisiste de Klee leur serait funeste, si, bénéficiant de la protection de certaines personnes compétentes, ce genre de peinture devait prendre pied dans notre pays. Ce serait une insulte à l'adresse du vrai art de la peinture, un avilissement du bon goût et des idées saines de la population en général', quoted from Frey 1990, p. 119. In further reports from November 4 and 9, 1939, the same policeman wrote that Klee's supporters were primarily of the 'Jewish race'. To the report of November 9, 1939 he attached a copy of Klee's watercolor 'Swiss Landscape', 1919, 46 (illustration 27). The picture shows cows, fir trees and a Swiss flag. The report-writer comments on how stupid these animals look: 'Ce tableau ne parlerait-il pas tout simplement, sans ambages, de ce que certains se plaisent à représenter sous la désignation de "Kuhschweizer"?', quoted from Frey 1990, p. 120. Something similar is mentioned by Otto Karl Werckmeister, in: Werckmeister 1987, p. 52, in reference to an article by Meta La Roche in 'Die Schweiz, Jean Arp, Paul Klee und ein geheimer Polizeirapport', St. Galler Tagblatt, July 13, 1957.

[68] Klee 1940, p. 14.

[69] The Zurich art historian Carola Giedion-Welcker visited Klee immediately after the appearance of the defamatory article: 'He [Klee] seemed angry and depressed by the critical gaffes by the press, which he thought could have a dangerous influence on his life in Switzerland, as they threatened to adversely affect his application to the Bern authorities for Swiss citizenship, or could even derail it completely. I found this out after I rather naively suggested that his inner circle would never pay any attention to such populist allusions to mental abnormalities.

He did not want to discuss this any more, as he really felt it was beneath him, but he dryly remarked that any suspicion of something like schizophrenia (Joyce and Arp also went through similar trials) would not exactly encourage the officials to help him with his resettlement plans'. (Giedion-Welcker 2000, p. 100 f.)

[70] Dr. Jakob Kehrli writes in his newspaper report of January 5, 1962 (see note 65): 'On January 15, 1940 Paul Klee's lawyer wrote to the Municipal Council to apply for citizenship of the Bern municipality (Bern Police Headquarters, Department of Citizenship). On March 12, 1940 Paul Klee handed in an additional form that was required, and as early as March 15 the police filed an application with the Municipal Council, asking them to grant the applicant citizenship of Bern. This application was forwarded to the Municipal Citizenship Commission with a recommendation for acceptance on March 28. The Commission is made up of town councillors and is responsible for considering applications made to the Municipal Council. The Commission decided, as a matter of caution, to ask the applicant why, at the age of 61, he was applying for Swiss citizenship. They felt this question was justified in light of the general opinion that naturalization should be suspended while the war was on, and that it was in the best interests of the applicant. As the latter was not in Bern at the time, and so could not be interviewed personally by the Commission, he was asked by letter. Paul Klee sent his reply from the Clinica Sant' Agnese in Muralto Locarno on the June 19, 1940: "After completing my professional studies in 1902, I lived for several years in Bern. It became clear to me that I would need to undertake further studies and work abroad.

Like many artists at that time I was more inclined to travel.

As a result of my marriage in 1906 in Bern, I had the opportunity to move to Munich. I gradually started to enjoy some professional success. As a result of my later appointments in Weimar, Dessau and Düsseldorf, I worked for 15 years as a teacher at the respective art schools and the Academy of Fine Arts. Upon the termination of my employment, I broke all ties with the German state. I returned to Bern and as soon as possible began the process of applying for naturalization.

Yours respectfully, (signed) Paul Klee."

This letter, dictated by Paul Klee and written by his wife, was as clear as it was revealing. The artist had no reason to apply for Swiss citizenship before 1933 as he was working in the German Reich.

On June 28, 1940 – one day before he died – Paul Klee dictated another letter to the Municipal Citizenship Commission in order to further strengthen his position: "In response to your esteemed letter, I would like to inform you that, after my return to Switzerland, I made every possible attempt to set my application for citizenship in motion. The application was, however, declined. I received the residence permit in May 1939. At this point I instructed my lawyer, Dr. Fritz Trüssel, to file my application for citizenship.

Yours respectfully (signed) Paul Klee." [...]'

[71] Extract from the minutes of the meeting of the Bern Municipal Council of July 5, 1940: '[...] Item 1. Applications for citizenship. Application no. 44. The President of the Citizenship Commission, Dr. La Nicca (fr. [member of the Free Democratic Party]) withdraws applications nos. 1, [...] and 11, Klee Ernest Paul, until further notice. No. 1 for further checking and application no. 11 because the applicant has recently died and it is to be checked whether the application can be transferred to his widow.' (Bern Municipal Archive.)

Early Signs of Systemic Sclerosis on the Gums

[178] This information is from communications between Dr. med. dent. Franziska Früh-von Arx, CH–3800 Interlaken (Bern) and the author, Interlaken, April 18, 2002, and between Dr. med. dent. Karl Dula, Head of the Department of Dental Radiology at the Clinic for Oral Surgery and Stomatology, University of Bern, and the author, Bern, April 29, 2002, as well as in a summary of clinical and radiological symptoms of systemic sclerosis in the mouth, jaw and facial areas by Dr. med. dent. Jochen Jackowski, Head of the Department of Dental Surgery of the Free University D-Witten/Herdecke GmbH, given to the author, Witten, June 28, 2002. Jackowski explains: 'Stafne and Austin (1944) were the first to report X-ray evidence of widening of the periodontal space, the so-called Stafne signs, in patients with systemic sclerosis. This is considered one of the early symptoms of the disease and pathognomonic for diagnosing the disease. The uniform enlargement of the periodontal space is the distinguishing radiological criterium that allows a diagnostic differentiation between this disease and changes in the area of the alveolar socket and the root of the tooth caused by periodontal disease. Occlusal stress, which can also cause a uniform widening of the periodontal space, has to be ruled out using a dedicated occlusion analysis. The affected teeth show no or only limited mobility (Stafne and Austin 1944, Fuchsbrunner 1963) and exhibit no pockets that can be probed (Fuchsbrunner 1963). [...] The results (from Hornstein and Gerdes 1971) confirm the data from other examinations, which show that premolars and molars are more often affected than the front region (Stafne and Austin 1944, Gores 1957, Green 1962, White et al. 1977).' I am very grateful for this information!

Composition of and Medical Indicators for the Drug 'Theominal'

[103] I would like to thank pharmacist Markus Ryser, CH–3652 Hilterfingen (Bern) for information on the composition of 'Theominal' and on its manufacturer (Bayer, Leverkusen) as well as for information on theobromine (Hagers Handbuch der Pharmazeutischen Praxis, 5th ed., Springer 1991, pp. 847 f) and phenobarbital (Luminal; Arzneistoff-Profile, Gobi, Frankfurt, Ext. edition November 1983, pp.1 f), letter to the author, Hilterfingen, December 23, 2003. I would like to thank Professor Hartmut Porzig, Deputy Director of the Institute of Pharmacology, University of Bern, for additional written details about 'Theominal', Bern, December 30, 2003 (From: Meyer/Gottlieb, Experimentelle Pharmakologie als Grundlage der Arzneibehandlung, 8th ed., 1933): 'It is a mixture of theobromine and luminal (10:1) for the treatment of "general hypertension and localized vasospasms". It is further explained in this text that theobromine affected the blood vessel walls directly, making them insensitive to vasomotor impulses, while luminal was attributed a relaxant and vasodilating effect, both centrally and peripherally.'

Composition of and Medical Indicators for the Drug 'Arsen-Triferrol'

[292] 'Arsen-Triferrol' (Gehe and Co., Dresden) is a phosphorous-containing arsenic iron compound of paranucleinic acid. Iron content 0.3%, arsenic content 0.002%. In bottles up to 300 g. Use: as a blood-building agent and stomachicum (remedy for stomach problems). In: Hagers Handbuch der Pharmazeutischen Praxis, vol. II, p. 1374, Springer 1930. I would like to thank pharmacist Markus Ryser, CH–3652 Hilterfingen (Bern) for this information, Hilterfingen, December 23, 2003. I would like to thank Professor Hartmut Porzig, Deputy Director of the Institute of Pharmacology, University of Bern, for additional details about this drug, Bern, December 30, 2003: 'At that time arsenic was popular as a roborantium (pick-me-up). As an anti-anemicum (anti-anemia drug) arsenic was used in the form of As_2O_3 (arsenic trioxide). [...] However, the effectiveness of arsenic compounds for blood building was contentious even in 1933.'

Composition of and Medical Indicators for the Drug 'Campolon'

[294] I would like to thank pharmacist Markus Ryser, CH–3652 Hilterfingen (Bern) for information on the composition of 'Campolon' and on its manufacturer (Bayer, Leverkusen), as well as on indicators for its use, Hilterfingen, December 13, 2004: 'Campolon ampules', 5 ml, active ingredient: liver extract up to 5 ml, 'Campolon forte ampules', 2 ml, active ingredients: liver extract with additional 30 µg vitamin B12/ml, total 60 µg vit. B12/ampule, 'Campolon forte ampules', 10 ml, active ingredients: liver extract with additional 30 µg vit. B12/ml, total 300 µg vit. B12/ampule. Indicators: 'pernicious and other serious forms of anemia, ulcerative colitis, liver disease, agranular cytosis' (information given directly to Markus Ryser by Bayer). I would like to thank Professor Hartmut Porzig, Deputy Director of the Institute of Pharmacology, University of Bern, for additional information on 'Campolon', Bern, December 30, 2003: '"Campolon" was a non-standardized, concentrated liver extract, with normally 1 ml of extract taken from 10–20 g of liver. Pernicious anemia was given as the main indicator (Möller, Pharmakologie als theoretische Grundlage einer rationellen Pharmakotherapie, 3rd ed., 1947).'

Wassily and Nina Kandinsky's Efforts to Have Paul Klee Treated by an Acupuncturist in Paris

[423] Kandinsky 1976, pp. 199–201: 'When Kandinsky became aware of Klee's illness, incurable scleroderma, he did everything he could to help [erratum: as it has been shown that the first reference to a diagnosis of scleroderma was made after Paul Klee's death, Kandinsky could not have had any knowledge of it.] Hermann Rupf wrote to us in Paris that Klee was getting visibly thinner and did not have much longer to live. Kandinsky tried to encourage his friend to come to Paris to be treated by a famous acupuncturist. Rupf was to act as intermediary and to start by convincing Mrs. Klee of the extraordinary skill of this particular doctor.' The acupuncturist in question was Soulié-de-Mourant, who had lived for 25 years in China, where he had studied acupuncture. Although he had a doctor's diploma, he was not officially allowed to practise in Paris. He treated his patients, including Wassily and Nina Kandinsky, Jean Arp and Jean Cocteau, at the practice of a female doctor friend of his. Lily Klee evidently reacted positively to this recommendation. Nina Kandinsky continued: 'After we asked Rupf to intercede he informed us shortly thereafter that Klee was already too weak to travel to Paris and that his condition was deteriorating further. As Soulié-de-Mourant's reputation was also known in Switzerland, Kandinsky pushed Rupf: "I would have thought you could speak to Klee's doctor and ask him for his opinion. The doctor could write to Soulié-de-Mourant and describe the case. If he thinks that a visit would be necessary, he could perhaps be asked to go to Bern." All efforts were in vain. In December [1936] we received very, very grave news from Bern. Kandinsky was devastated. "We are thinking about both our friends and don't know for which of them this inevitable end is worse – for him or his wife", he wrote to Rupf. Kandinsky made one last attempt. He called Soulié-de-Mourant and tried once more to encourage him to help Klee but had to accept that it was too late. "He robbed me of this last hope. He simply said '"aucune chance"'. I asked him if he might possibly travel to Bern to make one last attempt. In reply he said that he was powerless in this case and that nothing would help."'

Details of Paul Klee's Flu Illnesses

[479] Letter from Lily Klee to Gertrud Grohmann, Bern, January 24, 1937 (AWG): 'Unfortunately, he [Paul Klee] came down with flu 10 days ago and wasn't able to get up until today. Unfortunately this bout of flu has set him back and given me more cause for concern', and letter from Lily Klee to Will Grohmann, Bern, March 29, 1939 (AWG): 'My husband has had a relatively good winter, apart from a touch of flu.'

[480] Klee Diary, no. 923: 'Shortly after New Year [1914] Felix went down with flu. I was next, a devilish cold turned into a highly interesting discharge from the sinuses. Professor Lindt, a first-rate specialist[,] was summoned. I couldn't travel back before the end of January. In Munich an encore in the bronchial tubes. Finally an end to it all and full recovery.' Cf. also Castenholz/ML 2000, p. 83, note 113.

[481] During his military service in Landshut Paul Klee remarked on March 23, 1916: 'Heavy catarrh from last Monday cleared quickly but still have something in my larynx. Bit of a temperature at night.' (Klee Diary, no. 978). On March 24 he went on: 'Unfortunately I have a fever, a mouth infection. But I'm not going to report to the medic otherwise I'll get bed-rest instead of leave. Result: I'm currently on duty with a fever' (ibid., no. 979). On March 27 he made a note: 'The medic noticed that I have a fever and so now I'm allowed to stay in my nice room, Gabelsbergerstrasse 12 II. I only have to report for meals, that's clearly understood. But on Thursday it's back to business. By then I would like to be healthy again. [...] Bit of a temperature "38", convinced the medic to prescribe 3 days of bed-rest' (ibid., nos. 980 f.). On March 28 he noted: 'Slept more peacefully during the night. Recovery?' (ibid., no. 982). And on March 30 he concluded: 'The first fever-free evening. Played music valiantly. No technical problems. On the other hand, the bed-rest stops tomorrow. Still, it's better to be healthy here' (ibid., no. 983). Cf. Castenholz/ML 2000, p. 83, note 114.

[482] Klee Diary, no. 1132. I would like to thank Erasmus Weddigen, former chief restorer at the Bern Museum of Fine Arts, for pointing this out, Bern, September 4, 1998.

Paul Klee and Lily Klee and the National Socialists

[40] Cf. Grohmann 1965, p. 77. Klee was also described as 'one of the clearest examples of intellectual decadence of the individualistic cultural era' (Scholz, Robert, Kunstgötzen stürzen, in: Deutsche Kutur-Wacht, iss. 10, 1933, p. 5, quoted from Frey 1990, p. 111).

'Der Schweizerische Beobachter', Glattbrug, 18/1990, p. 52, reported: '"He [Klee] is a typical Galician Jew [...] paints ever more demented pictures, baffling, bewildering. Leaves his students wide-eyed and speechless." This no-holds-barred characterization is to be found in the 'Deutsche Volksparole' of March 1, 1933. It refers to Paul Klee – painter and professor at the Düsseldorf Academy of Fine Arts. [...] Not long after the Nazis seized power the artist was already being accused of "not being German enough". There was talk of "Klee's ridiculous scribbles". He was summarily dismissed for being a representative of "decadent German art".'

[41] Cf. Frey 2003, p. 282. See also Klee 1990/1, n. pag. [p. 22]: 'After this trip [Paul Klee's trip to Venice] he once again had to go back and forth between Dessau and Düsseldorf. Lily accompanied him sometimes to Düsseldorf to look for a house on the Rhine, though she did not like any of them as much as their fine master's house on the Elbe. The Nazi Party had now become powerful in Anhalt, and during her absence from Dessau, they took the opportunity to search the Klee house, confiscating letters and stealing several articles of value.'

[518] Letter from Lily Klee to Will Grohmann, February 2, 1932 (AWG): 'In Anhalt there is a National Socialist majority in the newly elected State Assembly. It doesn't look good. Even Prussia has moved significantly to the right', and May 5, 1932 (AWG): 'It is sad about the Bauhaus. It doesn't look like there is much hope. The malice, narrow-mindedness, stupidity and fanaticism from the election have joined together to form an alliance that will destroy everything intellectual and cultural'; August 22, 1932 (AWG): 'Thus they closed this thriving institute that offered so much hope [the Bauhaus] out of party hatred (murdered it more like). Threw the students out on the street and sacked the teachers like unqualified servants 5 weeks before the 1st of October. It couldn't have been done in a more cowardly or boorish way. But you can see what you're going to get from a National Socialist government. They only see the interests of the party. Everything intellectual or spiritual or edifying is alien and hostile to them', and May 26, 1933 (AWG): 'I hear all sorts of opinions and voices. But I can't share their optimism. There's no sense of reality. – I'm deeply worried about the fate of my homeland in the hands of such amateurs. I spoke to 2 Christian business people: the boycott of the Jews is proving to be more and more catastrophic for the economy. Has apparently already cost us billions and is a terrible thing. It has resulted in complete isolation abroad and lost us any vestige of sympathy. ... Spiritual and intellectual people now need to stand together against this evil. In times of great danger we need to form a kind of chain.' See also letter from Paul Klee to Lily Klee, April 6, 1933.

[519] Letter from Lily Klee to Will Grohmann, April 26, 1946 (AWG): 'You know how he [Felix] had to suffer under the regime as Paul Klee's son and that he earned so little that I always had to support him. He hated the appalling Hitler regime that had persecuted his father.'

[523] Cf. for example the following additional drawings: 'Revival of manly discipline', 1933, 71, 'Fool's party', 1933, 134, 'Child murder', 1933, 113, 'When the soldiers degenerate', 1933, 72, 'What an order!', 1933, 132, 'At the burial mound', 1933, 152, 'A curse on them!', 1933, 157, 'Already stiff!', 1933, 139, 'Prisoner has visitors', 1933, 336, 'Double murder', 1933, 211, 'Gunfight' 1933, 131, 'One error after another', 1933, 352, 'Catastrophes', 1933, 368, 'Sees it coming', 1933, 387, 'Hampered defence' 1934, 184, 'She devoured our children', 1934, 173, 'Arches of the bridge stepping out of line', 1937, 111, as well as the following additional paintings: 'Barbarian general', 1932, 1, 'Struck from the list', 1933, 424, 'Secret judge' 1933, 463, 'Europa', 1933, 7, 'Tragodia', 1933, 31, 'Double face', 1933, 383, 'Fear', 1934, 202, 'They all run after him!' 1940, 325. For Klee during the year of the National Socialists' seizure of power, please see the seminal exhibition in: Munich et al. 2003/2004.

The Mutual Appreciation between Paul Klee and Pablo Picasso

[630] Ju Aichinger-Grosch made the following comments on Picasso's visit to Paul and Lily Klee in Bern on November 28, 1937: 'He [Picasso] had apparently said some very significant and nice things about Klee's pictures, because Klee was beaming and reported "he liked them very much, but it's important for me to watch out that I don't subconsciously start to imitate him, because he has a big and very powerful personality, and it's too easy to adopt ways that you admire without even thinking, but everybody must find their own way."' (Aichinger-Grosch 1959, p. 54). Grohmann wrote of Klee's relationship with Picasso: 'His [Picasso's] admiration is spontaneous and genuine and Klee is very happy because he considers Picasso to be the greatest living painter. There were times when he couldn't bring himself to go to his exhibitions because he found his works so overwhelming.' (Grohmann 1965, p. 86). Glaesemer depicted Klee's affinity with Picasso's work as follows: 'The impulsiveness of expression in the drawings [of Klee from 1933] reminds you now and then of the works of Picasso, who Klee admired all his life as an almost forbidding role-model. Didn't Picasso possess that immediacy of creative expression, which Klee himself had always longed for? Only in his later works did the immediate flow-

ing pulse of spontaneous linear composition become a natural form of self-expression for him too.' (Glaesemer 1979, p. 31). Klee describes to Lily his visit to the Picasso exhibition at the Kunsthaus Zürich (Museum of Fine Arts) on October 6, 1932: '[…] the Picasso exhibition was a new affirmation and the latest very colorful pictures a big surprise. He has even incorporated Matisse. The formats are mostly bigger than you think. The humor in many of the bathing pictures is achieved by the subtlety of the painting. All in all, he is the painter of today.' (Klee 1979, p. 1189).

[631] Grohmann 1965, p. 87: 'Picasso was for his part very impressed by Klee's "miniatures" whenever he came across them.'

Acclaim for 'Paul Klee und seine Krankheit' / 'Paul Klee et sa maladie'

Aljoscha Klee
In the Preface

I welcome this book as an important and sensitive contribution towards the appreciation of Klee's later work.

Stefan Frey
Freelance art historian, secretary of the Klee family collection and Paul Klee's Estate, Bern

It is the first publication on the subject of Klee's illness to be carefully researched, and at the same time it is the most thorough. All the available documentation has been meticulously evaluated and the analyses are firmly grounded in scientific fact.

Prof. emeritus Alfred Krebs
University Dermatology Clinic, Bern

Hans Suter's study is without a doubt the most major and comprehensive academic work on Paul Klee's illness to date. It is unlikely to be surpassed by future researchers in this field.

Prof. emeritus Ernst G. Jung
University Dermatology Clinic, Mannheim/Heidelberg
In: Aktuelle Dermatologie 3/2007, Georg Thieme Verlag KG

Hans Suter has proceeded carefully and cautiously, affectionately and almost devoutly, following all the traces and sifting through all the medical, familial and artistic sources. After a thorough critical evaluation, he has knit them together to create an overall picture of the scleroderma which finally led to Paul Klee's death. It is a book full of documents and pictures which cannot fail to fascinate the reader.

Prof. Jean Cabane
Université Pierre & Marie Curie, Paris
In the Foreword to the French edition 2007

Dr. Hans Suter was the only person who could rise to the challenge of rolling back time and spending decades on a meticulous investigation which has finally led to this exhaustive synthesis of medical and artistic themes. I have been President of the Groupe Français de Recherche sur la Sclérodermie (French Scleroderma Research Group) since its inception. The Group was immediately keen to promote this work due to its exceptional quality and because it contains a mass of new information not only for doctors but also for lovers of art in general and of Paul Klee in particular.

Dr. Hans Christoph von Tavel, PhD
Former Director of the Bern Museum of Fine Arts

The book is absorbing for many reasons: the author's meticulous medical and historical research into the nature and course of Klee's illness; his accurate knowledge of art history; his critical review of previous academic works on the topic; and his very human empathy with the nature of the illness and with the artist and his family, his doctors and contemporaries.

Alice Henkes
In: Der Bund, October 26, 2006

The book reads like a thriller, with Hans Suter searching through old documents in his quest for evidence. He writes in clear and simple language which renders the medical glossary in the appendices largely superfluous.

Marc Peschke
In: Neue Zürcher Zeitung, November 26, 2006

This is a wonderful clearly-written book which not only fills a gap in our knowledge about one of the major artists of the 20th century but which is also an excellent example of a truly interdisciplinary approach.

PD Monika Harms
In: Dermatologica Helvetica 5/2007

An initial reaction to this book: it is a very interesting and special kind of art book which is an absolute 'must read' for doctors and lovers of art.

Maja Rehbein
In: Deutsches Ärzteblatt 104, February 23, 2007

This study is not only a recommended read for dermatologists who have an interest in art and for medical specialists in other fields, but also for the layman. It conveys Suter's passion for Klee, whose 'poetic art is magical and mystical – and yet ultimately so human.'

Detlev Rüsch
In: amazon.de, reviews, May 15, 2007

This book's impressive treatment of Paul Klee's personality, illness, work, life and companions makes it a true masterpiece.

Emma Margarete Reil
In: Sklerodermie, Selbsthilfe e.V., issue no. 78/79, I/II 2007, Heilbronn

This is the nicest book I have ever seen on Paul Klee. For me it is a book which is really enlightening, which imparts knowledge and which opens up new perspectives. It appeals to one's own sense of courage and hope; it is challenging and yet at the same time so beautiful to look at.

Acknowledgements

The author would like to thank the following:

For the preface
  Aljoscha Klee-Coll

For the foreword
  Dr. Hans Christoph von Tavel

For help during the research
  Aljoscha Klee-Coll
  Dr. Felix Klee
  Stefan Frey
  Prof. Alfred Krebs
  Sister Virginia Bachmann
  Dr. Michael Baumgartner
  Diana Bodmer
  Prof. Urs Boschung
  Dr. Gabriele Castenholz
  Prof. Brigitta Danuser
  Dr. Karl Dula
  Dr. Matthias Frehner
  Heidi Frautschi
  Dr. Bendicht Friedli
  Susanne Friedli
  Dr. Franziska Früh-von Arx
  Lic. phil. Walter J. Fuchs
  Dr. Jürgen Glaesemer
  Prof. Josef Helfenstein
  Dr. Christine Hopfengart
  Prof. Max Huggler
  Prof. Ernst G. Jung
  Theodor Künzi
  Gerold Lotmar
  Osamu Okuda
  Prof. Hartmut Porzig
  Heinrich Rohrer
  Prof. Beat Rüttimann
  Markus Ryser
  Lic. phil. Anna M. Schafroth
  Marie-Louise Stössel-Schorer
  Dr. Hans Christoph von Tavel
  Prof. Peter Vock
  Sister Liobina Werlen
  Kathi Zollinger-Streiff

For valuable medical advice
  Prof. Urs Boschung
  Prof. Jean Cabane
  Prof. Brigitta Danuser
  Prof. Edgar Heim
  Prof. Alfred Krebs
  Prof. Peter M. Villiger

For translation
  Gill McKay
  Neil McKay

For coordinating the publication
  Urs Gerber, Gerber Druck AG, Steffisburg (Bern)

For publishing the book
  Karger Publishers, Basel
  Dr. Thomas Karger
  Peter Roth
  Angela Weber
  Deborah Lautenschlager
  Jacqueline Dürring
  Erika Brunner

For advice on graphic design
  Eugen Götz-Gee, Bern

For the prepress
  Gerber Druck AG, Steffisburg (Bern)
  Urs Gerber
  Olivier Maier
  Sebastian Schmid

For printing
  Stämpfli Publikationen AG, Bern
  Dr. Rudolf Stämpfli
  Daniel Moosberger

For bookbinding
  Buchbinderei Schumacher AG, Schmitten (Fribourg)

For the loan of documents and photos as well as for bibliographical details
  Paul Klee's Estate, Bern
  Aljoscha Klee-Coll
  Stefan Frey
  Klee Family Donation, Zentrum Paul Klee, Bern
  Livia Klee Donation, Zentrum Paul Klee, Bern
  Zentrum Paul Klee, Bern
  Dr. Juri Steiner
  Dr. Michael Baumgartner
  Heidi Frautschi
  Fabienne Eggelhöfer
  Kunstmuseum Bern
  Dr. Matthias Frehner
  Hermann und Margrit Rupf-Stiftung, Kunstmuseum Bern
  Dr. Matthias Frehner
  Susanne Friedli
  Kunstmuseum Basel
  Kunstmuseum Winterthur
  Kunsthaus Zürich
  Hamburger Kunsthalle
  Sprengel Museum, Hannover
  Kunstsammlung Nordrhein-Westfalen, Düsseldorf
  ProLitteris, Zurich
  Yolanda Canonica
  Keystone, Zurich
  Prof. Hans Bietenhard (Steffisburg)
  PD Jochen Jackowski (Witten, Germany)
  Fernand Rausser, Bolligen (Bern)

  Dermatology Clinic, University of Bern
  Prof. Lasse R. Braathen
  Prof. Thomas Hunziker
  Fritz Schweizer

  Pediatric Clinic, University of Bern,
  Dept. of Childhood Communicable Diseases
  Prof. Christoph Aebi

  Rheumatology Clinic, University of Bern
  Prof. Peter M. Villiger
  Prof. Michael Seitz
  Dr. Stephan Gadola

  Institute of Medical History, University of Bern
  Prof. Urs Boschung

  Institute and Museum of Medical History, University of Zurich
  Prof. Beat Rüttimann
  Prof. Christoph Mörgeli
  Lic. phil. Walther J. Fuchs

  Swiss Federal Archive, Bern
  Lic. phil. Simone Chiquet

  Swiss Literary Archive, Bern
  Dr. Thomas Feitknecht

  Bern Municipal Archive, Bern
  Emil Erne

  Bern Police Headquarters, Bern
  Department of Citizenship

  Bauhaus Archive, Berlin
  Sabine Hartmann

  Archive Will Grohmann, Stuttgart
  Ilona Lütken

For other kind assistance
  World Scleroderma Association
  Prof. Alan Tyndall

And for all other assistance after the book was printed

I would particularly like to thank the following people who were such a pleasure to work with:
  Dr. Thomas Karger, Basel
  Peter Roth, Basel
  Angela Weber, Basel
  Deborah Lautenschlager, Basel
  Jacqueline Dürring, Basel
  Erika Brunner, Basel
  Gill McKay, Stuttgart
  Neil McKay, Stuttgart
  Urs Gerber, Steffisburg (Bern)
  Olivier Maier, Steffisburg (Bern)
  Sebastian Schmid, Steffisburg (Bern)
  Dr. Rudolf Stämpfli, Bern
  Daniel Moosberger, Bern
  Aljoscha Klee-Coll, Muri (Bern)
  Stefan Frey, Bern
  Dr. Juri Steiner, Bern
  Dr. Michael Baumgartner, Bern
  Heidi Frautschi, Bern
  Fabienne Eggelhöfer, Bern
  Prof. Alan Tyndall, Basel

Fahrni, February 2010

Dr. Hans Suter

World Scleroderma Association

There are an estimated 2.5 million individuals worldwide who suffer from scleroderma, with the majority being women of childbearing age. The cause is unknown and effective overall treatments are lacking.

Research is active on many fronts and recent progress has been considerable. Effective treatments have been developed for some of the complications, including kidney involvement and some forms of lung involvement. Progress is hampered by the extraordinary clinical diversity of the disease. No two patients are truly alike. Critically important research is underway in several areas including the biology of scar tissue formation, the mechanisms of blood vessel damage and attempting to better understand the central role of the immune system in triggering tissue damage.

From the perspective of the patients, the burden of disease is high and quality of life is affected in nearly all of them. Universal symptoms of pain, fatigue and malaise have a major influence on quality of life, particularly social life and interaction.

Dry statistics on prevalence and incidence fail to portray the daily human suffering experienced by patients with scleroderma and their families. Apart from the omnipresent fear of early death, mutilating changes in hands, face and other organs conspire to cause a humiliating loss of self-esteem and even deny the simple pleasures of physical affection and social intercourse.

However, although human suffering is universal, not all of us are gifted with the creative talent to express such emotions; we are therefore grateful to Hans Suter for this splendid book in which we share this anguish through the eyes of a creative genius, Paul Klee. In one of his last pictures, 'Tod und Feuer' (Death and fire), one sees the tight, ashen face of the scleroderma sufferer facing his imminent demise.

Despite the challenges of scleroderma, a spontaneous international collaboration has developed in recent years, inspired by years of dedicated commitment from people such as Dame Carol Black, Daniel Furst, James Seibold, Marco Matucci Cerinic, Alan Tyndall, Maureen Mayes, Virginia Steen, Thomas Medsger, John Varga and many others. This has resulted in the formation of the World Scleroderma Association, legally constituted in Basel, Switzerland, on November 12, 2009. We regret that some of the early pioneers and dear friends such as Gerald Rodnan, E. Carwile LeRoy and Joe Korn are no longer with us to share our excitement.

The World Scleroderma Association is dedicated to initiating and supporting research in scleroderma in all its aspects across all regions of our planet. Our commitment is to facilitate patient-oriented research independently, but also in collaboration with other existing organisations and learned societies working in this field. Support will be given in the form of project grants, expert advisory panels and knowledge dissemination platforms. Patient groups as well as allied health professionals will form an integral part of the association structure. Our association will liaise with society, industry and government in an open and dynamic fashion, whilst nonetheless remaining independent of regional, political and industrial pressures. The World Scleroderma Association is committed to improving the quality of life for scleroderma sufferers and their families.

Any person or organisation involved with scleroderma may be a member of the association on approval of the board.

We are grateful to Alexander Klee and his family for graciously consenting to act as patrons of our association, and together we intend to raise awareness and resources to further research and overcome this disease. We are in a new and optimistic era of targeted molecular, biological and cellular therapies, which have already impacted on other autoimmune diseases and give hope to our scleroderma patients.

Let us take the star from 'Dieser Stern lehrt beugen', metaphorically translated as 'This star teaches us to bow', as not just an acceptance of the inevitable, but also as a 'star of hope' for the future.

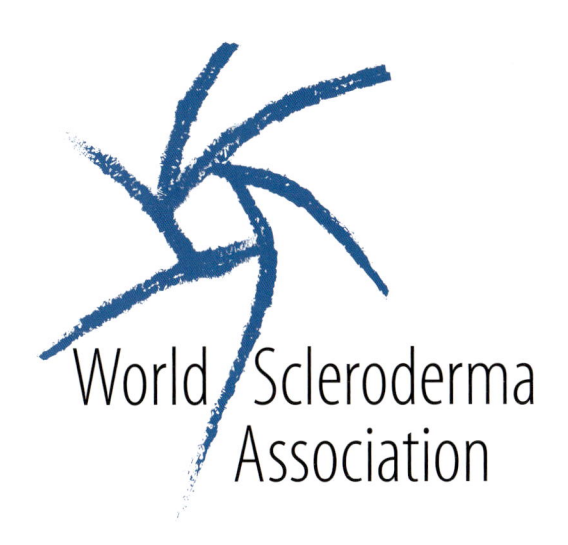

Founding Members

Marco Matucci Cerinic, President
Alan Tyndall, Secretary
Daniel Furst, Treasurer

Carol Black
Christopher Denton
James Seibold
Maureen Mayes
Steffen Gay
Loic Guillevin
Ulf Mueller-Ladner
Paul Emery

Copyright © 2010 English Edition by S. Karger AG, P.O. Box, CH–4009 Basel (Switzerland)
www.karger.com

Printed in Switzerland on acid free paper by Stämpfli Publikationen AG, CH–3006 Bern (Switzerland)

ISBN 978-3-8055-9381-6
e-ISBN 978-3-8055-9382-3

Copyright illustrations of works of art: ProLitteris, Zurich (Switzerland)
Copyright illustrations of documents and photos (when not otherwise stated):
Klee Estate Administration, Bern (Switzerland)
In all other cases copyright is vested in the relevant person/institution or their registered office/rights holders.

Despite intensive research the author could not locate all copyright holders. He is however happy to compensate all legal claims as customary and appropriate upon receipt of relevant notification. Some publishing houses that produced certain publications no longer exist.

All rights reserved. No part of this publication may be translated into other languages, reproduced or utilized in any form or by any means either electronically or mechanically, including photocopying, recording, microcopying, or by any information storage and retrieval system, without written consent from the publisher.

The German original edition entitled 'Hans Suter: Paul Klee und seine Krankheit' (ISBN 978-3-7272-1106-5) was published in 2006 by Stämpfli Verlag AG, Bern (Switzerland).

The French edition entitled 'Hans Suter: Paul Klee et sa maladie' was published in 2007 by Dr. Hans Suter and is available through the author:
Dr. Hans Suter, Lueg, CH–3617 Fahrni (Switzerland)
Tel. +41 33 437 59 51, Fax +41 33 437 59 52, E-Mail info@sammlung-suter.ch
www.sammlung-suter.ch

Library of Congress Cataloging-in-Publication Data

Suter, Hans, 1930-
  [Paul Klee und seine Krankheit. English]
  Paul Klee and his illness : bowed but not broken by suffering and adversity / Hans Suter ; translated from the German by Gillian McKay and Neil McKay.
       p. ; cm.
  Includes bibliographical references and index.
  ISBN 978-3-8055-9381-6 (hard cover : alk. paper)
  1. Klee, Paul, 1879-1940--Health. 2. Artists--Diseases--Switzerland--Biography. 3. Artists--Switzerland--Biography. 4. Systemic scleroderma--Patients--Switzerland--Biography. I. Title.
  [DNLM: 1. Klee, Paul, 1879-1940. 2. Famous Persons--Switzerland--Biography. 3. Scleroderma, Systemic--Switzerland. 4. Art--Switzerland. WZ 313 S965p 2010a]
  N6888.K55S8813 2010
  760.092--dc22
  [B]
                       2009049891

Author, concept, choice of pictures, book design and execution:
Dr. Hans Suter, Fahrni, Thun (Switzerland)

Translation: Gill McKay and Neil McKay, Stuttgart (Germany)

Publishing: S. Karger AG, Basel (Switzerland)
Editing: S. Karger AG, Basel (Switzerland)

Layout, type-setting, image processing, coordination:
Gerber Druck AG, Steffisburg (Switzerland)

Font: FF DIN (title), Frutiger Light/Frutiger Bold (text, notes)
Binding: Buchbinderei Schumacher AG, Schmitten (Switzerland)

Frontispiece: Paul Klee, 1939, photo by Charlotte Weidler, New York, N.Y. (USA)
Embossed illustration: Paul Klee, 'ecce ....', 1940, 138